Manter and Gatz's

Essentials of Clinical Neuroanatomy and Neurophysiology

Edition 9

Manter and Gatz's

Essentials of Clinical Neuroanatomy and Neurophysiology

Edition 9

Sid Gilman, M.D.
Professor and Chair
Department of Neurology
The University of Michigan Medical School
Ann Arbor, Michigan

Sarah Winans Newman, Ph.D.
Professor Emerita of Anatomy and Cell Biology
University of Michigan
Ann Arbor, Michigan
Visiting Scholar in Psychology
Cornell University
Ithaca, New York

Illustrations by Margaret Croup Brudon

 F. A. DAVIS COMPANY • Philadelphia

F. A. Davis Company
1915 Arch Street
Philadelphia, PA 19103

Printed in Canada

Last digit indicates print number: 10 9 8 7 6 5 4 3 2

Acquisitions Editor: Robert W. Reinhardt
Developmental Editor: Bernice M. Wissler
Production Editor: Jessica Howie Martin
Cover Designer: Louis J. Forgione

As new scientific information becomes available through basic and clinical research, recommended treatments and drug therapies undergo changes. The authors and publisher have done everything possible to make this book accurate, up to date, and in accord with accepted standards at the time of publication. The authors, editors, and publisher are not responsible for errors or omissions or for consequences from application of the book, and make no warranty, expressed or implied, in regard to the contents of the book. Any practice described in this book should be applied by the reader in accordance with professional standards of care used in regard to the unique circumstances that may apply in each situation. The reader is advised always to check product information (package inserts) for changes and new information regarding dose and contraindications before administering any drug. Caution is especially urged when using new or infrequently ordered drugs.

Library of Congress Cataloging-in-Publication Data

Gilman, Sid.
  Manter and Gatz's essentials of clinical neuroanatomy and neurophysiology. — Ed. 9 / Sid Gilman, Sarah Winans Newman ; illustrations by Margaret Croup Brudon.
       p. cm.
    Includes bibliographical references and index.
    ISBN 0-8036-0144-1 (pbk.)
    1. Neuroanatomy. 2. Neurophysiology. I. Newman, Sarah Winans.
II. Manter, John Tinkham, 1910–   . III. Gatz, Arthur John, 1907–   .
IV. Title.
    [DNLM: 1. Nervous System—anatomy & histology. 2. Nervous System—physiology. WL 100 G487m 1996]
    QM451.G47   1996
    612.8—dc20
    DNLM/DLC
    for Library of Congress   95-49487

PREFACE TO THE NINTH EDITION

The expansion of information in both basic and clinical neuroscience in the past several decades has continued at a rapid rate since the last edition of this book. Much of this information is important to neuroscientists and clinicians, including those in training programs in these fields. The present revision was undertaken to keep this book up to date with the many recent developments in neuroanatomy, neurophysiology, neuropharmacology, and clinical neurology. To that end, we have thoroughly revised each chapter. This resulted in major changes in the chapters on the basal ganglia, optic reflexes and eye movements, and chemical neuroanatomy. We have also reorganized and consolidated the material previously in Chapters 7 and 8 into a single chapter on proprioception, touch, and tactile discrimination. Finally, we have preserved and updated the chapter entitled Clinical Evaluation of Patients with Neurologic Disorders, which was introduced in the eighth edition. Responses to that edition suggested that this material was, as we had intended, useful to medical students making the transition from basic science to clinical studies. These extensive revisions required replacement of some illustrations and the addition of several new ones, as well as expansion of the index and the suggested reading list. The reading list is restricted to current textbooks and monographs and is intended only to provide a guide to the literature for students interested in obtaining further information about the topics covered.

In this edition, we continue to emphasize physiologic concepts within the context of the anatomic organization of the nervous system and to point out systematically the clinical relevance of the major anatomic structures. We have again adhered to Dr. Manter's original objective of providing a short but comprehensive survey of the human nervous system. The book is written for the student who wishes a brief, clinically oriented overview of neuroanatomy and neurophysiology that summarizes the material in more comprehensive textbooks. It is also intended to be helpful to house officers in neurology, neurosurgery, psychiatry, and physical medicine and rehabilitation who wish to update their knowledge. We also hope that it will be useful to physical therapists, speech pathologists, and nurses.

Sid Gilman, M.D.
Sarah Winans Newman, Ph.D.

v

PREFACE TO THE FIRST EDITION

This book has been written with the object of providing a short, but comprehensive survey of the human nervous system. It is hoped that it will furnish a unified concept of structure and function which will be of practical value in leading to the understanding of the working mechanisms of the brain and spinal cord. Neither of these two aspects—structure and function—stands apart from the other. Together they furnish the key to the significance of the abnormal changes in function that go hand in hand with structural lesions of the nervous system. The viewpoints of three closely dependent sciences—neuroanatomy, neurophysiology, and clinical neurology—are combined and used freely, not with the intent of covering these fields exhaustively, but in the belief that a more discerning approach to the study of the nervous system can be attained by bringing together all three facets of the subject.

To suit the needs of the medical student, or the physician who wishes to review the nervous system efficiently, basic information is presented in concise form. Consequently, it has not been feasible to cite published reports of research from which present concepts of the nervous system have evolved. The planning and arrangement of the chapters are such that whole topics can be covered rapidly. Presenting the subject material to classes in this form allows more time for discussion and review, or, if the teacher desires, for lectures dealing with advanced aspects, than would otherwise be permitted.

For the encouragement and valuable suggestions they have given me, I am indebted to my former colleague, Dr. William H. Waller, Jr., and to Dr. Lester L. Bowles. I am deeply grateful to Mr. A. H. Germagian for executing most of the drawings and diagrams, and to Mr. Richard Meyers for his special assistance with the illustrations.

John T. Manter

CONTENTS

CHAPTER 5
The Autonomic Nervous System

SECTION 3

Ascending and Descending Pathways ●●●●●●●●●

CHAPTER 6
Pain and Temperature

CHAPTER 7
Proprioception, Touch, and Tactile Discrimination

CHAPTER 8
The Descending Pathways

CHAPTER 9

Lesions of the Peripheral Nerves, Spinal Roots, and Spinal Cord

SECTION 4

Brain Stem and Cerebellum   • • • • • • • • •

CHAPTER 10

Anatomy of the Brain Stem: Medulla, Pons, and Midbrain

CHAPTER 11

Overview of the Cranial Nerves

CHAPTER 12

Cranial Nerves of the Medulla

SECTION 5

Higher Levels of the Nervous System • • • • • • • • •

CHAPTER 18
The Basal Ganglia

CHAPTER 19
Vision

CHAPTER 20
Optic Reflexes and Eye Movements

CHAPTER 21
The Thalamus

CHAPTER 22
The Hypothalamus and Limbic System

SECTION 7

Approaches to Patients with Neurologic Symptoms   • • • • • • • • •

CHAPTER 28
Clinical Evaluation of Patients with Neurologic Disorders

CHAPTER 29
Neurologic Diagnostic Tests

1

Basic Principles

CHAPTER

1

Introduction to the Nervous System

NERVE CELLS AND NERVE FIBERS

The **neuron** (nerve cell) is the primary functional and anatomic unit of the nervous system. Both central and peripheral neurons consist of a **cell body** (perikaryon) containing a nucleus and possessing one to several dozen processes (fibers) of varying lengths (Fig. 1A, B). **Dendrites** are branching processes that receive **stimuli** and conduct **impulses** generated by those stimuli **toward** the nerve cell body. These are **afferent** processes. The **axon (axis cylinder)** of a nerve cell is a single fiber extending to other parts of the nervous system or to a muscle or gland. The term **axon**, when used in a physiologic sense, applies to a fiber that conducts impulses **away** from a nerve cell body; thus, an axon is an **efferent** fiber or process. Any long fiber, however, may have the anatomic properties of an axon, regardless of the direction of conduction.

Peripheral and central nerve fibers may have a **myelin sheath**, but only peripheral nerve fibers have, in addition, a **neurolemma (sheath of Schwann)** outside the myelin. The myelin in peripheral neurons is actually a spiral wrapping of many layers of glial cell membranes from the same **Schwann cell** that forms the neurolemma on the outside. Each Schwann cell contributes myelin to one segment (or internode) of a myelinated axon. Between two adjacent myelinated segments is a small gap called the **node of Ranvier** (see Fig. 1E). Conversely, **unmyelinated fibers** are enfolded into adjacent Schwann cells by simple extensions of their cytoplasmic processes. There is no layering of Schwann cell membranes around an unmyelinated fiber.

The myelinated fibers in the white matter of the brain and spinal cord possess a myelin sheath but have no neurolemma because their myelin sheaths are formed by cytoplasmic extensions of oligodendrocytes, each of which contributes myelin to several nearby axons (see Fig. 1A).

3

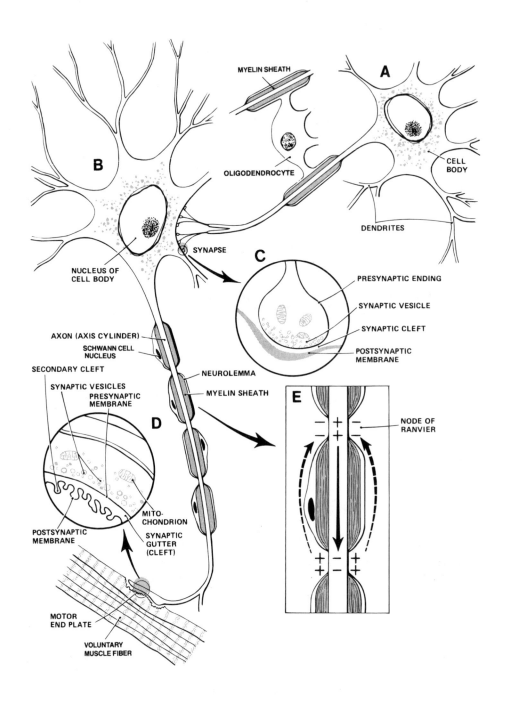

FIGURE 1

Neurons of the central nervous system (CNS). Neuron *A* is confined to the CNS and terminates on neuron *B* at a typical chemical synapse (*C*). Neuron *B* is a motor neuron; its axon extends to a peripheral nerve and innervates a striated (voluntary) muscle at the myoneural junction (motor end plate, *D*). In *E*, the action potential is moving in the direction of the solid arrow inside the axon; the dashed arrows indicate the direction of flow of the action current.

ORGANIZATION OF NERVE CELLS

• • • • • • • • •

Nerve cell bodies usually are located in groups. Outside of the brain and spinal cord, these groups are called **ganglia**. Within the brain and spinal cord, neurons form groups of various sizes and shapes known as nuclei. In this instance, the term **nucleus** has a meaning different from that of the nucleus of an individual cell. The laminated sheets of nerve cell bodies on the surface of the cerebrum and cerebellum are referred to as the cerebral cortex and cerebellar cortex. Regions of the brain and spinal cord that contain aggregations of nerve cell bodies comprise the **gray matter**, so called for its color in the fresh state. In gray matter the neuron cell bodies are surrounded by the ramifications of their dendrites and the terminal branches of axons. This delicate network surrounding the neuron cell bodies is known as **neuropil**. The remaining areas of the brain and spinal cord consist primarily of myelinated nerve fibers and compose the **white matter**.

Nerve fibers of the brain and spinal cord that have a common origin and a common destination constitute a **tract**. Although a tract occupies a definable position, it does not always form a compact bundle because there is some dispersion with intermingling fibers of neighboring tracts. However, a number of bundles of fibers in the brain are so anatomically distinct that they have been given distinct names such as **fasciculus**, **brachium**, **peduncle**, **column**, or **lemniscus**. These structures may contain only a single tract, or they may consist of several tracts running together in the same bundle. **Nerve**, **nerve root**, **nerve trunk**, **nerve cord**, and **ramus** are appropriate terms for bundles of nerve fibers outside the brain and spinal cord.

GLIA

• • • • • • • • •

The central nervous system contains three types of nonneuronal supporting (glial) cells: **oligodendrocytes**, **astrocytes**, and **microglia**. Oligodendrocytes form and maintain the myelin sheaths of fibers in the central nervous system. The functions of astrocytes are less well understood. Astrocytes function in a variety of ways as metabolic supporting cells for neurons. They cannot develop action potentials, but they are highly permeable to potassium ions (K^+) and become depolarized if the extracellular concentration of K^+ increases. Astrocytes are thought to take up extracellular K^+ during intense neuronal activity and thereby buffer K^+ concentration in the extracellular space. They also take up and store neurotransmitters and thus may regulate extracellular concentrations of neurotransmitters and store and transfer metabolites from capillaries to neurons. Astrocytes are sensitive to a wide variety of insults to central nervous system tissue. Depending on the noxious agent, astrocytes may respond to injury with cytoplasmic swelling, accumulation of glycogen, fibrillar proliferation within the cytoplasm, cell multiplication, or a combination of these reactions. They are frequently the cells that form a permanent scar or plaque after destruction of neuronal elements has occurred. Microglia are phagocytic cells that form part of the nervous system's defense against infection and injury.

PERIPHERAL NERVOUS SYSTEM

• • • • • • • • •

The 12 pairs of cranial nerves and 31 pairs of spinal nerves, with their associated ganglia, compose the human **peripheral nervous system (PNS)**. There are two types of motor (or efferent) fibers of peripheral nerves: **somatic motor fibers**, which terminate in **skeletal muscle**, and **autonomic fibers**, which innervate **cardiac muscle**, **smooth muscle**, **glands**, and **adipose tissue (fat)**. The termination of the somatic motor fiber on a skeletal muscle fiber occurs at the **motor end plate** or **myoneural junction**, which resembles a synapse (see Fig. 1D). The transmitter released by the vesicles of the motor end plate is acetylcholine.

The sensory (or afferent) nerve fibers of the PNS transmit signals from receptors of various types. Each afferent fiber conducts impulses toward the spinal cord and brain from the particular receptor type with which it is connected.

CENTRAL NERVOUS SYSTEM

• • • • • • • • •

The **central nervous system (CNS)** consists of the brain and the spinal cord. The brain of a young man averages 1380 g in weight, and the brain of a young woman averages 100 g less. The adult brain is divided into three gross parts: the **cerebrum**, the **cerebellum**, and the **brain stem**.

Cerebrum

The left and right cerebral hemispheres are incompletely separated by a deep **medial longitudinal fissure**. The surface of each hemisphere is wrinkled by the presence of eminences, known as **gyri**, and furrows, which are called **sulci** or **fissures**. The **cerebral cortex** consists of a layer of gray matter that varies from 1.3 to 4.5 mm in thickness and covers the expansive surface of the cerebral hemisphere. This cortex is estimated to contain 14 billion nerve cells.

There are two major grooves on the lateral surface of the brain (Fig. 2). The **lateral fissure (of Sylvius)** begins as a deep cleft on the basal surface of the brain and extends laterally, posteriorly, and upward. The **central sulcus (of Rolando)** runs from the dorsal border of the hemisphere near its midpoint obliquely downward and forward until it nearly meets the lateral fissure. For descriptive purposes, the lateral surface of the hemisphere is divided into four lobes. The **frontal lobe** (approximately the anterior one third of the hemisphere) is the portion that is rostral (anterior) to the central sulcus and above the lateral fissure. The **occipital lobe** is that part lying behind, or caudal to, an arbitrary line drawn from the parietooccipital fissure to the preoccipital notch. This lobe occupies a small area of the lateral surface but has more extensive territory on the medial aspect of the hemisphere (Fig. 3), where it includes all cortex posterior to the parietooccipital fissure. The **parietal lobe** extends from the central sulcus to the parietooccipital fissure and, on the lateral surface, is separated from the temporal lobe below by an imaginary line projecting from the horizontal portion of the lateral fissure to the middle of the line demarcating the occipital lobe. The gyri within each lobe are separated by sulci whose patterns show considerable individual variation.

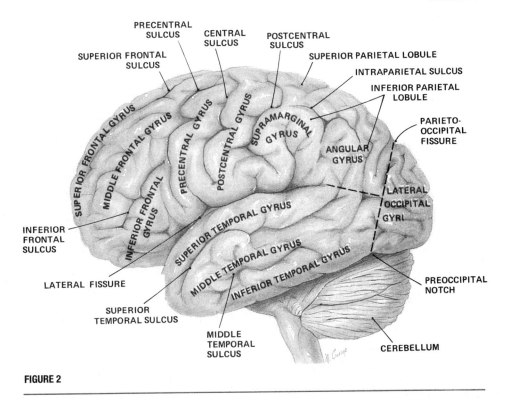

FIGURE 2

• • • • • • • • •

Lateral view of the left cerebral hemisphere, cerebellum, and brain stem.

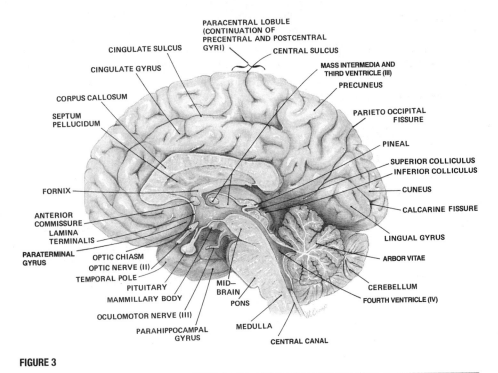

FIGURE 3

• • • • • • • • •

Medial (midsagittal) view of the right cerebral hemisphere, cerebellum, and brain stem of a hemisected brain.

Figure 3 depicts the structures that are located on the medial (midsagittal) surface of the brain. This surface is exposed by cutting the brain in half on a plane through the medial longitudinal fissure. This cut severs the **corpus callosum**, **brain stem**, and **cerebellum**, and it exposes a portion of the ventricular system within the brain (Fig. 4). On the medial surface of the cerebral cortex, the gyri and sulci of the frontal, parietal, occipital, and temporal lobes are continuous with those seen on the lateral surface. The central sulcus sometimes extends a short distance over the dorsal crest of the hemisphere onto the medial side, marking the boundary between the frontal and parietal lobes. The parietooccipital fissure, as its name implies, separates the parietal and occipital lobes. Only the temporal pole region of the temporal lobe can be seen on this medial section through the whole brain. With the brain cut in this manner, part of the fifth lobe can be seen on the cerebral cortex. This is the **limbic lobe**, a ring (or limbus) of cortical tissue consisting primarily of the **paraterminal gyrus**, the **cingulate gyrus**, and the **parahippocampal gyrus**, which is partially hidden by the brain stem. The ventral surface of the brain provides a more complete view of the parahippocampal gyrus (Fig. 5). This view also shows the cranial nerves exiting from the brain stem.

A sixth lobe, the **insular lobe**, cannot be seen in any of these figures. It consists of the cortical tissue that forms the floor of the deep lateral fissure and can be seen only when the lips (opercula) of this fissure are separated or coronal sections of the brain are made (see Fig. 56A in Chap. 18).

Cerebellum

The cerebellum is attached to the dorsal surface of the brain stem at the level of the pons. Its surface, like that of the cerebral hemispheres, is a layer of gray matter, the cerebellar cortex, which is arranged in ridges and grooves. In the cerebellum, the eminences of gray matter are called **folia**. On the midsagittally cut brain (see Fig. 3), a core of white matter, the **arbor vitae**, can be seen under the cortex of the cerebellar folia.

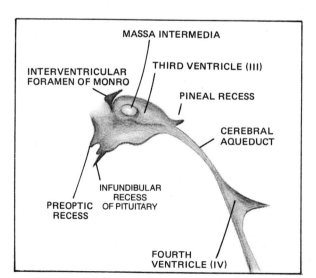

MASSA INTERMEDIA

THIRD VENTRICLE (III)

INTERVENTRICULAR
FORAMEN OF MONRO

PINEAL RECESS

CEREBRAL
AQUEDUCT

INFUNDIBULAR
RECESS
OF PITUITARY

PREOPTIC
RECESS

FOURTH
VENTRICLE (IV)

FIGURE 4

• • • • • • • • •

Components of the ventricular system as seen on the midsagittal section of the brain (compare with Fig. 3).

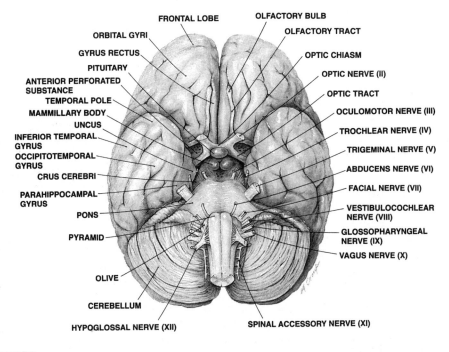

FIGURE 5

Ventral surface of the brain.

Brain Stem

The brain stem consists of the **medulla, pons**, and **midbrain**. This region is described in Chapter 10.

Ventricles, Meninges, and Cerebrospinal Fluid

Cavities within the brain, called the **ventricles,** are filled with **cerebrospinal fluid (CSF)** (see Fig. 4; also see Fig. 80 in Chap. 27). CSF is formed primarily by specialized tissue in the ventricles, called the **choroid plexus**. The ventricular system opens to the space outside of the brain at three sites in the brain stem. Through these three openings, CSF flows from the ventricles into the **subarachnoid space**, which surrounds the brain and spinal cord. This space is located between the pia mater and the arachnoid, two layers of the three connective-tissue membranes that enclose the CNS. The **pia mater** is intimately attached to the surface of the brain and spinal cord. Fine strands of connective tissue, the trabeculae, stretch across the subarachnoid space between the pia mater and the **arachnoid**. Outside the arachnoid, the tough **dura mater** lines the bony cranial cavity around the brain and the vertebral canal around the spinal cord. Together, the pia mater, arachnoid, and dura mater constitute the **meninges**. Additional details on the meninges and CSF can be found in Chapter 27.

Spinal Cord

The human spinal cord is a slender cylinder less than 2 cm in diameter. It is closely surrounded by the pia mater and anchored through the arachnoid to the dura mater by paired lateral septae of pia. These septae are called the **denticulate ligaments**. From its rostral junction with the medulla to its caudal end, the spinal cord is divided arbitrarily into five regions: **cervical, thoracic, lumbar, sacral**, and **coccygeal**. The spinal cord is enlarged in the lower cervical region and in the lumbosacral region, where nerve fibers supplying the upper and lower extremities are connected.

Spinal nerves are attached to the spinal cord in pairs; there are 8 cervical, 12 thoracic, 5 lumbar, 5 sacral, and 1 coccygeal pair of spinal nerves (Fig. 6). Each nerve is formed by the union of a **dorsal root**, composed of sensory or afferent fibers, and a **ventral root**, composed mostly of motor or efferent fibers. The sensory fibers of the dorsal roots are processes of special sensory cells in the dorsal root ganglia. The motor fibers in the ventral root are axons of cells in the spinal cord (see Fig. 13 in Chap. 3 and Fig. 15 in Chap. 4). The spinal cord does not extend to the lowest bony vertebral canal, but rather ends at the level of the lower border of the first lumbar vertebra. Its tapered end is called the **conus medullaris**. The pia mater continues caudally as a connective tissue filament, the **filum terminale**, which passes through the subarachnoid space to the end of the dural sac (level of vertebra S1, see Fig. 6), where it receives a covering of dura and continues to its attachment to the coccyx. Because the cord is about 25 cm shorter than the vertebral column, the lower segments of the spinal cord are not aligned opposite corresponding vertebrae. Thus, the lumbar and sacral spinal nerves have very long roots, extending from their respective segments in the cord to the lumbar and sacral **intervertebral foramina**, which are openings in the bony vertebral canal where dorsal and ventral roots join to form the spinal nerves. These roots descend in a bundle from the conus, and because of its resemblance to the tail of a horse, this formation is known as the **cauda equina**.

In describing the spinal cord, the terms **posterior** and **dorsal** are used interchangeably. Similarly, the terms **anterior** and **ventral** are interchangeable. Sections of the spinal cord cut perpendicular to the length of the cord (i.e., transverse sections) reveal a butterfly-shaped area of gray matter surrounded by white matter (Fig. 7). The white matter consists mainly of nerve fibers that run longitudinally through the cord and therefore are cut in cross section in a transverse section of the cord. Midline grooves are present on the dorsal and ventral surfaces and are known as the **dorsal median sulcus** and the **ventral median fissure**. The lateral surface shows a **dorsolateral** and a **ventrolateral sulcus**, which correspond to the dorsal root zone and the ventral root zone, respectively. These markings divide the white matter of the spinal cord into **dorsal, lateral**, and **ventral funiculi**. The dorsal root zone is interposed between the dorsal and lateral funiculi, and the ventral root zone lies between the lateral and ventral funiculi. The gray matter of the cord contains dorsal and ventral enlargements known as the **dorsal horns** and the **ventral horns**. Small **lateral horns** also are present in the thoracic and upper lumbar segments of the spinal cord (see Fig. 7). The ventral horns are larger in the cervical and lumbosacral enlargements than in the thoracic segments. This is because the muscle mass of the limbs is greater than that of the trunk, and these horns are made up largely of cell bodies of neurons that innervate skeletal muscles. Accordingly, the ventral horn of the lumbosacral enlargement is more massive than that of the cervical enlargement because of the greater muscle mass in the lower limbs. In addition, there is more white matter than gray matter at cervical levels than in the lumbosacral region (see Fig. 7). This is because the white matter in the cervical region is made

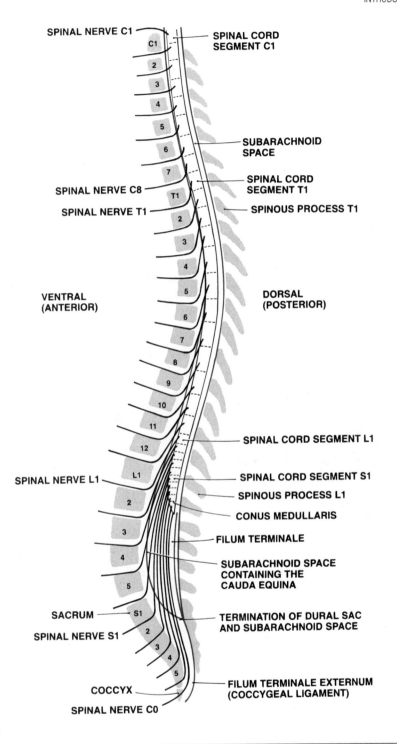

SPINAL NERVE C1

SPINAL CORD
SEGMENT C1

C1

2

3

4

5

6

SUBARACHNOID
SPACE

7

SPINAL NERVE C8

T1

SPINAL CORD
SEGMENT T1

SPINAL NERVE T1

SPINOUS PROCESS T1

2

3

4

VENTRAL
(ANTERIOR)

5

6

DORSAL
(POSTERIOR)

7

8

9

10

11

SPINAL CORD SEGMENT L1

12

SPINAL NERVE L1

L1

SPINAL CORD SEGMENT S1

2

SPINOUS PROCESS L1

CONUS MEDULLARIS

3

FILUM TERMINALE

4

SUBARACHNOID SPACE
CONTAINING THE
CAUDA EQUINA

5

SACRUM

S1

TERMINATION OF DURAL SAC
AND SUBARACHNOID SPACE

SPINAL NERVE S1

2

3

4

5

FILUM TERMINALE EXTERNUM
(COCCYGEAL LIGAMENT)

COCCYX

SPINAL NERVE C0

FIGURE 6

● ● ● ● ● ● ● ● ●

Diagram of the relation of the spinal cord segments and spinal nerve roots to the dural sac and vertebrae of the spinal column. The bodies of the individual vertebrae on the ventral side of the spinal cord are numbered. The spinous processes of the vertebrae are dorsal to the cord. The dural sac, filum terminale, and filum terminale externum (coccygeal ligament) are shown in color.

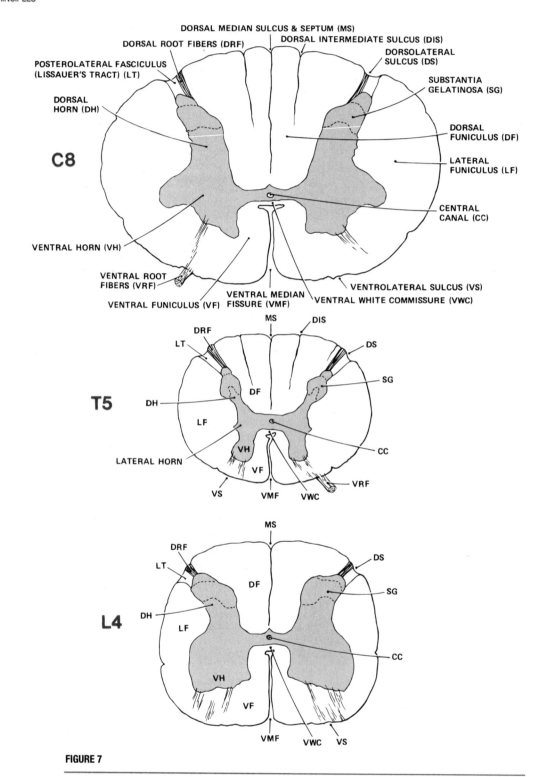

FIGURE 7

• • • • • • • • •

Cross sections of the spinal cord at approximately the eighth cervical (C8), fifth thoracic (T5), and fourth lumbar (L4) segmental levels.

up of fibers connecting the entire cord with the brain, whereas the white matter of the lumbosacral cord contains only fibers serving the caudal part of the cord.

In a transverse section of the cord, the gray matter can be subdivided into groups of perikarya that are called **nuclei**. When the spinal cord is cut along its length, these nuclei are seen to be cell columns, or laminae. Rexed divided the cord into 10 laminae (Fig. 8). Each **lamina** extends the length of the cord. Lamina I is the most dorsal part of the dorsal horn; lamina IX is the most ventral part of the ventral horn; and lamina X surrounds the central canal. Laminae I through VI are confined to the dorsal horn. Cells in these laminae receive and transmit information concerning sensory input from the spinal nerve afferents. Fiber pathways from other cord levels and the brain also influence cells in these laminae. Within laminae I to VI are found several classically defined nuclei or cell columns of the cord. For example, lamina II corresponds to the **substantia gelatinosa**, which receives information from pain and temperature afferents.

Lamina VII is located in the intermediate gray area and extends into the anterior horn. It contains the **nucleus dorsalis** and the **intermediolateral** and **intermediomedial gray columns**. The connections and functions of the nucleus dorsalis are described in Chapter 7, and those of the other two cell groups are described in Chapter 5. Lamina VIII is located in the ventral horn and contains many neurons that send **commissural** axons to the opposite side of the cord. Lamina IX consists of several columns of cells that are restricted to the ventral horn. These cell columns contain the **alpha**, **beta**, and **gamma motoneurons**, which send axons into the ventral roots of the spinal nerves and innervate the skeletal muscles.

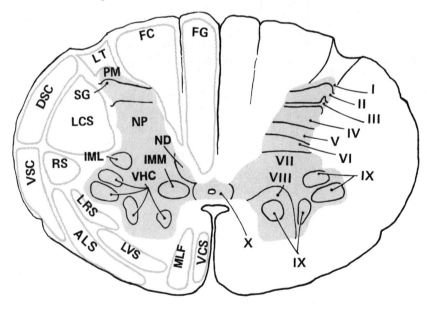

FIGURE 8

• • • • • • • • • •

Cross section of the spinal cord at approximately the C8–T1 segmental level. Tracts and nuclei of the cord are illustrated on the left; Rexed's laminar organization of the gray matter is illustrated on the right. ALS = anterolateral system; DSC = dorsal spinocerebellar tract; FC = fasciculus cuneatus; FG = fasciculus gracilis; IML = intermediolateral cell column; IMM = intermediomedial cell column; LCS = lateral corticospinal tract; LRS = lateral reticulospinal tract; LT = Lissauer's tract; LVS = lateral vestibulospinal tract; MLF = medial longitudinal fasciculus; ND = nucleus dorsalis; NP = nucleus proprius; PM = posteromarginal nucleus; RS = rubrospinal tract; SG = substantia gelatinosa; VCS = ventral corticospinal tract; VHC = ventral horn cell columns; VSC = ventral spinocerebellar tract.

DEVELOPMENT OF THE NERVOUS SYSTEM

• • • • • • • • •

Neural Tube

The adult human nervous system is derived from the ectoderm of the embryo. Initially, a rostrocaudal groove appears in the midline of the embryo. This **neural groove** is flanked by **neural folds**, which then close to form a **neural tube** (Fig. 9). The rostral end of this tube develops into the brain, and the remainder differentiates into the spinal cord. The tube closes first at the level destined to become the upper cervical region of the spinal cord. From this point, closure proceeds both rostrally and caudally. The closure of the **anterior and posterior neuropores** normally occurs during the fourth week of embryonic life. Thus, the final form of the early CNS is a hollow tube that is closed at both ends. Partial or complete failure of closure of the posterior neuropore results in **spina bifida**, a common developmental abnormality.

The tissue comprising the neural tube contains several different types of cells. **Neuroblasts**, the primordial neurons, and **glioblasts**, the primordial astrocytes and oligodendrocytes, compose most of this structure. The single layer of cells lining the tube is a precursor of the **ependyma**, which lines the ventricles of the adult brain.

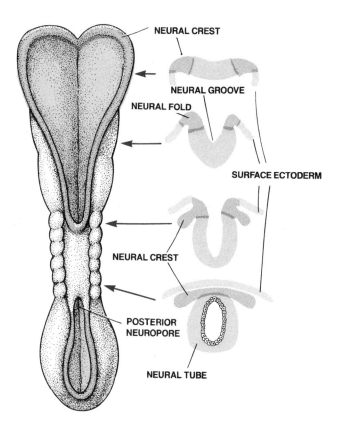

FIGURE 9

• • • • • • • • •

(*Left*) A dorsal view of the CNS in a human embryo at the end of the third week of development. (*Right*) Histologic sections through the CNS at the levels of the arrows.

Neural Crest and Ectodermal Placodes

Ectodermal tissue lateral to the neural tube is also important in the development of the nervous system. This structure is known as the **neural crest** (see Fig. 9), a collection of cells that differentiate into the neurons and glia of the PNS as well as a variety of nonneural structures including melanocytes, chromaffin cells of the adrenal medulla, and mesenchymal derivatives in the head. The crest-derived elements ultimately give rise to most of the autonomic and sensory ganglia of the head and body (Fig. 10; see Fig. 13 in Chap. 3), as well as Schwann cells, which produce myelin in peripheral nerves.

Other sources of neural structures in the embryo are the **ectodermal placodes** of the head. The nasal and otic placodes are precursors of the olfactory receptor neurons and the auditory and vestibular receptors and ganglia, respectively. In addition, a specialized group of neurons from the nasal placode, the gonadotropin-releasing hormone cells, actually migrates from the placode into the brain during embryogenesis.

Development of the Brain

Development of the brain begins with differentiation of three swellings, or **vesicles**, at the rostral end of the neural tube. These vesicles are the **prosencephalon**, **mesencephalon**, and **rhombencephalon** (see Fig. 10A, B). This stage quickly proceeds to a five-vesicle stage of development in which the brain consists of the embryonic **telencephalon**, **diencephalon**, **mesencephalon**, **metencephalon**, and **myelencephalon** (see Fig. 10C, D). The first three of these vesicles eventually differentiate into the cerebral hemispheres, the diencephalon (including the thalamus and hypothalamus), and the midbrain, respectively. The metencephalon becomes the cerebellum and pons, whereas the embryonic myelencephalon becomes the medulla oblongata. This basic arrangement of five vesicles is established by the time the embryo is 6 weeks of age. Thereafter, the major change in form that produces the adult human brain is a tremendous growth of the cerebral hemispheres and cerebellum relative to other parts of the brain.

The internal development of the neural tube results in two functionally distinct regions. Neurons in the ventral portion of the tube form the **basal plate**, which is a motor area; those in the dorsal part of the tube form the **alar plate**, which assumes sensory functions. This simple functional organization is maintained in the dorsal and ventral horns of the adult spinal cord, but is altered in the brain stem by the course of the long tracts connecting the brain and spinal cord and by the development of specialized interneuronal cell groups.

Histogenesis of the Nervous System

The gross embryologic development of the nervous system is the product of a complicated process including the migration of nerve cells, the growth of their axons and dendrites, and the establishment of synaptic connections. The factors controlling these processes are critical for the establishment of appropriate contacts between the various parts of the system. Although these factors are still only partially understood, chemical guidance is clearly of great importance in migration. Both neuron cell bodies and fibers migrate along chemically marked pathways and in response to chemical gradients. In some instances, however, the physical scaffolding on which this migration occurs has also been found to be important. For example, in the develop-

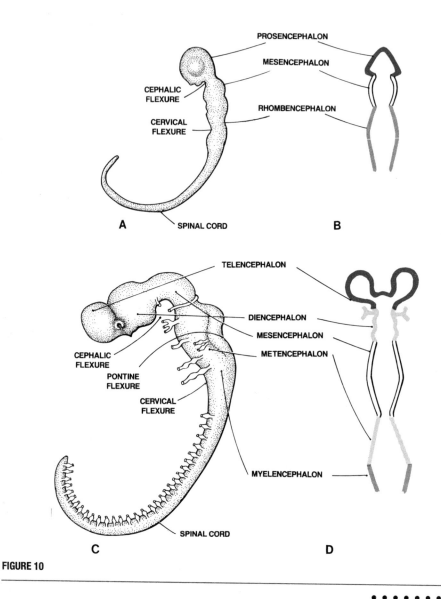

FIGURE 10

• • • • • • • • • •

(A) Lateral view of the CNS of a 4-week human embryo. (B) Dorsal view of a section through the three-vesicle brain in A. (C) Lateral view of the CNS and sensory ganglia in a 6-week human embryo. (D) Dorsal view of a section through the five-vesicle brain in C.

ing cerebral cortex and other laminated structures, the migrating neuron cell bodies follow the processes of radial glial cells to their place in the appropriate cell layer. Similarly, a neuroglial bridge of tissue between the developing cerebral hemispheres is a necessary substrate for the migration of fibers forming the corpus callosum.

Contacts between neurons are essential for normal development of the nervous system, as well as for its maintenance in the adult. Synaptic contacts provide a mechanism for exchange of trophic and regulatory influences for both the presynaptic and postsynaptic cells. In most cases, exchange of these factors prevents cell death of the presynaptic and postsynaptic neuron, but in some cases, this contact through active synapses actually appears to enhance cell death. Thus, cell contacts play a role in the control of cell death, which, like cell migration, is a fundamental process through which the adult form of the nervous system is achieved.

CHAPTER

2

The Physiology of Nerve Cells

THE RESTING MEMBRANE POTENTIAL

• • • • • • • • •

Neurons rely on both electrical (ionic) and chemical signals to communicate. In general, electrical signals are intraneuronal and chemical compounds are used as signals between neurons, but in some cases, interneuronal signals are ionic.

Nerve cells are bounded by membranes consisting of bilayers of lipoprotein. These cellular membranes maintain an electrical charge across the external and internal surfaces of the cell. At rest, nerve cells are positively charged on the outside and negatively charged on the inside. This electrical charge is termed the **resting membrane potential**. Arbitrarily, the outside of the cell is designated as zero, and because the inside of the cell is negative in relation to the outside, the resting membrane potential is a negative number. From direct measurements with microelectrodes, the resting membrane potential of various nerve cells has been found to be between -40 and -75 millivolts (mV) (a millivolt is one-thousandth of a volt). An increase in resting membrane potential, making it more negative, is termed **hyperpolarization**. A decrease in membrane potential, making it more positive, is called **depolarization**.

The resting membrane potential results from differences in the distribution of positive ions (cations) and negative ions (anions) over the intracellular and extracellular surfaces of the cell membrane. At rest, the nerve cell has an excess of positive charges on the outside of the membrane and an excess of negative charges on the inside. The membrane maintains this separation of charge because it acts as a barrier to the movement of these ions and because of energy-requiring pumps that maintain gradients of ions such as sodium and potassium (discussed later). Most of the fluid outside and inside nerve cells is electrically neutral; the separation of charges responsible for the resting membrane potential exists only in a very narrow region on either side of the membrane.

The ions principally responsible for the resting membrane potential include sodium

(Na$^+$) and chloride (Cl$^-$), which are concentrated outside the cell, and potassium (K$^+$) and organic anions (A$^-$), which are concentrated inside the cell. Organic anions are negatively charged amino acids and proteins. Nerve cells are variably permeable to Na$^+$, Cl$^-$, and K$^+$ but are impermeable to A$^-$.

The resting membrane potential of any cell can be determined by the **Nernst equation**. Developed originally to describe basic thermodynamic principles, it also applies to nerve cells at rest. According to this equation:

$$E = \frac{RT}{ZF} \ln \frac{C_2}{C_1}$$

where:

E = the difference in electrical potential between the inside and the outside of the cell (i.e., the resting membrane potential)

R = the universal gas constant

T = absolute temperature

Z = the valence of the ions under consideration

F = Faraday's constant (the electric charge per gram equivalent of univalent ions)

$\ln$ = the natural logarithm (this term can be replaced by $2.3 \times \log_{10}$)

C_2 = the concentration of ion outside the membrane

C_1 = the concentration of ion inside the membrane

The Nernst equation makes it possible to determine the resting membrane potential resulting from the concentrations of Na$^+$, K$^+$, and Cl$^-$ on the inside and outside of the cell.

For cells to maintain a steady resting membrane potential, the separation of charges across the membrane must be constant; that is, the influx of charge must be exactly balanced by the efflux of charge. Because of constantly open channels in the membrane and the differences in ion concentrations between the inside and outside of the cell, Na$^+$ constantly leaks into the cell and K$^+$ constantly leaks out of the cell. Opposing this migration is a **sodium-potassium pump**, which moves Na$^+$ out of the cell and K$^+$ into the cell and requires adenosine triphosphate as its energy source. Thus, metabolic energy is required to maintain the ionic gradients across the membrane. In contrast to Na$^+$ and K$^+$, Cl$^-$ is free to diffuse into or out of the cell, and in most cells, chloride is not pumped actively. Thus, Cl$^-$ is described as being **passively distributed** across the membrane, whereas Na$^+$ and K$^+$ are pumped and therefore are **actively distributed**.

THE ACTION POTENTIAL

• • • • • • • • •

The functions of various ion channels can disturb the resting membrane potential. These channels are multi-subunit proteins that span the cell membrane and are selectively permeable to ions. These channels fall into two broad classes, those that are opened or closed ("gated") by the presence or absence of neurotransmitters **(ligand-gated channels)** and those that open or close in response to changes in voltage across the membrane **(voltage-gated** or **voltage-sensitive channels)**. Specific types of channels are defined by characteristic physiologic behavior: their ion selectivity and pharmacology. These characteristics are conferred by the varieties of subunits available to assemble a channel protein. Finally, the activity of many of these channels is influenced by the various second-messenger systems within neurons. The processes by which neurotransmitters effect changes in neuronal activity via changes in ion channel activity is termed **signal transduction**.

The ion selectivity of neuronal channels is usually strict. The protein subunits that form the pore have sites that allow the passage of one or two ion species. In some instances, the ion, usually Na^+, K^+, Cl^- or Ca^{2+}, has only one function. For example, one type of K^+ channel (a passive or "leak" channel) is responsible for resting K^+ efflux, and a second type of voltage-sensitive K^+ channel is responsible for the K^+ efflux that participates in the action potential. In contrast, the acetylcholine-gated cation channel at the myoneural junction allows the influx of both Na^+ and K^+.

When a nerve cell is depolarized, for example, by application of an electrical stimulus or by a neurotransmitter (discussed later), voltage-sensitive Na^+ channels open and allow the influx of Na^+ ions. The greater the depolarization, the greater the fraction of open channels, resulting in a greater permeability to Na^+ and a net increase in positive charge flowing through the membrane. Positive charges thus accumulate inside the membrane, causing further depolarization (Fig. 11A). The increasing depolarization results in the opening of more voltage-gated Na^+ channels, resulting in a greater influx of positive charge, and thus increasing depolarization still further. Thus, a positive feedback cycle is established, driving the membrane potential toward the equilibrium potential of sodium, about +50 mV, which is the potential at which the electrical chemical gradients for Na^+ are exactly balanced inside and outside the cell.

Depolarization of a nerve cell membrane results in the opening of voltage-sensitive K^+ channels as well as Na^+ channels, but the opening of K^+ channels (see Fig. 11B) lags behind the opening of Na^+ channels (see Fig. 11D). Once they are open, however, these K^+ channels increase the efflux of K^+. Although depolarization continues, the Na^+ channels gradually become inactivated, and this, along with an increase in K^+ efflux, results in a net efflux of positive charge from the cell. The process continues until the cell repolarizes to its resting value (see Fig. 11B). The events described previously, influx of Na^+ followed by efflux of K^+, result in the development of an action potential (see Fig. 11C). The flow of current during the action potential is termed the **action current** (see Fig. 1E in Chap. 1). The action potential has characteristics determined only by the properties of the cell, independent of the characteristics of the exciting stimuli. The action potential can be propagated a very long distance along a nerve cell body or axon without variation of waveform and at a constant velocity.

Because of the ion selectivity of voltage-dependent channels, nerve cells can be modeled as electrical circuits. The electrical potential described previously as a resting potential can be viewed as the sum of different **electromotive forces** (i.e., batteries). The electromotive force components of nerve cells result from the concentration gradient of the ions distributed along the inside and outside of the nerve cell membranes. The channels themselves have the property of **(variable) conductance**, which is defined as the facility with which a current may flow. Conductance is the inverse of **resistance**, which is defined as the opposition to current flow. The conductance properties of nerve cells result from the individual characteristics of the proteins that form the ion channels. Nerve cells also have **capacitance**, which is the ability to store charges of opposite sign on two surfaces. Capacitance stems from the formation of the nerve cell membrane in a lipid bilayer.

In most nerve cells, action potentials are followed by a brief period of **hyperpolarization**, termed the **hyperpolarizing afterpotential**. This brief increase in the

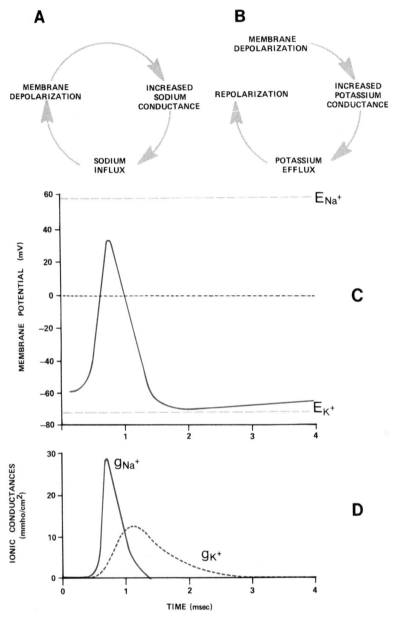

A

B

C

D

FIGURE 11

Events that occur during the action potential. (*A*) The depolarization phase of the nerve impulse has a regenerative aspect resulting from the positive feedback of membrane potential, sodium conductance, and sodium influx. (*B*) Membrane repolarization occurs when potassium efflux restores the internal negativity of the membrane. (*C and D*) Theoretical solution of the Nernst equation for changes in membrane potential (*C*) and sodium and potassium conductances (*D*) as a function of time.

negativity of the membrane potential occurs because the voltage-sensitive K⁺ channels that open during the late phase of the action potential do not all close immediately. It takes a few milliseconds for all of them to return to the closed state.

The action potential is also followed by a brief period of **refractoriness**, consisting of the **absolute** and **relative refractory periods**. The absolute refractory period comes immediately after the action potential, and during this interval, the cell cannot be excited to produce another action potential no matter how large a stimulating current is applied. The absolute refractory period is followed by the relative refractory period, an interval during which an action potential can be evoked by a stimulus that is stronger than the usual threshold stimulus necessary to evoke an action potential. Both periods of refractoriness result from the residual opening of K^+ channels and the residual inactivation of Na^+ channels.

Just as in nerve cell bodies, electrical stimulation of a peripheral nerve can evoke an action potential. In general, nerves with larger axons have lower stimulus thresholds for development of an action potential than do nerves with smaller axons. The conduction velocity of an action potential down an axon is proportional to the diameter of the axon. Thus, nerves with larger-diameter axons have greater conduction velocities than do nerves with smaller diameter axons. Conduction velocity is also substantially greater in **myelinated axons** than in **unmyelinated axons**. In unmyelinated fibers, nerve impulses are propagated by the continuous progression of the action potential along the length of the fiber. In myelinated fibers, during the propagation of the impulse, the transmembrane ionic current does not flow across the myelin sheath, but only flows across the cell membrane at the nodes of Ranvier (see Fig. 1E). The membrane at the nodes contains large numbers of voltage-dependent Na^+ and K^+ channels, whereas the intervening membrane has few channels. The action potential in effect jumps from node to node, a form of propagation termed **saltatory conduction**. This is an efficient method of transmitting action potentials because it results in maximum conduction velocities with a minimum amount of active-membrane and metabolic activity.

Electrical stimulation of a whole nerve consisting of large myelinated fibers produces in extracellular recordings a **spike potential**, followed by a **negative afterpotential**, followed by a **positive afterpotential** (Fig. 12). The negative afterpotential results from residual depolarization of nerve fiber membrane, and the positive afterpotential reflects hyperpolarization of the membrane.

SYNAPSES

Communication between neurons occurs at the **synapse**, which is the specialized contact zone where neurons communicate with each other. Two distinct types of synapses have been described: **electrical synapses** and **chemical synapses**. Electrical synapses have bridges interconnecting the cytoplasm of the presynaptic and postsynaptic cells. These synapses are called **bridged junctions** or **gap junctions**. The agent that mediates transmission at electrical synapses is ionic current, so there is little synaptic delay. Transmission across these synapses is limited only by the speed of electrical transmission across the short distance separating the presynaptic and postsynaptic elements. Electrical synapses can conduct in forward or backward directions equally well (i.e., from presynaptic to postsynaptic cell or from postsynaptic to presynaptic cell). In addition, channels between the two neurons at an electrical synapse allow for direct exchange of molecules between the cells. The human central nervous system (CNS) contains chiefly chemical synapses, though some electrical synapses have been described. For example, inferior olivary neurons contain electrical synapses.

Chemical synapses consist of presynaptic and postsynaptic neurons completely separated by a specialized synaptic cleft (see Fig. 1C in Chap. 1). The **presynaptic**

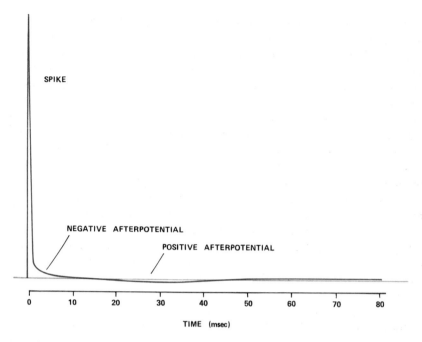

SPIKE

NEGATIVE AFTERPOTENTIAL

POSITIVE AFTERPOTENTIAL

TIME (msec)

FIGURE 12

• • • • • • • • •

Scale drawing of an action potential and related afterpotentials resulting from electrical stimulation, recorded extracellularly from the saphenous nerve of the cat. (Adapted from Erlanger, J and Gaser, HS: *Electrical Signs and Nervous Activity*. University of Pennsylvania Press, Philadelphia, 1938.)

terminal usually contains **synaptic vesicles**, which contain a chemical neurotransmitter. The **postsynaptic membrane active zone** contains specialized receptors, which are complex proteins that mediate the effect of the neurotransmitter. These synaptic agents, such as acetylcholine and norepinephrine, must diffuse across the synapse; thus, transmission is associated with a substantial **synaptic delay**, usually at least 0.3 millisecond (one-thousandth of a second) and sometimes up to 1 millisecond or even longer. This transmission can occur only in a single direction, from presynaptic cell to postsynaptic cell. Many single neurons of the CNS receive thousands of connections from other neurons. These are connected by chemical synapses, which can be excitatory or inhibitory.

A large number of chemical substances presumed to be excitatory neurotransmitters have been identified. The most common of these in the CNS is glutamate, which is thought to be a neurotransmitter in the cerebral cortex, hippocampus, subthalamic nucleus, and cerebellum. A smaller number of chemical substances thought to be inhibitory neurotransmitters have been identified. Gamma-aminobutyric acid (GABA) and glycine are the best characterized of these substances. GABA is distributed throughout the cerebral cortex, basal ganglia, and cerebellum and is inhibitory in all these sites. Glycine is found chiefly in the spinal cord, where it is inhibitory. Glycine is also found in small amounts within the cerebral cortex, where it has excitatory effects on glutamatergic synapses. Many other chemicals have been identified as putative neurotransmitters, including acetylcholine; monoamines such as dopamine, norepinephrine, and serotonin; and numerous peptides, including substance P, vasopressin, cholecystokinin, endorphin, and enkephalins. Only some of these have met the rigorous experimental criteria that establish them as neurotransmitters.

When an action potential moves down an axon and enters the axon terminal on the presynaptic side of the synapse, the opening of voltage-dependent Ca^{2+} channels allows the influx of Ca^{2+} ions, which initiate neurotransmitter release. As might be expected, Ca^{2+} channels are more abundant at presynaptic terminals than along the axons of nerve cells. Increasing extracellular Ca^{2+} concentration enhances transmitter release; decreasing Ca^{2+} concentration decreases release; and increasing magnesium (Mg^{2+}) concentration blocks release. There are several Ca^{2+} channel subtypes with different physiologic and pharmacologic properties; only some of these are coupled to transmitter release. After the transmitter is released, it diffuses across the synapse and binds to postsynaptic receptors.

Stimulation of a single presynaptic excitatory neuron evokes in the postsynaptic neuron an **excitatory postsynaptic potential (EPSP)**, which is a small, nonpropagated depolarization. The EPSP results from the opening of excitatory ligand-gated channels, usually cholinergic or glutamatergic channels. If increasing numbers of presynaptic neurons making connections with the same postsynaptic neuron are activated simultaneously, the EPSP progressively increases in amplitude until it brings the neuronal membrane to the threshold needed to generate an action potential. At this point, the postsynaptic neuron is depolarized, Na^+ channels have opened, and an all-or-nothing action potential is transmitted along the cell's axon.

Electrical stimulation of a single inhibitory presynaptic neuron contacting a single postsynaptic neuron results in the development of an **inhibitory postsynaptic potential (IPSP)**, which consists of a transient hyperpolarization of the postsynaptic membrane. The IPSP results from transient opening of transmitter-gated Cl^- and K^+ channels. Opening of Cl^- channels leads to movement of Cl^- into the cell; this hyperpolarizes the cell because it increases the negative charge intracellularly. Opening K^+ channels results in movement of K^+ out of the cell, decreasing the amount of positive charge within the cell and augmenting the hyperpolarization.

Neurotransmitters are released from presynaptic terminals in small packets termed **quanta**. A quantum of transmitter produces a small potential of fixed size in the postsynaptic neuron. This is known as a **unit potential**. Usually a **synaptic potential** is composed of many unit potentials. The amount of Ca^{2+} that enters the presynaptic neuron affects the number of quanta of transmitter that are released.

The processes of transmitter release, receptor activation, and the subsequent reuptake or chemical inactivation of the transmitter molecules are susceptible to the actions of chemicals at the synapses. Drugs and toxins, as well as endogenous enzymes, can interfere with presynaptic events, including the action potential; the synthesis of transmitter molecules and their release from vesicles; as well as the fate of the transmitter within the cleft and its influence on the postsynaptic membrane. All of these influence ion channel activity (and thus neuronal activity) indirectly, but some drugs, such as calcium channel blockers, also can directly influence ion channels.

All neurotransmitter receptors consist of proteins lodged in the cell membranes of either postsynaptic neurons or presynaptic terminals **(autoreceptors)**. Receptors act through two general mechanisms. In the first, the receptor is an integral part of a ligand-gated channel. Binding of a transmitter to its recognition site induces a conformational change in the channel, an associated ion flux, and either depolarization or hyperpolarization. This mechanism operates rapidly and underlies physiologic processes that require speed. Receptors of this type are called **ionotropic receptors**. The second mechanism involves a neurotransmitter–receptor interaction that leads to a signal mediated by second messengers. In this case, transmitter receptors are linked to other membrane-bound proteins called G proteins, which couple the receptor to its target inside the cell. The activated G protein may directly influence ion channel activity or may do so indirectly by a number of different biochemical pathways.

THE MYONEURAL JUNCTION

• • • • • • • • •

Communication from neuron to voluntary muscle occurs at the **motor end plate**, or **myoneural junction** (see Fig. 1D in Chap. 1). Here, the synaptic vesicles contain acetylcholine, which, upon release, activates the receptor channels in the postsynaptic membrane. The physiologic and molecular processes at the motor end plate are essentially identical to those at chemical synapses between neurons, and as at these neural junctions, drugs and toxins can affect function. For example, botulinum toxin inhibits the release of acetylcholine, thereby leading to loss of muscle activation. Clinically, this is seen as muscle weakness. If large amounts of the toxin have been ingested in inadequately processed food, weakness leads to a widespread paralysis that can be fatal.

The physiologic contact between neuron and muscle has long been recognized as a trophic and regulatory contact as well as a point of activation. Denervation of striated muscles leads to death of the muscle fibers and atrophy of the muscle. Research has demonstrated that this trophic function is also characteristic of contact between neurons in the CNS. If a neuron is deprived of its synaptic contacts as a result of injury or disease, rapid changes in metabolism, transmitter receptor production, and even the morphology (e.g., the dendritic structure) of the postsynaptic cell can occur.

SECTION

2

The Peripheral Nervous System

CHAPTER

3

The Spinal Nerves

The following terms are used to describe the nerves of the body. The fibers that innervate the muscles, joints, and skin of the body wall are termed **somatic**; those that innervate the internal organs of the body cavities and blood vessels throughout the body are termed **visceral**; sensory fibers are designated **afferent**; and motor fibers are designated **efferent**.

FUNCTIONAL COMPONENTS OF THE SPINAL NERVES

General Afferent Fibers

General afferent fibers are the sensory fibers that have their cells of origin in the **dorsal root ganglia**. These cells differ in shape from the neurons shown in Figure 1 in Chapter 1. Dorsal root ganglia cells are round and have only one process leaving the cell body. That process splits into a peripheral process, which enters the nerve, and a central process, which passes through the dorsal root to the spinal cord (Fig. 13).

General somatic afferent (GSA) fibers (Fig. 13A) carry exteroceptive information from receptors in the skin that mediate pain, temperature, and touch. **Exteroceptive** information is information received by an organism from its outer surface. GSA fibers also carry **proprioceptive** information from sensory endings in the muscles, tendons, and joints.

General visceral afferent (GVA) fibers (Fig. 13B) carry sensory impulses from receptors in the visceral structures, known as **interoceptive** information.

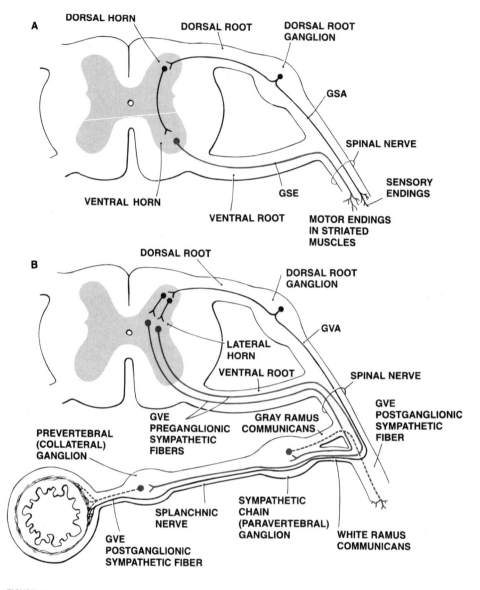

FIGURE 13

Functional components of a spinal nerve. (*A*) General somatic afferent (GSA) and general somatic efferent (GSE) components of a polysynaptic somatic reflex arc seen in two transverse sections through the spinal cord. (*B*) General visceral afferent (GVA) and general visceral efferent (GVE) components of visceral reflex arcs are also shown.

General Efferent Fibers

General efferent fibers are the motor fibers that have their cells of origin in the spinal cord (in the case of general somatic efferent and general visceral efferent preganglionic fibers) or in the autonomic ganglia (in the case of general visceral efferent postganglionic fibers).

General somatic efferent (GSE) fibers (Fig. 13A) consist of the motor fibers originating from the cell bodies of alpha, beta, and gamma motoneurons in lamina IX. These fibers innervate the striated skeletal muscles.

General visceral efferent (GVE) fibers (Fig. 13B) consist of the preganglionic and postganglionic autonomic fibers that innervate smooth muscle and cardiac muscle and regulate glandular secretion. **Preganglionic sympathetic** cell bodies are located in the intermediolateral cell column within lamina VII, which forms the lateral horn and extends only from segment T1 to segment L2 or L3 of the spinal cord. **Preganglionic parasympathetic** cell bodies are located in lamina VII in the sacral spinal cord (S2 to S4). In the sympathetic ganglia (and in parasympathetic ganglia in the pelvis), preganglionic fibers from the spinal cord synapse on the cell bodies of postganglionic autonomic neurons.

CLASSIFICATION OF NERVE FIBERS

• • • • • • • • •

Nerve fibers can be categorized according to fiber diameter, thickness of the myelin sheath, and speed of conduction of the nerve impulse. As mentioned in Chapter 2, in general, the larger the diameter of the fiber and the thicker the myelin sheath, the faster the conduction velocity. Two classifications of nerve fibers are in use (Table 1). One is an electrophysiologic classification based on the conduction velocities of motor and sensory nerve fibers. These velocities are revealed by peaks in the compound action potential when an entire compound nerve (i.e., a nerve containing many motor and sensory fibers) is stimulated electrically and recordings are made extracellularly. This action potential consists of the algebraic sum of the action po-

• • • • • • • • •

TABLE 1

CLASSIFICATION OF NERVE FIBERS

Sensory and Motor Fibers	Sensory Fibers	Largest Fiber Diameter	Fastest Conduction Velocity (m/sec)	General Comments	
Aα		22	120	Motor:	The large alpha motoneurons of lamina IX, innervating extrafusal muscle fibers
Aα	Ia	22	120	Sensory:	The primary afferents of muscle spindles
Aα	Ib	22	120	Sensory:	Golgi tendon organs, touch and pressure receptors
Aβ		13	70	Motor:	The motor neurons innervating both extrafusal and intrafusal (muscle spindle) muscle fibers
Aβ	II	13	70	Sensory:	The secondary afferents of muscle spindles, touch and pressure receptors, and Pacinian corpuscles (vibratory sensors)
Aγ		8	40	Motor:	The small gamma motoneurons of lamina IX, innervating intrafusal fibers (muscle spindles)
Aδ	III	5	15	Sensory:	Small, lightly myelinated fibers; touch, pressure, pain, and temperature receptors
B		3	14	Motor:	Small, lightly myelinated preganglionic autonomic fibers
C		1	2	Motor:	All postganglionic autonomic fibers (all are unmyelinated)
C	IV	1	2	Sensory:	Unmyelinated pain and temperature fibers

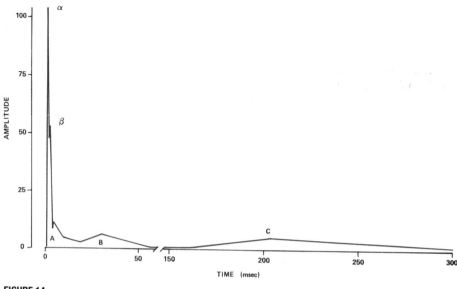

FIGURE 14

A complete compound action potential resulting from electrical stimulation of the sciatic nerve of a frog. Several components of the A group of fibers cannot be distinguished, because the time scale was chosen to illustrate the B and C fiber peaks. The amplitude of the action potential is plotted relative to the A peak. (Adapted from Erlanger, J and Gaser, HS: *Electrical Signs and Nervous Activity.* University of Pennsylvania Press, Philadelphia, 1938.)

tentials of the individual fibers within the nerve. In this classification, fibers fall into three groups: A, B, and C (Fig. 14). The A and B fibers are myelinated, and the C fibers are unmyelinated. The A fibers are further subdivided on the basis of mean conduction velocity, and hence fiber size, into several subgroups: alpha, beta, gamma, and delta. The A fibers contain separate motor components that innervate two types of muscle fiber. **Extrafusal muscle** is striated muscle outside the muscle spindles; it is innervated by the large-diameter **alpha fibers. Intrafusal muscle** consists of muscle fibers within the muscle spindles; it is innervated by the small-diameter **gamma fibers**. The intermediate-sized **beta** group has motor fibers innervating both types of muscle. The C fibers are subdivided into two classes: sC fibers (postganglionic efferent sympathetic C fibers) and drC fibers (afferent dorsal root C fibers). A second system of nerve fiber classification, pertaining only to sensory fibers, includes four groups that are differentiated chiefly on the basis of size but also according to fiber origin. Three important elements in this classification are as follows: group Ia afferents **(spindle primary afferents)**, which arise in muscle spindles; group Ib afferents, which originate in **Golgi tendon organs**; and group II afferents **(spindle secondary afferents)**, which also come from muscle spindles.

CHAPTER

4

Spinal Reflexes and Muscle Tone

SPINAL REFLEXES

Any reflex action consists of a specific, stereotyped response to an **adequate stimulus**. The adequate stimuli for somatic spinal reflexes involve input to the central nervous system (CNS) from peripheral receptors in muscles, skin, and joints. (Visceral reflexes are discussed in Chap. 5). The response involves contraction of striated skeletal muscle fibers (extrafusal fibers). A reflex response may be mediated by as few as two neurons, one afferent and one efferent, and in this case is termed a **monosynaptic reflex response**. Muscle stretch (deep tendon) reflexes such as the knee jerk are monosynaptic reflexes.

In most instances, a reflex response involves several neurons, called **interneurons** or **internuncial cells**, in addition to the afferent and efferent neurons. A reflex response mediated by more than two neurons is termed **polysynaptic** (see Fig. 13A in Chap. 3). A reflex may involve neurons in (1) just one or a few spinal cord levels, as in the case of segmental reflexes (those restricted to a single spinal cord segment); (2) several to many spinal cord levels, as in the case of intersegmental reflexes; or (3) structures in the brain that influence the spinal cord, as in the case of supraspinal reflexes.

MUSCLE SPINDLES

Muscle spindles are receptor organs that provide the CNS with information about the length and the rate of change in length of striated muscles. Thus, the muscle spindles are the afferent component of muscle stretch reflexes. These receptor organs are also equipped with a motor nerve supply that is capable of altering the sensitivity of the receptor to muscle length. Muscle spindles are encapsulated structures, found in most skeletal muscles of the body. They vary in length from 1 to 3 mm in small muscles, such as the lumbricalis, to 7 to 10 mm in large muscles. Muscle spindles also vary in number, or density, in different muscles of the body and are particularly numerous in the small, delicate muscles of the hand. Each spindle contains 2 to 12 thin muscle fibers of modified striated muscle. Because these fibers are enclosed within the capsule of the fusiform spindle, they are termed **intrafusal** muscle fibers to differentiate them from the large **extrafusal** fibers (Fig. 15). The muscle spindle is attached to the connective tissue septae that run between extrafusal fibers. Consequently, the entire muscle spindle structure is connected to the muscle's tendons in parallel with the extrafusal fibers, a fact that is important in the function of the muscle spindle. This parallel arrangement means that increases in force during muscle contraction induce modest lengthening of the tendon, which is accompanied by a relative reduction of spindle fiber length and a decline in spindle afferent firing. There are two distinct types of intrafusal fibers, as well as a third, intermediate type. The longest and largest type of intrafusal fiber contains numerous large nuclei closely packed in a central bag and hence is called a **nuclear bag** fiber (see Fig. 15). The other main type of intrafusal fiber is shorter and thinner and contains a single row, or chain, of central nuclei; this is known as a **nuclear chain** fiber (see Fig. 15). A third type of intrafusal fiber is intermediary in structure between bag and chain fibers and is termed bag$_2$ to differentiate it from the more conventional type of bag fiber, which is now termed bag$_1$.

Both bag and chain fibers are innervated by gamma motoneurons, which terminate in two types of endings: **plates** and **trails** (see Fig. 15). Plate endings occur chiefly on nuclear bag fibers and rarely on nuclear chain fibers. Trail endings occur mostly on nuclear chain fibers but are frequently found on bag fibers as well. Muscle spindles are amply supplied with sensory nerve endings of two types: primary endings derived from group Ia nerve fibers and secondary endings derived from group II fibers. Primary afferents arise in the central equatorial region of both bag and chain fibers. Secondary endings arise predominantly on nuclear chain fibers and lie to either side of the primary endings.

ALPHA, BETA, AND GAMMA MOTONEURONS

• • • • • • • • •

Muscle contraction in response to a stimulus involves activation of the alpha, beta, and gamma motoneurons of lamina IX. **Alpha motoneurons** are the largest of the anterior horn cells. They can be stimulated monosynaptically by (1) the Ia primary afferents and group II secondary afferents of the muscle spindles; (2) corticospinal tract fibers in primates (see Fig. 15); (3) lateral vestibulospinal tract fibers; and (4) reticulospinal and raphe spinal tract fibers. Although alpha motoneurons can be stimulated monosynaptically by muscle spindles and their descending tracts, in a vast majority of cases, they are influenced through interneurons in the spinal cord gray matter in response to activation of segmental, intersegmental, and supraspinal circuits. All descending tracts of the spinal cord ultimately influence the activity of these neurons. Each alpha motoneuron innervates a group of extrafusal muscle fibers within a specific muscle. The functional unit defined by this neuron and its muscle fibers is called a **motor unit**. Motor units in proximal muscles, which are used for

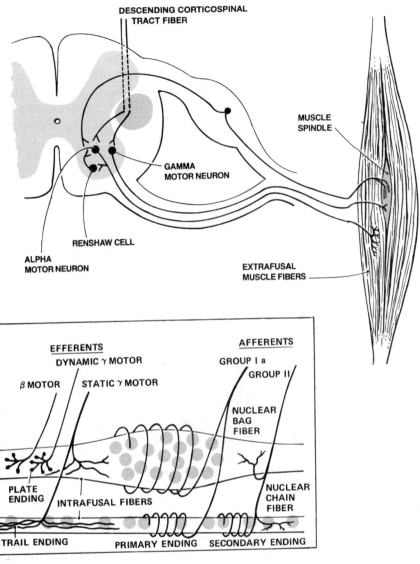

FIGURE 15

A cross section of the spinal cord shows a Ia afferent fiber originating in a muscle spindle, passing through a peripheral nerve, entering a dorsal root, and making synaptic connection with an alpha motoneuron. The axon of the alpha motoneuron emerges through the ventral root, passes through the peripheral nerve, and terminates in extrafusal muscle fibers. The axon of the gamma motoneuron terminates in intrafusal fibers within the muscle spindle. The inset shows an enlarged view of the **intrafusal fibers** within the muscle spindle and the principal nerve endings on the fibers.

postural control, are much larger (i.e., many muscle fibers are controlled by a single motoneuron) than motor units in distal limb muscles, which are used for finely controlled movements. Thus, in the muscles of the shoulder, for example, there may be hundreds of muscle fibers in each motor unit, whereas in an intrinsic muscle of the hand, each alpha motoneuron may innervate fewer than 10 muscle cells.

Alpha motoneurons innervate not only the large extrafusal skeletal muscle fibers but also interneurons in the ventral horn **(Renshaw cells)** through collateral fibers emerging from their axons (see Fig. 15). Renshaw cells have weak inhibitory synaptic actions on alpha motoneurons and can modify the probability of firing of these neurons.

Gamma motoneurons, which are also termed **fusimotor neurons**, innervate the intrafusal muscle fibers within the muscle spindles of skeletal muscle. They do not innervate extrafusal muscle fibers and consequently do not produce extrafusal muscle contraction. Gamma motoneurons differ from alpha motoneurons in other ways as well. Gamma motoneurons (1) are smaller; (2) are not excited monosynaptically by segmental inputs; (3) are not involved in inhibitory feedback mechanisms by Renshaw cells; and (4) tend to discharge spontaneously, often at high frequencies. Despite these differences between gamma and alpha motoneurons, both generally respond similarly to incoming stimuli. Most of the descending pathways of the spinal cord influence the activity of both types of neurons. The reticular system, cerebellum, and basal ganglia exert particularly strong control over the gamma motoneurons through descending pathways described in Chapter 8.

The axons of **beta motoneurons** are comparable in diameter to those of alpha motoneurons. Beta motoneurons innervate both extrafusal and intrafusal muscle fibers, and they provide a significant fraction of the innervation of muscle spindles.

THE STRETCH REFLEX

• • • • • • • • •

The **stretch (myotatic) reflex** is the basic neural mechanism for maintaining tone (i.e., a constant state of mild tension) in muscles. Aside from its role in keeping relaxed muscles slightly active, the stretch reflex is capable of increasing the tension of select muscle groups to provide a background of postural muscle tone on which voluntary muscle movements can be superimposed. The stretch reflex results from inputs to motoneuron pools from both group Ia excitatory afferents mediated monosynaptically and group II excitatory afferents mediated both monosynaptically and polysynaptically.

The **deep tendon reflex** is a manifestation of the stretch reflex that can be tested by tapping the tendon of a muscle. For example, tapping the patellar tendon stretches the extrafusal fibers of the quadriceps femoris muscle group. Because the muscle spindles are arranged in parallel with the extrafusal fibers of the quadriceps, the intrafusal fibers are also stretched. The stretching stimulates the sensory endings on the intrafusal fibers, particularly the primary afferents (group Ia fibers). The Ia afferents monosynaptically stimulate the alpha motoneurons that supply the quadriceps muscle and polysynaptically inhibit the alpha motoneurons of the antagonist muscle group (the hamstring muscles). Consequently, the quadriceps suddenly contracts and the hamstring muscles relax, causing the leg to extend at the knee.

Group Ia fibers innervating the primary endings in muscle spindles establish direct monosynaptic connections with alpha motoneurons innervating the same (homonymous) muscles and synergistic (heteronymous) muscles (see Fig. 15). Group II afferent fibers from muscle spindles excite homonymous alpha motoneurons monosynaptically.

The sensory function of the intrafusal fibers is to inform the nervous system of the length and rate of change in length of the extrafusal fibers. In the absence of any gamma motoneuron activation, the primary afferents respond to both the length of muscle and the rate of change in length of muscle. In contrast, the secondary endings respond chiefly to muscle length. Activation of gamma motoneurons makes the intrafusal muscle fibers contract and therefore makes the sensory portion of the muscle spindles more responsive to stretch. Because muscle spindles are located in parallel with extrafusal fibers, muscle spindles are passively shortened during muscle contraction, which results in cessation of discharge of the afferent nerve fibers. Gamma motoneuron activation, however, can prevent muscle spindles from ceasing to fire during extrafusal muscle contraction.

Two types of gamma motoneurons have been described. One type affects the afferent responses to phasic extension more than the responses to static tension. This type of neuron is called the **dynamic gamma motoneuron**. The other type of neuron increases the spindle response to static extension and thus is called the **static gamma motoneuron**. Dynamic gamma motoneurons are thought to terminate in plate endings solely on nuclear bag fibers, whereas static gamma fibers terminate in trail endings on both bag and chain fibers. Thus, gamma motoneurons can adjust the length of intrafusal fibers so that the spindle receptors can operate on a sensitive portion of their response scale. In addition, during a powerful contraction with considerable shortening, it may be advantageous for the spindle receptors to continue firing to reinforce the power of the contraction reflexly. This is referred to as the **servo-assisted** method of producing and controlling movement. Much of the information from spindles is used at high levels of the nervous system, particularly the cerebellum and cerebral cortex. Muscle spindles convey information needed for the conscious perception of limb position and movement. Moreover, these high levels of the nervous system can influence the descending pathways that facilitate and inhibit alpha and gamma motoneuron activity. Supraspinal, intersegmental, and segmental influences usually cause the discharge of both alpha and gamma motoneurons innervating a particular muscle. This phenomenon is known as **coactivation.**

GOLGI TENDON ORGANS

● ● ● ● ● ● ● ●

Golgi tendon organs are encapsulated structures attached in series with the large, collagenous fibers of tendons at the insertions of muscles and along the fascial covering of muscles. Within the capsule, sensory nerve endings (Ib afferents) terminate on small bundles of collagenous fibers of tendons. When muscle contraction occurs, shortening of the contractile part of the muscle stretches the noncontractile region where tendon organs are located. The result is vigorous firing of the afferent fibers innervating Golgi tendon organs. Thus, these receptors are primarily sensitive to muscle contraction. Their afferents project to the spinal cord, where they polysynaptically inhibit the alpha motoneurons innervating the agonist muscle and facilitate motoneurons of the antagonist muscle.

MUSCLE TONE

● ● ● ● ● ● ● ●

The term **muscle tone** indicates the resistance that an examiner perceives when passively manipulating the limbs of a patient. In a relaxed normal person, when a limb is manipulated at one of the joints, a certain amount of resistance is encountered in muscle; this resistance is not related to any conscious effort on the part of the patient. There are two general abnormalities of muscle tone: hypotonia and hypertonia. **Hypotonia** is a decrease of resistance to passive manipulation of the limbs, and **hypertonia** is an increase of resistance to passive manipulation of the limbs.

Hypotonia occurs in a limb at once if the ventral roots containing the motor nerve fibers to the limb are cut. It also results from transection of the dorsal roots that contain sensory fibers from the muscle. Thus, muscle tone is maintained and regulated in muscles by reflex activity of the nervous system and is not a property of isolated muscle. Hypotonia may also occur with disease that affects certain parts of the nervous system, particularly the cerebellum.

Hypertonia appears in one of two general forms: spasticity and rigidity. In **spasticity**, which usually results from disease of the corticospinal and corticobulbar pathways, there is a "clasp-knife" type of resistance to passive manipulation accompanied by an increase in the amplitude of the muscle stretch reflexes. The clasp-knife phenomenon indicates a marked increase in resistance to passive manipulation (in flexion or extension) during the initial portion of the manipulation. As the manipulation proceeds, the resistance suddenly decreases and disappears. The disappearance of resistance previously was thought to result from activation of Golgi tendon organs, but evidence indicates that group III and IV (Aδ and C) muscle afferents are responsible. Group III and IV afferents are those that respond to a variety of stimuli, including thermal, chemical, mechanical, and noxious stimuli. In **rigidity**, which usually results from disease of the basal ganglia, there is a plastic or "cogwheel" type of resistance to passive manipulation, often without changes in muscle stretch reflexes.

REFLEXES OF CUTANEOUS ORIGIN

• • • • • • • • •

The sensory receptors in skin and subcutaneous tissues respond to touch, pressure, temperature, and tissue damage. These receptors generate signals that have reflex effects on spinal motoneurons mediated by interneurons. The **flexor reflex** and **crossed extensor reflex** are examples of responses to aversive stimuli that permit a limb to be withdrawn from a source of injury and that allow a postural compensation to occur. A noxious stimulus to a limb results in flexion of the ipsilateral limb and extension of the contralateral limb. For example, when an individual steps on something very hot or sharp, a reflex withdrawal of the stimulated extremity occurs. This is the result of the polysynaptic facilitation of alpha motoneurons innervating the ipsilateral flexor muscles and inhibition of motoneurons innervating the extensor muscles of the same leg (the flexor reflex). Simultaneously, the opposite limb extends to support the weight of the body. The limb extension results from facilitation of motoneurons innervating extensor muscles and inhibition of motoneurons innervating flexor muscles (i.e., the crossed extensor reflexes).

CHAPTER

5

The Autonomic Nervous System

The autonomic nervous system (ANS) is the functional division of the peripheral nervous system that innervates **smooth and cardiac muscle** and the **glands** of the body. Although by its original definition the ANS consists only of motor **(general visceral efferent)** fibers, the sensory **(general visceral afferent)** fibers accompanying the motor fibers to the viscera are integrally related, both anatomically and functionally, with the motor fibers and must be considered part of the ANS. Only the efferent system is described here, and a brief discussion of the visceral afferent system is located in Chapter 6. Under ordinary circumstances, the ANS functions at the subconscious level. It acts to regulate the ongoing, reflexively driven activity of smooth muscle, cardiac muscle, and glands and integrates visceral systems with each other and with somatic motor function. The organs innervated by the ANS can carry out their most basic functions (e.g., cardiac contractions, peristalsis of the intestinal tract) without external regulation from the autonomic fibers. In situations that require rapidly fluctuating or extreme responses, however, the autonomic nerves are essential for proper visceral function.

Visceral motor neurons are controlled by visceral and somatic sensory inputs, as well as by integrative influences from the brain stem and hypothalamus. Unlike the somatic motor system, the peripheral ANS reaches its effector organs by a two-neuron chain.

The cell bodies and fibers of this chain are classified as follows:

1. The **preganglionic neuron**, the presynaptic or primary neuron, is located in the brain stem (cranial nerve nuclei III, VII, IX, X, and XI) or spinal cord (intermediolateral cell column in lamina VII).
2. The **postganglionic neuron**, the postsynaptic or secondary neuron, is located in an outlying ganglion and innervates the end organ.

DIVISIONS OF THE AUTONOMIC NERVOUS SYSTEM

• • • • • • • • •

The preganglionic fibers have their cell bodies of origin in three regions of the brain stem and spinal cord. The **thoracolumbar outflow** consists of the fibers that arise in the **intermediolateral cell column** of the 12 thoracic and the first 2 lumbar segments of the spinal cord. This is the **sympathetic division of the ANS**. The **cranial outflow** consists of fibers that arise in the nuclei of cranial nerves III, VII, IX, X, and XI. These fibers follow the cranial nerve branches to their destinations. The **sacral outflow** consists of fibers that arise from cell bodies in the intermediate cell column of sacral segments 2 through 4. These fibers form the pelvic splanchnic nerves (nervi erigentes). The cranial and sacral outflow share many anatomic and functional features and together form the **parasympathetic division of the ANS**.

The sympathetic and parasympathetic divisions of the ANS are differentiated not only by their sites of origin but also on the basis of the neurotransmitters released at the terminals of the postganglionic fibers. The terminals of the parasympathetic postganglionic fibers liberate acetylcholine and thus are classified as **cholinergic**. The terminals of the sympathetic postganglionic fibers release **norepinephrine** and thus are classified as **adrenergic**. An exception to this rule is found in the terminals of sympathetic fibers on sweat glands, which are cholinergic.

Many organs receive postganglionic innervation from both the sympathetic and parasympathetic systems. When this occurs, the fibers from the two systems frequently have opposing effects. For example, parasympathetic fibers to the stomach increase peristalsis and relax the sphincters, whereas sympathetic fibers have the opposite effect.

Although the neurotransmitters released by postganglionic fibers distinguish the sympathetic and parasympathetic divisions, the preganglionic neurons in both of these visceral efferent systems release acetylcholine.

THE SYMPATHETIC NERVOUS SYSTEM

• • • • • • • • •

The myelinated preganglionic fibers (B fibers) of the sympathetic system, which originate in the intermediolateral cell column of the thoracolumbar cord, leave the spinal cord with the motor fibers of ventral roots T1 to L2, but soon separate from the spinal nerves to form the **white rami communicantes**, which enter the **chain ganglia** of the **sympathetic trunks** (see Fig. 13B in Chap. 3). The trunks are the paired, ganglionated chains of nerve fibers that extend along either side of the vertebral column from the base of the skull to the coccyx. Some of the fibers of the white rami synapse with postganglionic neurons in the chain ganglion (also called **paravertebral ganglion**) nearest their point of entrance (see Fig. 13B in Chap. 3). Other preganglionic fibers pass up or down the chain to end in paravertebral ganglia at higher or lower levels than the point of entrance (not shown in Fig. 13 in Chap. 3). A third group of preganglionic fibers passes through the paravertebral ganglion into a thoracic **splanchnic nerve** and terminates in the **prevertebral ganglia** of the abdomen and pelvis (see Fig. 13B in Chap. 3).

Some of the nonmyelinated postganglionic fibers (C fibers) given off from the neurons in the sympathetic chain ganglia form the **gray rami communicantes** (see

Fig. 13B in Chap. 3). Each spinal nerve receives a gray ramus that delivers postganglionic fibers to be distributed to the blood vessels, erector pili muscles, and sweat glands of the body wall throughout the dermatome innervated by that nerve. Thus, there are 31 gray rami on each side of the body, one for each spinal nerve, but there are only 14 white rami. As mentioned previously, the white rami carry the preganglionic fibers from the thoracic and upper lumbar segments to the sympathetic chain (trunk). Therefore, the cervical, lower lumbar, and sacral ganglia of the chain receive preganglionic fibers that have traveled up or down the trunk from the thoracolumbar levels.

The **cervical part** of the sympathetic trunk consists of ascending preganglionic fibers from the first four or five thoracic segments of the spinal cord. Three ganglia are present: **superior cervical, middle cervical,** and **cervicothoracic** (stellate). The latter is formed by fusion of the inferior cervical and first thoracic ganglia. The superior cervical ganglion cells give rise to the **carotid plexus**, a network of postganglionic fibers that follow the ramifications of the carotid arteries and furnish the sympathetic innervation of the entire head. Some fibers end in blood vessels and sweat glands of the head and face; others supply the lacrimal and salivary glands. The eye receives sympathetic fibers that innervate the dilator muscles of the pupil and the smooth muscle fibers in the muscle that raises the eyelid. Sympathetic innervation to the neck and arms is provided by gray rami from the cervical ganglia to each of the cervical and the first thoracic spinal nerves. In addition, these same ganglia give rise to postganglionic fibers forming the **cardiac nerves** to the cardiac plexus.

The viscera of the thorax are supplied by the cardiac nerves from the cervical ganglia and by postganglionic fibers from the upper thoracic ganglia. These fibers enter the plexus of the heart and lungs.

The viscera of the abdominal and pelvic cavities are supplied by the **thoracic splanchnic nerves**. The greater, lesser, and least thoracic splanchnic nerves carry mainly preganglionic fibers from spinal cord levels T5 to T12, through the sympathetic trunk without synapsing, to the **prevertebral ganglia** (collateral) of the abdomen. The prevertebral ganglia include the **celiac, superior mesenteric,** and **aorticorenal** ganglia, which are located at the roots of the arteries for which they are named. The neurons in these ganglia give rise to postganglionic axons that travel along the arterial walls to reach most of the abdominal viscera. There are also **lumbar splanchnic nerves**, which carry the preganglionic fibers from the levels of the upper lumbar spinal cord. These lumbar splanchnic nerves terminate in the **inferior mesenteric** and **hypogastric ganglia**. The postganglionic fibers from these prevertebral ganglia follow the ramifications of the visceral arteries to reach the organs of the lower abdomen and pelvis.

Summary of Sympathetic Nervous System Anatomy

The preganglionic neurons of the sympathetic nervous system are all located in the thoracolumbar spinal cord gray matter. Their axons form the 14 pairs of white rami communicantes, which connect spinal nerves T1 to L2 with their corresponding chain ganglia. Postganglionic neurons are found in all ganglia of the sympathetic chain. The cervical ganglia receive their preganglionic input from cells in spinal cord segments T1 to T5. Axons of these cells enter the sympathetic chain in the thorax and ascend through the cervical trunk. The superior cervical ganglion supplies postganglionic fibers to structures of the head. The lower cervical ganglia supply the viscera of the neck. The thoracic viscera receive postganglionic innervation from cells in the upper thoracic chain ganglia. The heart also receives innervation from the cervical ganglia. The abdominal and pelvic viscera receive postganglionic input from cells of the prevertebral ganglia in the abdomen. These ganglia receive preganglionic innervation from cells in the lower thoracic and upper lumbar spinal cord. The preganglionic axons are conveyed to the ganglia through the thoracic splanchnic nerves (to the abdomen) and the lumbar and sacral splanchnic nerves (to the pelvis).

In addition to this visceral distribution, the blood vessels in the muscles and the blood vessels, sweat glands, and erector pili muscles in the skin of the entire body wall receive postganglionic sympathetic innervation. These postganglionic fibers arise entirely from the chain ganglia and reach each spinal nerve by way of a gray ramus communicantes. There are 31 gray rami on each side of the body. In regions of the body where there are not separate chain ganglia for each segment, more than one gray ramus arises from each ganglion (e.g., the large superior cervical ganglion provides postganglionic fibers in gray rami to cervical nerves 1 to 4 in addition to its postganglionic supply to the head).

Clinical Aspects of Sympathetic Function

Injury to the cervical portion of the sympathetic system produces **Horner's syndrome**. The **pupil** of the eye on the injured side is constricted (miotic) because its dilator muscle is paralyzed. There is partial ptosis of the eyelid because of denervation of the smooth muscle fibers in the levator palpebrae superioris muscle, but the lid can still be raised voluntarily through the action of the general somatic efferent fibers in cranial nerve III on the skeletal muscle fibers in the same muscle. An apparent enophthalmos (the eye appears to be sunken into its socket) may be noted as well. **Absence of sweating (anhidrosis)** and **vasodilatation** on the affected side cause the skin of the face and neck to appear reddened and feel warmer and drier than the normal side. Horner's syndrome may result from lesions that interrupt the central nervous system pathways descending ipsilaterally from the hypothalamus through the brain stem to the spinal cord. It can also occur when a lesion of the spinal cord destroys the preganglionic neurons at their origin in the upper thoracic segments. Horner's syndrome also can follow injury to the cervical sympathetic chain ganglia or the superior cervical ganglion and its postganglionic fibers.

Sympathetic fibers are known vasoconstrictors, and operations have been devised to increase circulation by interrupting this innervation. **Lumbar sympathectomy**, which is performed to increase circulation in the lower extremity, is the most common procedure.

Sympathetic Innervation of the Adrenal Gland

Stimulation of the sympathetic nervous system ordinarily produces generalized physiologic responses rather than discrete localized effects. This results in part from the wide dispersion of sympathetic fibers, but it is augmented by the release of epinephrine from the adrenal glands into the blood. Preganglionic fibers from the lesser and least splanchnic nerves supply the medulla of the adrenal gland, ending directly on the adrenal medullary cells without synapsing in an interposed ganglion. The chromaffin cells in the adrenal medulla are derivatives of the neural crest, as are the autonomic ganglia. Thus, in effect, the adrenal medulla constitutes a modified sympathetic ganglion. Pain, exposure to cold, and strong emotions such as rage and fear evoke sympathetic activity that mobilizes the body's resources for violent action. The functions of the gastrointestinal tract are suspended, and blood is shunted away from the splanchnic area. Heart rate and blood pressure increase, the coronary arteries dilate, and the bronchioles of the lungs widen. The spleen releases extra red cells to the blood. This activity has been described as the "fight or flight" phenomenon and is primarily the result of activation of the sympathetic nervous system and the adrenal medulla.

THE PARASYMPATHETIC NERVOUS SYSTEM

The preganglionic fibers of the parasympathetic system extend to the **terminal ganglia** located within, or very close to, the organs they supply. As a result, the postganglionic fibers are short.

The **cranial division** of the parasympathetic system originates in cranial nerves III, VII, IX, X, and XI. Parasympathetic innervation of the ciliary muscle and sphincter muscle of the pupil passes through the oculomotor nerve (III) and **ciliary ganglion**. Secretory preganglionic fibers from the nervus intermedius of cranial nerve VII synapse in the **pterygopalatine** and **submandibular ganglia**. Postganglionic fibers from the pterygopalatine ganglion innervate glands in the mucous membrane of the nasal chamber, the air sinuses, the palate and pharynx, and the lacrimal gland, whereas the fibers of the submandibular ganglion supply the sublingual and submandibular salivary glands. The **otic ganglion**, which receives preganglionic fibers of cranial nerve IX, supplies postganglionic fibers to the parotid gland. The vagus nerve (X) supplies the preganglionic fibers to the heart, lungs, and abdominal viscera. The latter organs have their postganglionic neurons in associated plexuses adjacent to or within the walls of the viscus. The cranial, or bulbar, part of cranial nerve XI also contributes to the preganglionic parasympathetic innervation of the heart.

The **sacral division** arises from parasympathetic preganglionic neurons in the intermediate gray column of lamina VII in spinal cord segments S2, S3, and S4. Axons of these cells form the **pelvic splanchnic nerves** and supply fibers to ganglia in the muscular coats of the urinary and reproductive tracts, the descending and sigmoid colon, and the rectum. In the pelvic region, the parasympathetic system is primarily concerned with mechanisms for emptying the bladder and rectum. Under strong emotional circumstances, these fibers may discharge along with a generalized sympathetic response and produce involuntary emptying of these organs.

Both the parasympathetic and sympathetic divisions of the ANS are needed for sexual activity. In women, the parasympathetic fibers are responsible for increased vaginal secretions, erection of the clitoris, and engorgement of the labia minora. In men, the parasympathetic fibers are responsible for penile erection, but stimulation by sympathetic fibers initiates the contractions of the ductus deferens and seminal vesicles to start the processes of emission and ejaculation. Final ejaculation through the urethral canal results from parasympathetic activity. Disease of the parasympathetic fibers, as in diabetic neuropathy, causes impotence, with failure of erection and ejaculation. Disease of the sympathetic fibers or drug treatment with adrenergic blocking agents can impair ejaculation. Sympathetic overactivity, often related to emotions, can cause weakness of erection and premature ejaculation. Loss of both libido and potency can be caused by cerebral lesions or the use of various drugs, including antihypertensives, diuretics, antidepressants, antipsychotics, and sedatives.

INNERVATION OF THE URINARY BLADDER

• • • • • • • • •

Motor control of the urinary bladder results primarily from parasympathetic function that is purely reflex in infants but is under voluntary regulation in normal adults. The preganglionic fibers of the parasympathetic nerves to the bladder have their cell bodies in the intermediate region of the gray matter of sacral cord segments 2, 3,

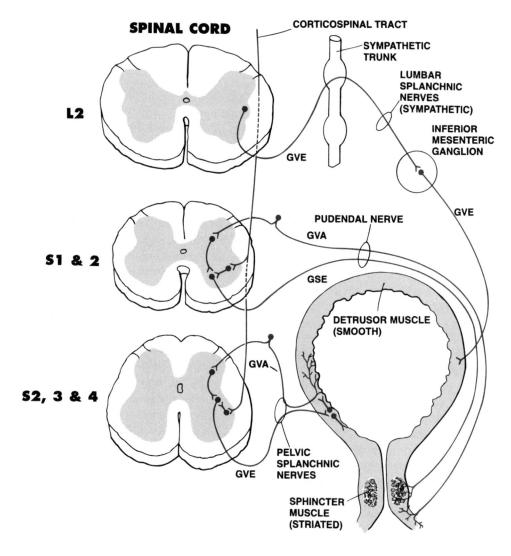

FIGURE 16

• • • • • • • • •

Autonomic innervation of the urinary bladder and associated somatic innervation of the sphincter.

and 4. They enter the pelvic splanchnic nerves, pass through the vesical plexus, and terminate on ganglia located in the wall of the bladder (Fig. 16). Short postganglionic fibers innervate the detrusor muscle, which forms the wall of the bladder. Stimulation of the parasympathetic nerves of the bladder contracts the detrusor muscle, opens the neck of the bladder into the urethra, and empties the bladder.

The **sympathetic** supply to the bladder originates in cells of the intermediolateral gray column of upper lumbar cord segments whose axons pass through the sympathetic trunk to reach the inferior mesenteric ganglion through the lumbar splanchnic nerves. Postganglionic fibers continue through the hypogastric and vesical plexuses to the wall of the bladder. The functions of the sympathetic nerves are uncertain. They may assist the filling of the bladder by relaxing the detrusor muscle, but they have little influence on emptying mechanisms. Cutting the sympathetic nerves to the bladder does not have a serious effect on its function.

The external sphincter of the urethra is composed of striated muscle and is innervated, along with other muscles of the perineum, by somatic motor fibers of the pudendal nerve. The external sphincter may be closed voluntarily, but it relaxes by reflex action as soon as urine is released into the urethra at the beginning of micturition.

The smooth muscle of the bladder responds to a stretch reflex operated by proprioceptors in its wall that send impulses to spinal cord segments S2, S3, and S4. The efferent reflex fibers return impulses over the pelvic splanchnic nerves to maintain tonus in the detrusor muscle while the bladder is filling. Reflex contraction of the detrusor muscle in response to bladder filling is called the **vesical reflex**. It can be evaluated clinically by **cystometry**, a procedure in which measured amounts of sterile fluid are placed into the bladder and the resulting pressure is measured. In infants, the uninhibited bladder fills to nearly its normal capacity, then a strong reflex response takes place, and it empties automatically. Voluntary suppression of urination depends on fibers that descend in the corticospinal tracts from the cortex of the paracentral lobules of the cerebral cortex. This system is described in Chapter 8. These fibers can inhibit the detrusor reflex. The sensation of increased bladder tension and the desire to void are conveyed by sensory impulses in the afferent fibers of the pelvic nerves and visceral afferent pathways deep to the lateral spinothalamic tracts in the lateral funiculus of the spinal cord. The sensations of urethral touch and pressure, however, may be mediated by the dorsal columns (see Chaps. 6 and 7).

Lesions of the dorsal roots of the sacral segments interrupt afferent reflex fibers and produce an **atonic bladder**. The bladder wall becomes flaccid, and its capacity is greatly increased. The sensation of fullness of the bladder is entirely lost. As the bladder becomes distended, incontinence and dribbling occur. Voluntary emptying remains possible, but emptying is incomplete, and some urine is left in the bladder. Lesions of the conus medullaris of the spinal cord interrupt the central connections of the same reflex system. Lesions of the cauda equina that destroy the second and third sacral roots interrupt both the afferent and efferent pathways of the reflex. Thus, all three of these lesions can cause an atonic bladder.

Injuries of the spinal cord above the level of the conus medullaris cause a derangement of the bladder reflexes that usually results initially in contraction of sphincter muscles and retention of urine. In the patient with acute transection of the spinal cord, the bladder becomes atonic and fails to empty when full. Constant or intermittent drainage through a catheter inserted through the urethra is needed to prevent overstretching of the bladder musculature. After several weeks, reflexes in the sacral segments of the cord may recover and begin to function so that an automatic bladder is established. In this condition, the bladder fills and empties, either spontaneously or after the skin over the sacral cutaneous area is stimulated by scratching.

AUTONOMIC REFLEXES

Many important reflexes, including pupillary, lacrimal, salivary, cough, vomiting, and carotid sinus reflexes, are mediated by the ANS. Most of these are described elsewhere in the book. Some of the other reflexes are listed below.

Rectal (defecation) reflex: Distention of the rectum or stimulation of rectal mucosa results in contraction of the rectal musculature. This reflex is mediated by sacral segments S2, S3, and S4.

Internal anal sphincter reflex: Contraction of the internal anal sphincter can be detected on introduction of the examiner's gloved finger into the anus. The reflex is mediated by postganglionic sympathetic fibers through the hypogastric plexus.

Bulbocavernosus reflex: Pinching the dorsum of the glans penis results in contraction of the bulbocavernosus muscle and the urethral constrictor. The contraction can be palpated by placing a finger on the perineum behind the scrotum, with pressure on the bulbous or membranous portion of the urethra. An accompanying contraction of the external anal sphincter can be detected with a gloved finger placed in the anus. The reflex is mediated by the third and fourth sacral nerves.

3

Ascending and Descending Pathways

CHAPTER

6

Pain and Temperature

Our contact with the external world occurs through specialized structures termed **sensory receptors**. There are three general types: (1) **exteroceptive receptors** respond to stimuli from the external environment, including visual, auditory, and tactile stimuli; (2) **proprioceptive receptors** receive information about the relative positions of the body segments and of the body in space; and (3) **interoceptive receptors** detect internal events such as changes in blood pressure. The somatic sensory system receives information primarily from exteroceptive and proprioceptive receptors. There are four major subclasses of **somatic sensation**: (1) **pain sensation** is elicited by noxious stimuli; (2) **thermal sensations** consist of separate senses of cold and warmth; (3) **position sense** is evoked by mechanical changes in the muscles and joints, but it includes the sensations of static limb position and limb movement (kinesthesia); and (4) **touch-pressure sensation** is elicited by mechanical stimulation applied to the body surface.

The sensations of pain, temperature, and simple touch (a sense of light contact with the skin associated with light pressure and a crude sense of tactile localization) are mediated by the **anterolateral system**, which consists of a diffuse bundle of fibers located at the junction of the anterior and lateral funiculi of the spinal cord. The cells of origin of the anterolateral system are activated by small-diameter, lightly myelinated and unmyelinated dorsal root afferents, including Aδ and C fibers, as well as larger myelinated cutaneous afferents. The system contains the **spinothalamic tracts** and the **spinoreticular tract**, which does not reach the thalamus and thus cannot be termed "spinothalamic." Axons of the anterolateral system arise from cells located in several layers of the dorsal horn. Most of these axons cross through the ventral commissure of the spinal cord and ascend, although a small number may ascend ipsilaterally. This system conveys itching and touch sensations in addition to pain and temperature. The touch components are discussed in Chapter 7.

DORSAL ROOTS

• • • • • • • • •

Essentially, all sensations from receptors below the level of the head are conveyed to the central nervous system by the dorsal roots, which consist almost entirely of sensory (afferent) nerve fibers. The area of skin supplied by one dorsal root is a **dermatome**, or skin segment. The approximate boundaries of human dermatomes are shown on the left side of Figures 17 and 18. A small number of sensory fibers have been discovered in the ventral roots. Many of these ventral root afferents respond to painful stimuli from superficial or deep tissues. The cell bodies of the dorsal root fibers are located in the spinal, or dorsal root, ganglia. Each pseudounipolar ganglion cell possesses a single nerve process that divides in the form of a T, with a central branch running to the spinal cord and a peripheral branch coming from a receptor organ or organs (Fig. 19). There are no synapses in a dorsal root ganglion. The area in which the dorsal root fibers enter the spinal cord, in the region of the dorsolateral sulcus, is called the **dorsal root entry zone**. The largest and most heavily myelinated fibers (Aα and Aβ) generally occupy the most medial position in this zone, and the small myelinated and unmyelinated fibers (Aδ and C), the most lateral.

The dorsal and ventral roots come together to form the **spinal nerves** (see Fig. 3 in Chap. 3). Peripheral to this union of the dorsal and ventral roots, a mixture of sensory and motor fibers from an individual spinal nerve separates into bundles or fascicles that join those of adjacent spinal nerves to form **peripheral nerves**. The cutaneous branches of each peripheral nerve therefore carry fibers from more than one spinal nerve, and the skin territory of each of these peripheral nerves covers portions of several dermatomes (see Figs. 17 and 18, right side).

PAIN-TEMPERATURE PATHWAYS

• • • • • • • • •

The peripheral receptors for pain are thought to be the naked terminals of small (Aδ and C) nerve fibers. Many of these may be specialized chemoreceptors that are excited by tissue substances released in response to noxious and inflammatory stimuli. A variety of substances have been implicated, including histamine, bradykinin, serotonin, acetylcholine, substance P, high concentrations of K^+, and substances involved in the arachidonic acid cascade, including products related to the cyclooxygenases. The concentration of H^+ in these substances is a critical factor in the activation of pain receptors. The stimulus that evokes pain is usually intense and may cause damage or destruction of tissue. Neural responses to noxious stimuli are mediated by Aδ and C peripheral nerve fibers. These fibers enter the spinal cord through the lateral part of the dorsal root zone and immediately divide into short ascending and descending branches that run longitudinally in the **posterolateral fasciculus (Lissauer's tract**, see Fig. 1a). Within one segment or two, these fibers leave Lissauer's tract to make synaptic connections with neurons in the dorsal horn, including neurons in laminae I (the posteromarginal nucleus), II **(substantia gelatinosa)**, III, IV, and V. Substance P is thought to be one of the neurotransmitters released by Aδ and C fibers at their connections with these neurons. Other substances implicated include calcitonin gene–related peptide, glutamate, and vasoactive intestinal peptide. Interneurons in laminae II through IV project to neurons in laminae V through VIII

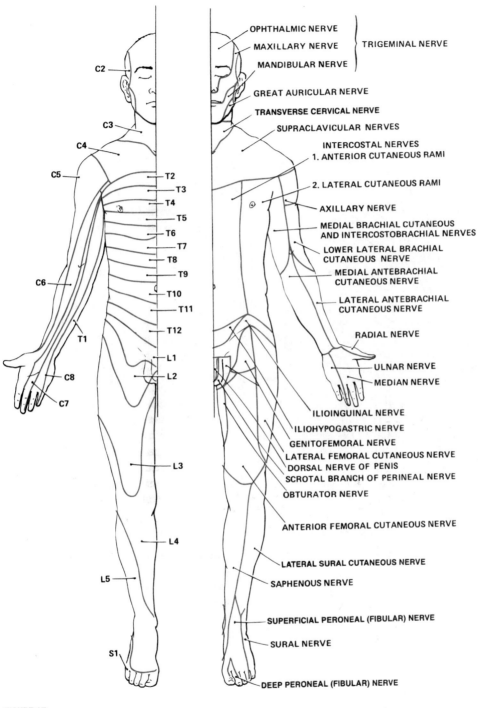

FIGURE 17

• • • • • • • • •

The innervation of the anterior surface of the body by dorsal roots (*left*) and peripheral nerves (*right*).

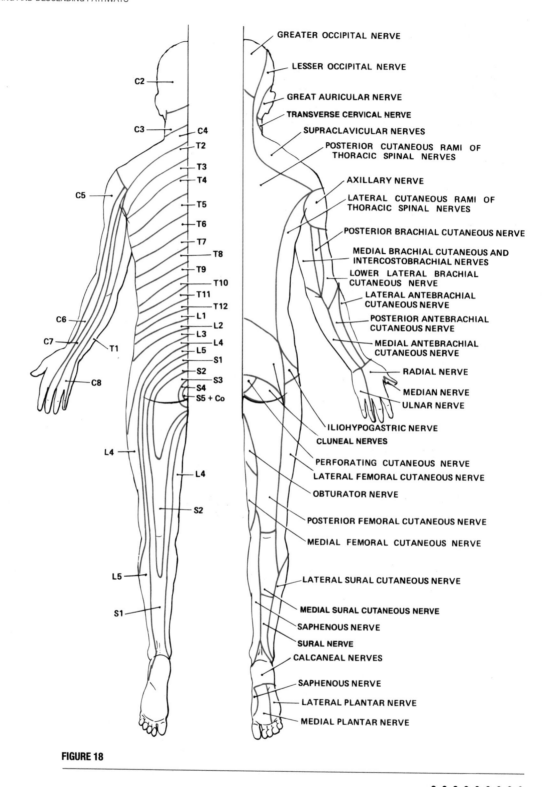

FIGURE 18

The innervation of the posterior surface of the body by dorsal roots (*left*) and peripheral nerves (*right*).

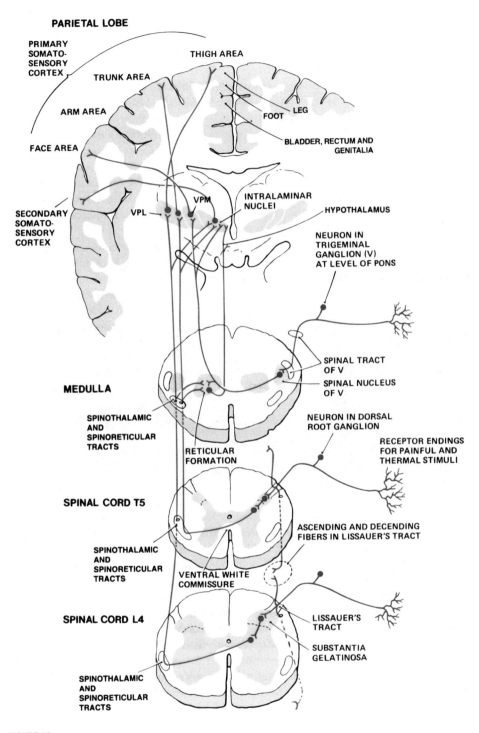

FIGURE 19

The central nervous system pathways that mediate the sensations of pain and temperature. VPL = ventral posterolateral nucleus; VPM = ventral posteromedial nucleus.

and there make synaptic connection on the cells of origin of the anterolateral system, including the spinothalamic tracts and the spinoreticular projections. Neurons in lamina I also give rise to fibers that contribute directly to the spinothalamic tracts (not shown in Fig. 19).

The axons of spinothalamic tract cells in laminae I and in laminae V through VIII cross anterior to the central canal in the **ventral white commissure** and then course rostrally in the **anterolateral funiculus**. The spinothalamic and spinoreticular tracts ascend through the spinal cord and brain stem, supplying inputs to other cord segments, the **reticular formation**, the **superior colliculus**, and **thalamic nuclei**, including the **intralaminar nuclei** and the **ventral posterolateral nucleus** (**VPL**). These areas are discussed in greater detail in Chapter 21. The VPL is considered to be part of the **ventrobasal complex**, in which activity mediated by the spinothalamic projections converges with activity carried by the lemniscal system (see Chap. 7). The projection of the anterolateral system to the VPL is organized somatotopically, so that the fibers carrying input from the upper body are located medial to those that carry input from the lower body (see Fig. 19). This somatotopic organization is maintained in the projections of fibers from the VPL nucleus conveying painful and thermal sensations to the **primary somatosensory cortex**—Brodmann's areas 3, 1, and 2 of the postcentral gyrus (see Fig. 19 and Figs. 67 and 68 in Chap. 24). Like the adjacent primary motor cortex, the primary somatosensory cortex is organized by body parts (i.e., somatotopically). The fibers from the upper parts of the body project to cortical areas near the lateral fissure, and the fibers conveying information from the lower limb and perineum terminate on the medial surface of the hemisphere in the paracentral lobule (see cortical area SI in Fig. 70 in Chap. 24). The postcentral gyrus and its connections with the posterior portions of the parietal lobe are responsible for localizing pain stimuli and integrating the pain modality with other types of sensory stimuli.

A portion of the anterolateral system that is phylogenetically old, the **paleo-spinothalamic tract**, projects to the medial portions of the thalamus (the intralaminar nuclei). The **neospinothalamic tract**, which is phylogenetically more recent, projects to the ventral posterolateral region of the thalamus. In conjunction with the spinoreticular projections, these two pathways constitute the anterolateral system. The anterolateral system is predominantly a slowly conducting, polysynaptic system. In humans, a small percentage of the fibers go directly from the spinal cord to the thalamus, but many synapse in the reticular formation throughout its length in the brain stem. Ascending reticular fibers then relay pain information to thalamic nuclei and to the hypothalamus and limbic system (see Chap. 22).

Pain fibers from the face, the cornea of the eye, the sinuses, and the mucosa of the lips, cheeks, and tongue are carried in the **trigeminal nerve** to its sensory ganglion, which is known as the **semilunar**, **trigeminal**, or **gasserian ganglion**. On entering the brain stem in the pontine region, the central processes of the trigeminal ganglion neurons form a descending tract, the **spinal tract of V**, which courses to the level of the upper cervical segments of the spinal cord. Along the course of this tract, terminals of its fibers form synapses in an adjacent nucleus, the **spinal nucleus of V**. Axons originating in the spinal nucleus of V cross to the opposite side and ascend to the **ventral posteromedial nucleus (VPM)** of the thalamus (see Fig. 19 and Fig. 44 in Chap. 13). This pathway also projects to the reticular formation and the medial and intralaminar thalamic nuclei that receive projections from the anterolateral system of the spinal cord. The cortical projections of the VPM are to the part of the somatosensory cortex closest to the lateral fissure. The areas of the body most sensitive to somatosensory stimuli (e.g., lips and fingers) have disproportion-ately large areas of neuronal representation in the somatosensory cortex.

Thalamocortical fibers from neurons in the intralaminar thalamic nuclei and parts of the VPL–VPM complex relay pain information to the **secondary somatic sen-sory area** of the cerebral cortex (see Fig. 19, and Fig. 70 in Chap. 24).

PERCEPTION OF PAIN

• • • • • • • • •

Although the clinical management of pain is a problem that continually confronts the physician, there are wide gaps in knowledge concerning the structure and func-tion of the receptors and central pathways mediating this modality. Pain is composed of a distinctive sensation, the individual's reaction to this sensation (including ac-companying emotional overtones), activity in both somatic and autonomic systems, and volitional efforts of avoidance or escape. Three types of pain sensation are gen-erally recognized. The first is **fast pain**, consisting of a sharp, pricking sensation that is accurately localized and results from activation of Aδ fibers, which are myelinated. The second is **slow pain**, a burning sensation that has a slower onset, greater per-sistence, and a less clear location. Slow pain results from the activation of C fibers, which are unmyelinated. The third type is **deep** or **visceral pain**, which is described as aching, sometimes with a burning sensation. Visceral pain results from stimula-tion of visceral and deep somatic receptors. These receptors are connected with nerve fibers running largely in sympathetic and somatic nerves consisting of both unmyelinated C fibers and Aδ-size myelinated afferent fibers.

There is no convincing evidence that separate central nervous system pathways mediate fast pain or slow pain. There is good evidence that the neospinothalamic pathway, projecting to the VPL of the thalamus and from there to the primary so-matosensory cortex, is essential for the spatial and temporal discrimination of painful sensations. The paleospinothalamic pathway and the spinoreticular pathways, with their connections to the secondary somatosensory cortex, hypothalamus, and lim-bic system, mediate the autonomic and reflexive responses to painful input, and probably the emotional and affective responses as well. Cortical activation patterns revealed using positron emission tomography indicate that the cingulate cortex is one of these limbic areas activated by pain.

Painful stimuli can be detected on the contralateral side of the body in patients with complete destruction of the somatosensory areas of cerebral cortex on one side of the brain provided the thalamus and lower structures remain intact. Destruction of the posterior and intralaminar nuclei of the thalamus has been found to relieve intractable pain. Such lesions may be effective only briefly, however, and pain may return. Lesions of the dorsomedial and anterior nuclei of the thalamus, or transec-tion of the fibers linking these nuclei to the frontal lobe and anterior cingulate cor-tex (i.e., **prefrontal leukotomy)**, can diminish the anguish of constant pain by changing the psychologic response to painful stimuli. Unfortunately, however, marked negative changes in personality and intellectual capacities occur after these lesions. Recently, bilateral section of the cingulum bundle (i.e., **cingulotomy)** has proved to be effective in relieving the patient's reaction to pain without causing the drastic personality changes that occur with prefrontal leukotomy.

TEMPERATURE SENSE

• • • • • • • • •

The receptors in the skin for the sensations of cold and warmth consist of naked nerve endings. The peripheral nerve fibers mediating these sensations consist of the thinly myelinated Aδ and some C fibers. Other types of C fibers mediate only the painful components of the extremes of heat and cold stimuli. The central nervous system pathway for thermal sensation appears to follow the same course as the pain pathway. The two systems are so closely associated in the central nervous system that they can scarcely be distinguished anatomically, and injury to one usually affects the other to a similar degree.

THE EFFECT OF CUTTING THE SPINOTHALAMIC TRACT

• • • • • • • • •

The lateral spinothalamic tracts are sometimes sectioned in the spinal cord of humans to relieve intractable pain. This surgical procedure is known as **tractotomy**. The cut is made in the anterior part of the lateral funiculus. There is usually some damage to the ventral spinocerebellar tract, and perhaps to certain extrapyramidal motor fibers, but no permanent symptoms develop except a loss of pain sensibility on the contralateral side beginning one or two segments below the cut (see Fig. 23 in Chap. 7). In some patients, pain relief occurs only temporarily, suggesting that other routes may be available or that the information is mediated by both crossed and uncrossed tracts. Bilateral tractotomy is usually necessary to abolish pain from visceral organs, because the tracts conveying visceral pain information to the brain from each dorsal horn ascend both ipsilaterally and contralaterally. These visceral sensory tracts are located adjacent to, but deep to, the spinothalamic tracts (i.e., they are close to the gray matter of the cord). Thus, attempts to relieve visceral pain surgically require cutting fibers close to the motoneurons in the ventral horn.

SENSORY EFFECTS OF DORSAL ROOT IRRITATION

• • • • • • • • •

Mechanical compression or local inflammation of dorsal nerve roots irritates pain fibers and commonly produces pain along the distribution of the affected roots. Pain distributed over an area that is consistent with the boundaries of one dermatome or more than one adjacent dermatome is known as **radicular pain**. Sensory changes other than pain may be associated with dorsal root irritation. There may be localized areas of **paresthesias**, which are spontaneous sensations of prickling, tingling, or numbness. Zones of **hyperesthesia**, in which tactile stimuli appear to be grossly exaggerated, may be present. If the pathologic process progresses and gradually destroys fibers, the dorsal roots will eventually lose their ability to conduct sensory impulses. There will then be **hypesthesia** (i.e., diminished sensitivity) and eventually **anesthesia** (i.e., complete absence of all forms of sensibility) in the affected territory. Essentially all areas of skin receive fibers from more than a single dorsal root; consequently, damage to a single dorsal root may cause little or no sensory loss.

VISCERAL AND REFERRED PAIN

• • • • • • • • •

The parenchyma of internal organs, including the brain itself, is not supplied with pain receptors. Pain receptors are contained within the walls of arteries, all peritoneal surfaces, pleural membranes, and the dura mater covering the brain, and these structures may be sources of severe pain, especially when they are subjected to inflammation or mechanical traction. Abnormal contraction or dilatation of the walls of hollow viscera, including blood vessels, also causes pain. Pain fibers from viscera are thought to follow the sympathetic nerves back to the spinal cord. Conversely, visceral afferents in the vagus and the parasympathetic nerves of the pelvis convey primarily nonpainful visceral sensations.

Pain of visceral origin is apt to be vaguely localized. It may be felt in a surface area of the body far removed from its actual source, a phenomenon known as **referred pain**. For example, the pain of coronary heart disease may be felt in the chest wall, left axilla, or down the inside of the left arm; inflammation of the peritoneum covering the diaphragm may be felt over the shoulder. In each case, the neurons that supply the skin area in which the pain is felt enter the same segment of the spinal cord as do the neurons that actually conduct the pain stimuli from the visceral organ. Spinal cord segments T1 and T2 receive sensory fibers from skin areas of the left upper extremity and from the heart; segments C3, C4, and C5 supply the skin of the shoulder area and also receive sensory fibers from the diaphragm. One of the many theoretical explanations of referred pain is that the visceral sensory fibers are discharging into the same pool of neurons in the spinal cord as the fibers from the skin, and an "overflow" of impulses results in misinterpretation of the true origin of the pain.

Pain may be referred from deep somatic as well as visceral structures. In the case of ligaments and muscles associated with the vertebral column, the referred area may be in a segmental distribution different from the level of origin of the painful stimuli.

Visceral afferents conveying pain stimuli synapse in the dorsal horn and intermediate gray matter, including the intermediomedial nucleus of lamina VII (see Fig. 8 in Chap. 1). The pathways through which pain from the viscera is transmitted to the brain stem and thalamus are the bilateral spinoreticular tracts. These fibers travel deep to the spinothalamic tracts and form part of the anterolateral system. Many of these fibers terminate in the reticular formation. Those that extend beyond the brain stem project primarily to intralaminar thalamic nuclei and the hypothalamus.

ENDOGENOUS ANALGESIA

• • • • • • • • •

Studies in animals, principally rats, have shown that analgesia results from electrical stimulation of peripheral nerve fibers or of discretely distributed loci in the brain, particularly in an irregular series of sites along the medial periventricular and periaqueductal axis, including the **midline raphe nuclei** of the brain stem. The raphe nuclei are found throughout the brain stem. These nuclei are densely populated with neurons that produce the neurotransmitter serotonin. The axons of the caudal raphe nuclei descend to the spinal cord through the dorsolateral fasciculus (see Chap. 8). These axons terminate in the dorsal horn, where they attenuate the responses of spinothalamic and other dorsal horn cells to spinal nerve afferents mediating noxious stimuli. The analgesia produced by electrical stimulation of the central nervous system probably results primarily from the release of opioid peptides, although other nonopioid neurotransmitters such as serotonin, dopamine, and norepinephrine also mediate analgesia. Enkephalin, beta-endorphin, and dynorphin represent the three families of the opioid peptides, which are naturally occurring substances that bind to the same receptors in the central nervous system as do opiate drugs. Opioid peptides have been found to be neurotransmitters in specific systems of the brain (see Chap. 25). These neurotransmitters and their opioid-binding receptors are found in the brain structures involved in the modulation of pain transmission. One of these neurotransmitter systems is concentrated densely in the dorsal horn, particularly in laminae I through III. The effect of opioid release and binding on opioid receptors is suppression of the activity of neurons in the immediate vicinity. Thus, painful sensations can be modulated at the first synaptic connection in the dorsal horn. This is thought to be a way in which pain may be suppressed through intrinsic, endogenous central nervous system mechanisms.

CHAPTER

7

Proprioception, Touch, and Tactile Discrimination

Tactile sensations are complex in nature because they involve a blending of light cutaneous contact and variable degrees of pressure, depending on the intensity of the stimuli. Cutaneous mechanical stimuli are either static or dynamic with respect to space and time. In the normal individual, even light tactile stimuli that reach threshold can be localized with precision. From the clinical perspective, touch sensibility is divided into **light touch** and **tactile discrimination**. Light touch involves a sense of contact with the skin. Tactile discrimination involves perception of the size and shape of objects. Tickling and itching sensations are related to pain sense.

The method of testing light touch is contacting the skin with a wisp of cotton wool. Von Frey hairs are used for experimental work. These are a series of fine hairs of graduated stiffness used to apply stimuli at calibrated intensities to the skin. Tactile discrimination is tested by having the patient, with the eyes closed, identify common small objects placed in his or her hand **(stereognosis)**, determine whether one touch stimulus or two simultaneous stimuli have been applied to the skin **(two-point discrimination)**, and identify numbers or letters written on the surface of the skin with a blunt object **(complex tactile discrimination)**.

The sense of flutter-vibration is also an important component of tactile sensation. The sense of **flutter** is a feeling of repetitive movement, and the sense of **vibration** is a more diffuse and penetrating feeling of "humming" when the base of a vibrating tuning fork is held in contact with a bony prominence of the body.

Proprioceptive sensation includes both the sense of **static limb position** and **kinesthesia** (i.e., the sense of movement). Proprioception is tested by asking the patient, with the eyes closed, to identify the position of a distal joint at rest and after the examiner has moved the joint to a new position.

PATHWAYS

• • • • • • • • •

Two different sets of sensory pathways provide essential information to the brain about muscle action, joint position, and the objects with which a person is in contact. The pathways in one of these groups project to the cerebellum, where the information is used for the coordination of movement but not for conscious perception. This group includes four named pathways: the dorsal and ventral spinocerebellar tracts, the cuneocerebellar tract, and the rostral spinocerebellar tract. The second set of pathways includes three tracts that project to the cerebral cortex by way of the thalamus, and this information can be perceived consciously. These pathways are the spinal lemniscus, the spinothalamic tract, and the lateral cervical system. Collectively, the sensory pathways in both sets begin with the mechanoreceptors.

Mechanoreceptors

Mechanoreceptors in the muscles, joints, and skin mediate the various separate and integrated sensations of proprioception and touch and tactile discrimination. Mechanoreceptors include muscle spindles, Golgi tendon organs, Pacinian corpuscles, Meissner's corpuscles, and other encapsulated receptors, as well as free nerve endings, in muscles, tendons, ligaments, joint capsules, and skin. Information about static limb position comes chiefly from **muscle spindle** afferents. Kinesthetic (joint movement) sensation is not mediated solely by the **joint receptor** afferents, which appear to play a minor role, but by a combination of receptors in the skin, muscles, and joints. **Pacinian corpuscles** detect vibration; they are found in the skin and connective tissues surrounding the bones and joints. **Meissner's corpuscles** mediate superficial phasic touch sensation. In addition, the movement of hairs, detected by **free nerve endings** in hair follicles, conveys a sense of touch. Most of the mechanoreceptors, with the exception of free nerve endings, are innervated by large-diameter myelinated fibers. The cell bodies of these peripheral nerve fibers are in the dorsal root ganglia, and their central processes enter the medial side of the dorsal root zone.

After entering the spinal cord, afferent fibers from mechanoreceptors distribute to three different sites: (1) interneurons and motoneurons in the ventral horn of the spinal cord; (2) neurons of origin of the ascending pathways, which are in the dorsal and intermediate gray areas of the spinal cord; and (3) the medulla, where they synapse in the dorsal column nuclei.

Mechanoreceptor Reflexes

Afferent fibers from muscle spindles make excitatory monosynaptic connections on alpha motoneurons innervating the muscles of origin of the respective spindle afferents. These connections form the basis of the myotatic (deep tendon) reflex (see Fig. 15 in Chap. 4). Afferent fibers from muscle spindles also make inhibitory polysynaptic connections with motoneurons innervating the physiologic antagonists of the muscles of origin of the spindles.

Golgi tendon organ afferents synapse on interneurons that inhibit motoneurons innervating the muscles of origin of these tendon organs. They also make excitatory polysynaptic connections with motoneurons of antagonist muscles.

Pathways to the Cerebellum

Some proprioceptive fiber collaterals, especially from Golgi tendon organs, as well as fibers conveying other sensory modalities such as pressure and pain, synapse with neurons in the intermediate gray area and the base of the posterior horn of the spinal cord (Fig. 20, left side). At lumbar and, to a lesser extent, sacral levels of the cord (but not at more rostral levels) these neurons give rise to the primarily crossed **ventral spinocerebellar tract**, the most peripheral tract in the ventral margin of the lateral funiculus.

The nucleus dorsalis, or Clarke's nucleus, is located at the base of the posterior horn in spinal segments T1 through L2. The neurons of this nuclear column receive Ia and Ib afferents from muscle spindles, cutaneous touch receptors, and joint receptors. Axons of these neurons ascend rostrally on the ipsilateral side in the **dorsal spinocerebellar tract**, which is located just posterior to the ventral spinocerebellar tract in the lateral funiculus (see Fig. 20, right side), whereas the Ia and Ib afferents from dorsal roots T1 to L2 synapse in the nucleus dorsalis at the level where they enter the cord. These afferents from dorsal roots L3 to S5 ascend in the fasciculus gracilis of the dorsal funiculus to reach the nucleus dorsalis, where they synapse in the lowest part of this nuclear column at segmental levels L1 and L2. Thus, both the dorsal and ventral spinocerebellar pathways carry information to the cerebellum from the lower limbs.

Mechanoreceptor information from the upper limbs reaches the cerebellum through two additional pathways, the cuneocerebellar pathway and the rostral spinocerebellar pathway. Afferent fibers from C2 to T5 travel up the dorsal funiculus in the fasciculus cuneatus to synapse with neurons in the **accessory cuneate nucleus** (see Fig. 20, right side) in the lower medulla. This nucleus is the upper-extremity counterpart of the nucleus dorsalis and gives rise to the ipsilateral **cuneocerebellar tract** (dorsal arcuate fibers). This pathway mediates information chiefly from cutaneous receptors, joint afferents, and muscle spindles.

The **rostral spinocerebellar tract** is the upper-limb equivalent of the ventral spinocerebellar tract. It originates in the cervical enlargement from cells of the intermediate zone of the spinal cord gray area (see Fig. 20, left side). Axons of these cells decussate and project to the cerebellum with the fibers of the ventral spinocerebellar tract.

The ascending fibers of the dorsal spinocerebellar and cuneocerebellar pathways enter the cerebellum through the inferior cerebellar peduncle, whereas those in the ventral and rostral spinocerebellar tracts continue through the pons and ascend into the cerebellum through the superior cerebellar peduncle. All four of these tracts terminate primarily in the midline (vermis and intermediate zone) portions of the cerebellum, especially in the anterior lobe, and are concerned with processes that govern standing and walking.

Pathways to the Cerebrum

The **spinal lemniscal system** carries proprioceptive information from receptors for position sense and kinesthesia, and in addition, information necessary for tactile discrimination, to the cerebral cortex. Two other pathways also mediate tactile sensation. The **spinothalamic tract** of the anterolateral system subserves light touch sensation in addition to pain and temperature. This pathway is described in Chapter 6. Finally, the **lateral cervical system** (spinocervicothalamic pathway) is thought to mediate touch sensations as well as vibratory and proprioceptive senses.

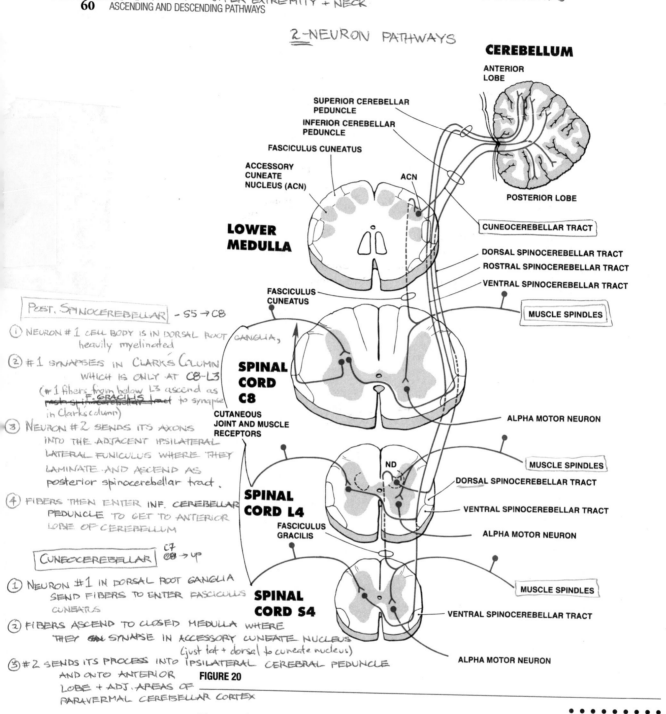

2-NEURON PATHWAYS

CEREBELLUM

ANTERIOR LOBE

SUPERIOR CEREBELLAR PEDUNCLE

INFERIOR CEREBELLAR PEDUNCLE

FASCICULUS CUNEATUS

ACCESSORY CUNEATE NUCLEUS (ACN)

ACN

POSTERIOR LOBE

CUNEOCEREBELLAR TRACT

LOWER MEDULLA

DORSAL SPINOCEREBELLAR TRACT
ROSTRAL SPINOCEREBELLAR TRACT
VENTRAL SPINOCEREBELLAR TRACT

FASCICULUS CUNEATUS

MUSCLE SPINDLES

POST. SPINOCEREBELLAR — S5 → C8

① NEURON #1 CELL BODY IS IN DORSAL ROOT GANGLIA, heavily myelinated

② #1 SYNAPSES IN CLARK'S COLUMN WHICH IS ONLY AT C8-L3 (#1 fibers from below L3 ascend as ~~post spinocerebellar tract~~ F. GRACILIS to synapse in Clark's column)

③ NEURON #2 SENDS ITS AXONS INTO THE ADJACENT IPSILATERAL LATERAL FUNICULUS WHERE THEY LAMINATE AND ASCEND AS posterior spinocerebellar tract.

④ FIBERS THEN ENTER INF. CEREBELLAR PEDUNCLE TO GET TO ANTERIOR LOBE OF CEREBELLUM

SPINAL CORD C8

FASCICULUS CUNEATUS

CUTANEOUS JOINT AND MUSCLE RECEPTORS

ALPHA MOTOR NEURON

MUSCLE SPINDLES

CUNEOCEREBELLAR   C7 C8 → up

① NEURON #1 IN DORSAL ROOT GANGLIA SEND FIBERS TO ENTER FASCICULUS CUNEATUS

② FIBERS ASCEND TO CLOSED MEDULLA WHERE THEY ~~can~~ SYNAPSE IN ACCESSORY CUNEATE NUCLEUS (just lat + dorsal to cuneate nucleus)

③ #2 SENDS ITS PROCESS INTO IPSILATERAL CEREBRAL PEDUNCLE AND ONTO ANTERIOR LOBE + ADJ. AREAS OF PARAVERMAL CEREBELLAR CORTEX

SPINAL CORD L4

ND

FASCICULUS GRACILIS

DORSAL SPINOCEREBELLAR TRACT

VENTRAL SPINOCEREBELLAR TRACT

ALPHA MOTOR NEURON

SPINAL CORD S4

MUSCLE SPINDLES

VENTRAL SPINOCEREBELLAR TRACT

ALPHA MOTOR NEURON

FIGURE 20

The central nervous system pathways that convey information from mechanoreceptors in the muscles, joints, and skin to the cerebellum. ND = nucleus dorsalis.

THE SPINAL LEMNISCAL SYSTEM

Fibers from muscle spindles (Ia fibers), Golgi tendon organs (Ib fibers), and mechanoreceptors in the joints and skin project through the spinal lemniscal system to the thalamus and cortex and contribute to conscious position and movement sense. Other fibers in this system convey information about touch, pressure, and flutter–vibration. Many of these fibers are dorsal root afferents that ascend in the posterior funiculi, without synapsing in the spinal cord, to relay nuclei in the lower part of the medulla. Other fibers in this system are axons of dorsal horn cells, which receive synapses from mechanoreceptor afferents. Fibers from the leg ascend adjacent to the dorsal median septum and form the **fasciculus gracilis** (Fig. 21). Fibers from the arm ascend lateral to the leg fibers and constitute the **fasciculus cuneatus**. Both fasciculi ascend to the lower medulla, where they terminate in the **nucleus gracilis** and **nucleus cuneatus**, respectively. Clinicians often refer to these tracts as the posterior, or dorsal, column pathways and to the nuclei as the dorsal column nuclei. Additional fibers of the spinal lemniscal system travel within the dorsal part of the lateral funiculus, accompanying the lateral cervical system (Fig. 22). Thus the term **dorsolateral pathway** can be used for the entire lemniscal pathway in the spinal cord. Fibers from the cells of the dorsal column nuclei form the **internal arcuate fibers** (see Fig. 34 in Chap. 10). These fibers promptly cross to the opposite side in the decussation of the medial lemniscus, and they then ascend as the **medial lemniscus** to the thalamus and terminate in the **ventral posterolateral nucleus** (VPL). In both the medial lemniscus and the VPL, a somatotopic organization is maintained. In the medial lemniscus of the medulla, the fibers from the nucleus gracilis, conveying information from the leg, are ventral to fibers from the nucleus cuneatus. In the pons and midbrain, these gracile fibers are lateral to the cuneate fibers. In contrast to the anterolateral system discussed in Chapter 6, few if any of the fibers in this system synapse in the reticular formation.

Thalamocortical fibers from the VPL continue to the postcentral gyrus of the parietal lobe. The band of the cortex that receives these terminals is the primary somesthetic area, or **primary somatosensory area** (see Fig. 21), where topographic representation of the body areas is similar to that of the motor strip that lies parallel to it on the opposite side of the central sulcus. The primary somatosensory area includes Brodmann's areas 3, 1, and 2 (see Figs. 67 and 68 in Chap. 24).

This lemniscal system is responsible for the sense of limb position and movement, including the sense of steady joint angles, the sense of motion produced by active muscular contraction (kinesthesis) or passive movement, the sense of tension exerted by contracting muscles, and the sense of effort. The conscious recognition of body and limb posture requires cortical participation. In addition, the lemniscal pathway is important for providing information about the place, intensity, and temporal and spatial patterns of neural activity evoked by mechanical stimulation of skin, particularly moving stimuli on the skin. Thus, this pathway to the cerebral cortex is necessary for discriminative tactile sensation. It also appears to be important in recognition of flutter–vibration.

LATERAL CERVICAL SYSTEM

Almost all cells of the lateral cervical system are sensitive to light mechanical stimulation of the skin of the ipsilateral side of the body, but a few are activated by noxious stimuli. Peripheral nerve fibers entering this system make synaptic connections in the dorsal horn, primarily in lamina IV, throughout the length of the spinal cord. Heavily myelinated axons from the second-order neurons arise in this lamina and ascend ipsilaterally in the most dorsal corner of the lateral funiculus to terminate in the **lateral cervical nucleus**. This nucleus is located just lateral to the dorsal horn of the first four cervical segments (see Fig. 22). The axons of these cells cross the spinal cord in the ventral white commissure to join the contralateral medial lemniscus and, with this lemniscus, terminate within the thalamus. Projections from the thalamus reach the somatic sensory areas of the cerebral cortex. The fibers of the entire lateral cervical system conduct very rapidly.

POSTERIOR WHITE COLUMN : DISCRIMINATIVE SENSORY INFORMATION
i.e. touch, pressure, tactile localization, 2-pt tactile discrimination, joint + mov't sense, vibratory sense

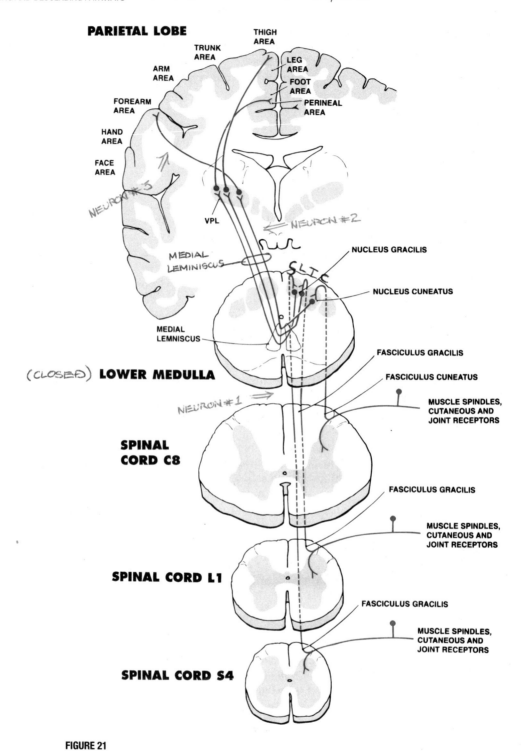

FIGURE 21

The fasciculus gracilis and fasciculus cuneatus of the spinal lemniscal system mediate proprioception, flutter–vibration, and tactile discrimination. VPL = ventral posterolateral nucleus.

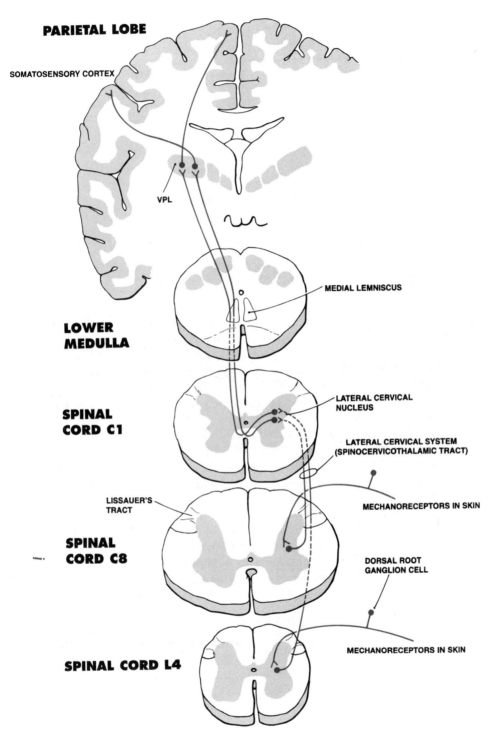

PARIETAL LOBE

SOMATOSENSORY CORTEX

VPL

MEDIAL LEMNISCUS

LOWER MEDULLA

SPINAL CORD C1

LATERAL CERVICAL NUCLEUS

LATERAL CERVICAL SYSTEM (SPINOCERVICOTHALAMIC TRACT)

LISSAUER'S TRACT

MECHANORECEPTORS IN SKIN

SPINAL CORD C8

DORSAL ROOT GANGLION CELL

MECHANORECEPTORS IN SKIN

SPINAL CORD L4

FIGURE 22

The lateral cervical system (spinocervicothalamic tract) mediates touch sensation. VPL = ventral posterolateral nucleus.

THE EFFECT OF SPINAL CORD LESIONS ON TOUCH SENSATION

• • • • • • • • •

Of all types of skin sensibility, simple touch is least likely to be impaired by lesions of the spinal cord. Although a lesion of the dorsal column usually abolishes tactile discrimination such as the ability to detect the direction of movement of a cutaneous stimulus, light-touch sensation may be decreased only slightly or not at all on the ipsilateral side by such a lesion. After destruction of the spinothalamic tracts, pain perception is lost on the opposite side of the body, but light touch generally persists because the dorsolateral pathways also can mediate this function.

PHYSIOLOGIC ASPECTS OF TACTILE DISCRIMINATION

• • • • • • • • •

In the various relay nuclei of the pathways mediating tactile discrimination, each neuron receives synaptic input from many afferent fibers, and each afferent cell ends on many relay cells. Thus, the relay cells receive sensory information that undergoes both **convergence** and **divergence**. Furthermore, afferent fibers reaching relay nuclei activate not only relay cells but also excitatory and inhibitory interneurons. Consequently, sensory information is not merely transmitted along the pathway; the information can be transformed into different patterns of activity.

In the somatic sensory system, there is no synaptic inhibition in the peripheral receptor; inhibitory processes can occur only at the first synaptic site in the dorsal horn or dorsal column nuclei and then in subsequent synaptic sites along the relay pathway. Two types of inhibitory processes have been described: (1) **local feedback inhibition** and (2) **distal feedback inhibition**. Local feedback inhibition consists of the inhibition of surrounding dorsal horn and dorsal column relay cells by collaterals of relay cells activated by incoming volleys. Distal feedback inhibition consists of the inhibition of presynaptic activity **(presynaptic inhibition)** in axons reaching neurons in dorsal horn and dorsal column nuclei. This inhibition comes from the axons of neurons in the motor and somatosensory areas of the cerebral cortex and in the brain stem. The first of these inhibitory processes limits the extent of excitation among adjacent neurons, thereby functionally decreasing the divergence of excitation and sharpening the localization of signals. The second process allows higher levels of the nervous system to determine how much information is transmitted upward.

Neurons in each of the nuclei along the lemniscal pathway, including the dorsal column nuclei, the VPL, and the somatosensory area of the cerebral cortex, have specific **receptive fields**. The receptive field of each neuron is the area on the body surface that, when touched, will either excite or inhibit that neuron. The receptive fields of individual neurons vary considerably. The tips of the fingers and the tongue are the regions of skin that are most sensitive to touch. These regions have the largest areas of representation in the postcentral gyrus. In addition, the neurons in these areas of the postcentral gyrus have the smallest receptive fields. Stimulation of skin in the receptive field of a neuron usually excites the neuron, and stimulation of skin surrounding the excitatory area usually inhibits the neuron. This is termed **inhibitory surround**. As with other inhibitory processes in the somatosensory system, the inhibitory surroundings can enhance the information being received from a particular area of skin by blocking out less intense stimulation received from nearby sites.

The somatosensory cortex is organized into narrow vertical columns of neurons that extend from the cortical surface to the white matter. Each neuron within a single column responds to the same modality of sensory stimulus. Thus, some columns are activated by touch, some by joint position, and some by movement of hair on the skin. Neurons within each column also have almost identical receptive fields. Moreover, there are specific cutaneous, direction-sensitive (spatial discrimination) and displacement frequency (temporal discrimination)–sensitive neurons in the somatosensory cortex. These cortical neuronal response properties reflect the integration of multiple inputs from lower levels of sensory processing. The existence of modality-specific columns indicates that each sensory modality is transmitted through the nervous system in a specific communication line.

DISTURBANCES OF SENSATION FOLLOWING INTERRUPTION OF THE DORSOLATERAL PATHWAYS

Complete loss of proprioceptive sensation from a spinal lesion requires bilateral interruption of the dorsolateral pathway (both dorsal columns and the lateral cervical system in the dorsal part of the lateral columns). The results of lesions in this location are deficits in position sense, vibration sense, and tactile discrimination. The symptoms occur prominently on the same side of the body after unilateral injury of a dorsolateral funiculus (Fig. 23A). Symptoms of varying degrees are also found with lesions of the gracile and cuneate nuclei, the medial lemniscus, the thalamus, and the postcentral gyrus. Lesions of the lemniscal pathway leave preserved the sensations of pain and temperature. Interruption of the dorsal columns without injury to the lateral columns results in loss of detection of the direction of a moving stimulus on the skin, but appreciation of touch and movement of joints remains intact.

Clinical signs of injury to the lemniscal (dorsolateral) pathways, which are frequently tested in a neurologic examination, include the following:

1. Inability to recognize limb position. The patient is unable to say, without looking, whether a joint is put in a position of flexion or extension. The patient also cannot detect the direction of limb displacement during a movement.
2. Astereognosis. There is loss or impairment of the ability to recognize common objects, such as keys, coins, blocks, and marbles, by touching and handling them with the eyes closed.
3. Loss of two-point discrimination. There is loss of the normal ability to distinguish two points of stimuli applied simultaneously to the skin from a single stimulus point. The two points of a compass may be used for testing, although the tips should be blunt.
4. Loss of vibratory sense. The normal person perceives as a mild tingling the sensation evoked by a vibrating tuning fork applied to the base of a bony prominence. When this sensory ability is lost, the patient cannot differentiate a vibrating fork from a silent one.
5. Positive Romberg sign. In this test, the patient is asked to stand with the feet placed close together. The amount of body sway when the patient's eyes are open

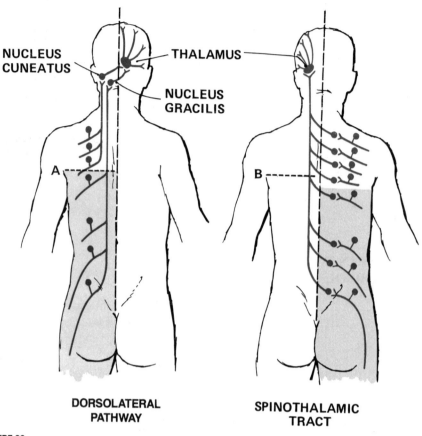

NUCLEUS
CUNEATUS

THALAMUS

NUCLEUS
GRACILIS

A

B

**DORSOLATERAL
PATHWAY**

**SPINOTHALAMIC
TRACT**

FIGURE 23

• • • • • • • • •

The effects of lesions on the left side of the spinal cord. The shaded regions show the body surface areas affected by interrupting the dorsolateral pathway in the diagram on the left at level A and the spinothalamic tract in the diagram on the right at level B. In lesion A, the sensory disturbance is on the ipsilateral side of the body, because the ascending fibers cross above the level of the lesion, in the medulla, where fibers from the nuclei cuneatus and gracilis cross to form the medial lemniscus. In lesion B, the sensory loss is on the contralateral side of the body and one or two segments below the level of the lesion, because fibers entering the spinothalamic tract ascend one or two segments as they cross to the opposite side of the body.

is noted. This amount is then compared with the degree of sway present when the patient's eyes are closed. An abnormal accentuation of sway or an actual loss of balance with the eyes closed is a positive result. Visual sense is able to compensate in part for a deficiency in conscious recognition of muscle and joint position; therefore, patients may be able to maintain their balance if they are allowed to keep their eyes open but lose their balance when they close their eyes.

CHAPTER

8

The Descending Pathways

MOTOR AREAS OF THE CEREBRAL CORTEX

Based on differences in cytoarchitecture in the cerebral cortex, Brodmann designated 52 anatomic areas. The **primary motor area**, **Brodmann's area 4**, is located in the precentral gyrus of the frontal lobe. It extends from the lateral fissure upward to the dorsal border of the hemisphere and a short distance beyond on the medial surface of the frontal lobe in the rostral aspect of the paracentral lobule (see Figs. 2 and 3 in Chap. 1 and Figs. 67 and 68 in Chap. 24). The left motor strip controls the right side of the body, and the right strip controls the left side. The larynx and tongue are influenced by neurons in the lowest lateral part of this strip, followed in upward sequence by the face, thumb, hand, forearm, upper arm, thorax, abdomen, thigh, leg, foot, and the muscles of the perineum. The neurons controlling leg, foot, and perineal muscles are in the paracentral lobule (see Fig. 69 in Chap. 24). In humans, areas for the hand, tongue, and larynx are disproportionately large, conforming with the development of elaborate motor control of these muscle groups. A functional map of the motor cortex resembles a distorted image of the body turned upside down and reversed left for right. This functional map is termed a **homonculus**.

Immediately rostral to the primary motor area is the **premotor cortex**, which consists of **Brodmann's area 6** on the lateral surface of the hemispheres (see Fig. 67 in Chap. 24). The premotor area contains a homonculus similar to the one in area 4. The most medial aspect of area 6 can be observed on a midsagittal section of the brain just rostral to the paracentral lobule (see Fig. 68 in Chap. 24). This is the location of the **supplementary motor area**, which also contains a functional map of body movements.

Additional regions of cortex from which movement can be influenced are Brodmann's areas 3, 1, and 2 on the **postcentral gyrus** and the **secondary motor area**, located on the most ventral aspect of both the precentral and postcentral gyri and the lateral fissure. This latter area overlaps the **secondary somatosensory cortex** (see Fig. 70 in Chap. 24). Brodmann's area 8 in the middle frontal gyrus is also related to motor control. This region, referred to as the **frontal eye fields**, contains neurons that specifically influence eye movements.

Movements result from the actions of networks of neurons at many different levels of the nervous system. Central nervous system pattern generators for complex movements such as locomotion and other rhythmic activities are laid down at low levels, including the spinal cord. The descending pathways of the nervous system have the important task of interacting with and controlling lower-level neuronal patterns of discharge in a hierarchical manner. At the level of the cerebral cortex, individual neurons appear to be capable of controlling contractions of individual muscles and of determining the force of these contractions. It appears, however, that **populations** of motor cortical neurons act together to specify the **direction** of movements and the force of movements. These functions pertain not only to neurons in the primary motor cortex but also to those in the premotor, supplementary, and postcentral regions. The premotor and supplementary motor areas appear to be important in planning movements. The supplementary motor area probably has a special role in integrating movements performed simultaneously on both sides of the body.

DESCENDING FIBERS FROM THE CEREBRAL CORTEX AND BRAIN STEM THAT INFLUENCE MOTOR ACTIVITY

• • • • • • • • •

Skeletal muscle activity results from the net influence of higher nervous system structures on the motoneurons of the spinal cord and the motor components of the cranial nerve nuclei. Collectively, these spinal cord and brain stem neurons provide the final direct link with muscles through myoneural junctions (motor end plates). These neurons are referred to as **lower motoneurons (LMNs)**. Their cell bodies reside within the central nervous system, and their axons make synaptic contact with extrafusal and intrafusal muscle fibers of somatic and branchiomeric origin. **Somatic** muscle fibers derive from true somites in the developing embryo. **Branchiomeric** muscles stem from segments of the head and neck, which develop into gill arches in water-dwelling vertebrates. These branchiomeres are not true somites, but the muscles that develop from them, like somatic muscles, are striated and under voluntary control. They include the muscles of mastication, the muscles of facial expression, and the muscles of the pharynx and larynx.

A number of descending motor pathways regulate LMN activity. These descending pathways are controlled directly or indirectly by the cerebral cortex, cerebellum, or basal ganglia. In the strictest sense, the neurons in all such pathways should be termed **upper motoneurons (UMNs)**. UMNs synapse directly, or through interneurons, on alpha, beta, and gamma motoneurons in the spinal cord and cranial nerve nuclei. They are contained completely within the central nervous system. Clinicians usually use the term UMN only when referring to the corticospinal tract or, to a lesser extent, the corticobulbar tract (Fig. 24).

Corticospinal Tract

The corticospinal tract, also termed the pyramidal tract, was once considered to be the pathway that initiated and controlled all "voluntary" muscular activity. It is

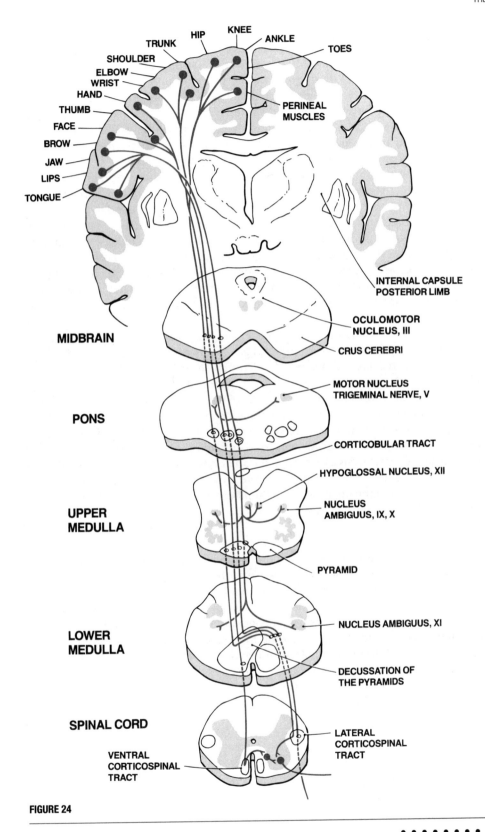

TRUNK
HIP
KNEE
ANKLE
SHOULDER
ELBOW
WRIST
HAND
THUMB
FACE
BROW
JAW
LIPS
TONGUE
TOES
PERINEAL
MUSCLES

INTERNAL CAPSULE
POSTERIOR LIMB

MIDBRAIN

OCULOMOTOR
NUCLEUS, III
CRUS CEREBRI

PONS

MOTOR NUCLEUS
TRIGEMINAL NERVE, V

CORTICOBULAR TRACT

HYPOGLOSSAL NUCLEUS, XII

UPPER
MEDULLA

NUCLEUS
AMBIGUUS, IX, X

PYRAMID

LOWER
MEDULLA

NUCLEUS AMBIGUUS, XI

DECUSSATION OF
THE PYRAMIDS

SPINAL CORD

LATERAL
CORTICOSPINAL
TRACT

VENTRAL
CORTICOSPINAL
TRACT

FIGURE 24

The corticospinal pathways and some parts of the corticobulbar pathways of the central nervous system.

now known to be concerned primarily with skilled movements of the distal muscles of the limbs and, in particular, with facilitation of the alpha, beta, and gamma motoneurons that innervate distal flexor musculature. Approximately one third of the axons in the corticospinal tract arise from the primary motor cortex in areas 4 and 6, and about 3 percent of these fibers originate from unusually large pyramidal cells called Betz cells, which are located in the fifth layer of this cortex. Another one third of the fibers in the corticospinal tract arise from the premotor and supplementary motor regions in area 6, and the remaining one third of the fibers originate from the parietal lobe, primarily areas 3, 1, and 2 of the postcentral gyrus.

The corticospinal tract passes through the posterior limb of the internal capsule and the middle of the crus cerebri (see Fig. 24). It then breaks up into bundles in the basilar portion of the pons and finally collects into a discrete bundle, forming the pyramid of the medulla. This pathway was originally named the pyramidal tract because of its passage through the medullary pyramid, not because of its origin from pyramidal cells in the cortex. In the lower levels of the medulla, most of the corticospinal tract crosses (decussates) to the opposite side. This region is referred to as the level of the motor or pyramidal tract decussation. Approximately 90 percent of the fibers cross at this level and descend through the spinal cord as the **lateral corticospinal tract**, which passes to all cord levels in the lateral funiculus and synapses in the lateral aspects of laminae IV through VIII. Many of the cells in these laminae are interneurons that synapse on alpha and gamma motoneurons in lamina IX. In primates, a small percentage of the fibers (perhaps those arising from Betz cells) synapse directly on the alpha, beta, and gamma motoneurons in lamina IX. These motoneurons innervate the muscles in the distal parts of the extremities (i.e., hands and feet).

The 10 percent of corticospinal fibers that do not decussate in the medulla descend in the anterior funiculus of the cervical and upper thoracic cord levels as the **ventral corticospinal tract**. At their levels of termination, however, most of the fibers in this pathway decussate through the anterior white commissure (ventral white commissure; see Fig. 7 in Chap. 1) before synapsing on interneurons and motoneurons of the contralateral side. The number of fibers in both lateral and ventral corticospinal tracts decreases in successively lower cord segments as more and more fibers reach their terminations.

The corticospinal tract sends fibers to synapse on interneurons in laminae IV, V, and VI of the spinal cord. These interneurons can influence local reflex arcs and cells of origin of ascending sensory pathways. Thus, through this system, the cerebral cortex can control motor output and can also modify sensory input reaching the brain.

The corticospinal tract exerts both facilitating and inhibitory influences on the spinal interneurons and motoneurons it contacts. Activation of the corticospinal tract generally evokes excitatory postsynaptic potentials in interneurons and motoneurons of flexor muscles and inhibitory postsynaptic potentials in those of extensor muscles. The facilitating effects of the corticospinal tract are thought to be mediated by the amino acid neurotransmitter glutamate, and the inhibitory effects, at least in part, through glycinergic interneurons.

Corticobulbar Tract

The fibers of the corticobulbar tract arise from neurons in the ventral part of area 4 on the lateral surface of the hemisphere and from area 8. The axons start out in company with the corticospinal tract but take a divergent route at the level of the midbrain. The fibers of this pathway terminate in the brain stem, where they influence the motor nuclei of cranial nerves III (oculomotor); IV (trochlear); V (trigeminal); VI (abducens); VII (facial); IX (glossopharyngeal); X (vagus); XI (accessory); and XII (hypoglossal). Fibers from cortical area 8 in the middle frontal gyrus, the frontal eye fields, influence eye movements indirectly by synapsing on cells in the superior colliculus, pretectal nuclei, and accessory optic nuclei of the midbrain. These areas project directly, or by way of another relay in the pontine reticular formation, to the nuclei of cranial nerves III, IV, and VI (see Chap. 20). Corticobulbar fibers from the facial region of areas 4 and 6 terminate on interneurons adjacent to the motoneurons that innervate the remaining (nonextraocular) striated skeletal musculature, either of somatic or branchiomeric origin. (Some of these connections are shown in Fig. 24.) The cranial nerve motor nuclei are innervated bilaterally, and in most cases, the muscles they control cannot be contracted voluntarily on one side only. Both the lower facial nucleus, which innervates facial musculature below the eye, and the hypoglossal nucleus receive innervation from the opposite cerebral cortex that is much heavier than the innervation from the ipsilateral cortex. Thus, these muscles can be controlled rather independently on the two sides, and a lesion of one cerebral hemisphere results in weakness primarily on the contralateral (opposite) side.

Like the corticospinal tract, the corticobulbar tract contains fibers that terminate on sensory "relay" neurons. In the brain stem, these relay nuclei include the nuclei gracilis and cuneatus, the sensory trigeminal nuclei, and the nucleus of the solitary tract.

Corticotectal and Tectospinal Tracts

Some authors have used the term **corticomesencephalic tracts** to identify the pathways that arise from cerebral cortical areas in the occipital and inferior parietal lobes and project to the upper parts of the brain stem to influence extraocular muscle activity. These fibers are referred to in this text as the **corticotectal tract**. Many of these fibers synapse in the superior colliculus, the interstitial nucleus of Cajal, or the nucleus of Darkschewitsch. These nuclei project through the pontine reticular formation and the medial longitudinal fasciculus (MLF) to synapse upon the oculomotor, trochlear, and abducens nuclei. Other cortical fibers may first synapse in various regions of the reticular formation that influence the extrinsic eye muscle nuclei directly (see Fig. 62 in Chap. 20).

Corticotectal fibers also make connections in the deep layers of the superior colliculus with neurons that give rise to the **tectospinal tract**. Axons of these cells cross the midline in the **dorsal tegmental decussation** (see Fig. 39 in Chap. 10) and descend through the brain stem in a position ventral to the medial longitudinal fasciculus (MLF) (see Figs. 34 through 37 in Chap. 10). In the spinal cord, the tectospinal tract travels through the ventral funiculus as part of the medial longitudinal fasciculus (MLF) (see Fig. 8 in Chap. 1), which is described later in this chapter. The tectospinal tract extends only through the cervical segments of the cord, where it influences neurons innervating muscles of the neck, including the neurons of the spinal accessory nucleus (cranial nerve XI).

The corticotectal projections are concerned with turning movements of the head and eyes, possibly combined with reaching movements of the arm. Corticotectal fibers have a greater influence on reflexive than on voluntary eye movements.

Corticorubral and Rubrospinal Tracts

The corticorubral and rubrospinal tracts represent an indirect route from the cerebral cortex to the spinal cord. Fibers originating from the same cortical areas that give rise to the corticospinal tract form the corticorubral tract. This tract projects to the ipsilateral red nucleus in the tegmentum of the midbrain. The red nucleus gives rise to the **rubrospinal tract**, the fibers of which cross the midline in the **ventral tegmental decussation** (see Fig. 39 in Chap. 10) and descend through the lateral tegmentum of the pons, midbrain, and medulla (see Fig. 27 in Chap. 9 and Figs. 34 through 38 in Chap. 10). In the spinal cord, this crossed pathway is found just anterior to the lateral corticospinal tract in the lateral funiculus (see Fig. 8 in Chap. 1). Its fibers synapse at all cord levels in the lateral aspect of laminae V, VI, and VII and thus overlap part of the termination of the corticospinal tract. The rubrospinal tract is functionally similar to the corticospinal tract in that generally it facilitates flexor and inhibits extensor alpha, beta, and gamma motoneurons, particularly those innervating the distal parts of the arms. The red nucleus also forms a synaptic relay between the cerebellum and the ventral lateral nucleus of the thalamus.

Corticoreticular and Reticulospinal Tracts

The reticular formation, a matrix of nuclei in the core of the brain stem, receives a large input from **corticoreticular fibers**, which accompany the corticospinal and corticobulbar fibers. Like the majority of the corticobulbar fibers, the corticoreticular fibers from each hemisphere terminate bilaterally in the brain stem. Two areas of the reticular formation send major projections into the spinal cord. The pontine reticular formation gives rise to the uncrossed **pontine (medial) reticulospinal tract**. In the brain stem, this pathway travels just ventral to the MLF. In the spinal cord, the pontine pathway passes through the ventral funiculus to all cord levels. In its passage through the cervical and highest thoracic segments of the cord, it is incorporated into the MLF. Its fibers synapse in laminae VII and VIII. The pontine tract is mainly excitatory for extensor alpha motoneurons, particularly those innervating the midline musculature of the body and the proximal parts of the extremities (see Fig. 27 in Chap. 9). It also provides an important input to gamma motoneurons.

The medial aspect of the medullary reticular formation gives rise to the **medullary (lateral) reticulospinal tract**, which is primarily uncrossed but has a small crossed component. This tract passes to all cord levels in the lateral funiculus immediately anterior to the rubrospinal tract (see Fig. 8 in Chap. 1). It synapses in laminae VII and IX. The tract conveys **autonomic information** from higher levels to the preganglionic sympathetic and parasympathetic neurons to influence respiration, circulation, sweating, shivering, and dilation of the pupils, as well as the function of the sphincteric muscles of the gastrointestinal and urinary tracts. Autonomic functions, particularly cardiovascular functions, are also influenced directly by hypothalamic projections to the spinal cord from the paraventricular and other hypothalamic nuclei.

Raphe-Spinal and Ceruleus-Spinal Projections

The raphe nuclei are a special subgroup of the nuclei that constitute the reticular formation. Projections from the raphe nuclei are serotonergic. Fibers arising from neurons within the caudal raphe nuclei, particularly the nucleus raphe magnus, project to the spinal cord. These fibers pass through the dorsolateral funiculus of the spinal cord and terminate within laminae I, II, V, and VII. In laminae I and II, these fibers have an important influence over the transmission of pain information from the peripheral nerves. In lamina VII, the raphe-spinal projections end on preganglionic sympathetic neurons.

The nucleus locus ceruleus and nucleus subceruleus give rise to a projection descending into the spinal cord through the ventrolateral funiculus and terminating in laminae I, II, V, VII, IX, and X. This projection is noradrenergic.

Although the role of the raphe-spinal and ceruleus-spinal projections in motor function has not been clearly defined, these systems are thought to exert a facilitating action on motoneurons, and thus they may function as a gain-setting system that determines the overall responsiveness of the motoneurons. These pathways may be used to modulate the responsiveness of the motor system in different phases of sleep-waking cycles and with various changes in emotional state.

Vestibulospinal Tracts

The two vestibulospinal tracts are also discussed in Chapter 16. Both of these tracts pass into the anterior funiculus and synapse on cells in laminae VII and VIII. The **lateral vestibulospinal tract** extends the entire length of the cord. The **medial vestibulospinal tract** extends through the MLF only to upper thoracic levels. Stimulation of the lateral vestibulospinal tract evokes excitatory postsynaptic potentials (EPSPs) in extensor motoneurons innervating the neck, back, forelimb, and hindlimb muscles. These EPSPs are monosynaptic for neck motoneurons and some back and leg motoneurons. Stimulation of the lateral vestibulospinal tract evokes reciprocal inhibition in flexor motoneurons through disynaptic or polysynaptic connections. Stimulation of the medial vestibulospinal tract evokes monosynaptic inhibition and excitation in neck and back motoneurons but does not influence limb motoneurons. The vestibulospinal pathways are concerned with postural adjustments of the body accompanying head movements and with the maintenance of postural tone.

Medial Longitudinal Fasciculus

The MLF is not a single tract but a bundle of several tracts in the brain stem, some of which project into the ventral funiculus of the spinal cord. This "descending portion" of the MLF in the spinal cord contains the **pontine (medial) reticulospinal tract** and the **medial vestibulospinal tract**, which have been discussed. The **interstitiospinal tract**, which arises from the interstitial nucleus of Cajal (an accessory oculomotor nucleus), is also part of the MLF. The interstitiospinal tract supplies only the upper cervical levels, where it synapses in laminae VII and VIII. In the spinal cord, the MLF also contains the **tectospinal tract**. This tract arises from the superior colliculus, crosses to the opposite side in the dorsal tegmental decussation (near the oculomotor nucleus), and passes caudally. In the brain stem, this tract lies anterior to the MLF, but in the cord, its fibers become part of the MLF, which does not extend below the upper thoracic cord segments. The MLF is concerned with reflex movements of the head and neck in response to visual and vestibular stimuli.

THE INFLUENCE OF DESCENDING PATHWAYS ON THE SPINAL CORD

• • • • • • • • •

The distribution of fibers to the spinal cord that control movement and visceral function is summarized in Figure 25. The motor system pathways arising in the cerebral cortex and brain stem that reach the spinal cord are illustrated on the left of this

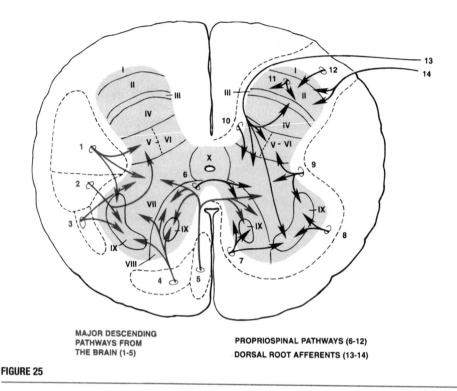

MAJOR DESCENDING PATHWAYS FROM THE BRAIN (1-5)

PROPRIOSPINAL PATHWAYS (6-12)
DORSAL ROOT AFFERENTS (13-14)

FIGURE 25

Afferents to the spinal cord gray matter. (*Left*) Major descending pathways from the brain: 1, lateral corticospinal tract; 2, lateral brain stem system (rubrospinal tract and pontine tegmentum projections); 3, lateral reticulospinal tract; 4, ventromedial brain stem system (interstitiospinal, tectospinal, medial reticulospinal, and vestibulospinal tracts); 5, ventral corticospinal tract. (*Right*) Propriospinal fibers: 6, commissural; 7, ventromedial; 8, ventrolateral; 9, dorsolateral propriospinal fibers; 10, cornucommisural tract; 11, propriospinal fibers within the substantia gelatinosa; 12, posterolateral fasciculus, or Lissauer's tract. Dorsal root afferents: 13, large diameter (Aα and Aβ) afferents; 14, small-diameter (Aδ and C) afferents.

figure. As described previously in this chapter, the **lateral and ventral corticospinal tracts** provide the capacity for control of finely fractionated movements, such as independent movements of the fingers. The remaining pathways that regulate movement can be described as two general projection systems from the brain stem: ventromedial and lateral.

The **ventromedial brain stem system** consists of fibers arising in the interstitial nucleus of Cajal; the superior colliculus; the mesencephalic, pontine, and some of the medullary reticular formation; and the vestibular nuclei. The tracts formed from these fibers terminate in the ventral and medial aspects of the anterior horn of the spinal cord, including laminae VII, VIII and IX, where motoneurons innervating the axial and girdle musculature are found. The ventromedial pathways are particularly concerned with maintenance of erect posture, integrated movements of the body and limbs, and progression movements of the limbs. These pathways generally facilitate the activity of motoneurons projecting to extensor muscles and inhibit the activity of motoneurons projecting to flexor muscles.

The **lateral brain stem system** consists of fibers arising in the contralateral magnocellular red nucleus, which project to the spinal cord through the rubrospinal tract; and additional fibers from the ventrolateral portion of the contralateral pontine tegmentum, which project through the lateral column of the spinal cord. This lateral pathway terminates in the dorsal and lateral aspect of the dorsal and ventral horns of the spinal cord, including laminae V, VI, VII, and IX. Like the corticospinal tracts, the lateral brain stem system is concerned with fine manipulative, independent movements of the limbs, particularly of the hands and feet. This pathway generally facilitates the activity of motoneurons projecting to flexor muscles and inhibits the activity of motoneurons projecting to extensors.

The final descending system illustrated in Figure 25 is the **lateral reticulospinal system**, which is predominantly concerned with regulation of the autonomic motoneurons in the intermediolateral cell column of lamina VII.

In addition to these major descending pathways from the brain, **propriospinal pathways** play an essential role in spinal cord function. These intersegmental projections arise from both dorsal and ventral horn neurons. Their axons travel in the white matter immediately surrounding the gray matter, linking both nearby and distant segments of the cord to facilitate integrated body movements and visceral function (see Fig. 25, right). Exceptions to this pattern are the projections of neurons in the substantia gelatinosa (lamina II) and in lamina VIII, whose axons travel within the gray matter.

Lesions of the Peripheral Nerves, Spinal Roots, and Spinal Cord

DEGENERATION AND REGENERATION OF NERVE CELLS AND FIBERS

When a peripheral nerve fiber is transected or permanently destroyed, the part that has been separated from the nerve cell body degenerates completely and, in the process, loses its myelin sheath. This process is called **wallerian degeneration**. Degenerated fibers can be studied histologically by obtaining a series of microscopic sections, staining them appropriately, and reconstructing the course of the fibers.

In addition to causing permanent destruction of the disconnected portion, severing a cell's axon has a harmful effect on the nerve cell body itself. For several weeks after the injury, the cell's Nissl bodies (chromophilic substance) undergo **chromatolysis**, a process in which the ribosomes (RNA) lose their staining characteristics and seem to dissolve in the surrounding cytoplasm. Some of the affected cells disintegrate, but others recover with restoration of Nissl substance. Those that recover participate in the process of regeneration.

A completely severed peripheral nerve has some capacity to repair itself. Schwann (neurolemma) cells that previously formed the myelin of the central end of the nerve stump proliferate and attempt to bridge the gap with the distal end of the nerve. The axis cylinders in the central end of the cut nerve divide longitudinally and soon begin to sprout from the end of the nerve. Many sprouting axons go astray in random directions, but some of them cross the gap and enter neurolemmal tubes leading to the peripheral endings. Their growth rate is normally 1 to 2 mm per day. Chance apparently determines whether a regenerating motor fiber enters a neurolemmal tube leading to a motor or to a sensory terminal. If suitably matched, connections can be reestablished and function restored.

When nerve fibers in the brain and spinal cord are completely severed, they do not regenerate effectively. However, injuries to these fibers in the spinal cord vary in degree. Some are sufficient to prevent conduction of nerve impulses without causing irreversible fiber degeneration. The pressure of tumors, herniated intervertebral discs, blood clots, or swelling and edema following wounds may produce spinal cord symptoms that are later alleviated by treatment. The prospect of recovery depends on the severity and duration of the pressure.

LESIONS OF PERIPHERAL NERVES

• • • • • • • • •

Injury of an individual peripheral nerve (see Fig. 26, lesion 1) is followed by paralysis of muscles and loss of sensation distal to the lesion, involving only muscles and skin areas supplied by the injured nerve. The paralyzed muscles are **flaccid** (i.e., severely hypotonic) and gradually undergo severe atrophy. All forms of sensation, including proprioception, are lost. Recognition of peripheral nerve lesions is based on knowledge of the course and distribution of such nerves (see right sides of Figs. 17 and 18 in Chap. 6).

Polyneuropathy is a term used to describe the clinical syndrome resulting from diffuse lesions of peripheral nerves. The lesions often occur bilaterally, and the effects are usually more prominent in the distal than in the proximal parts of the extremities. Muscular weakness and atrophy accompanied by sensory loss in the distal portions of the extremities (often in a "glove-and-stocking" distribution) are characteristic of this disorder. The muscle stretch reflexes usually are diminished or absent in the affected portions of the limbs. Frequent causes of polyneuropathy include diabetes mellitus, alcoholism, vitamin B_{12} deficiency, carcinoma, and the Guillain-Barré syndrome.

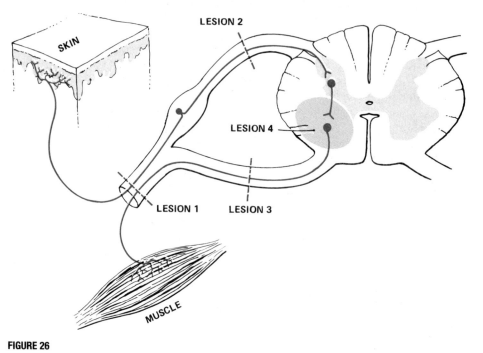

FIGURE 26

• • • • • • • • •

A cross section of the spinal cord, dorsal and ventral roots, and peripheral nerve. Lesion 1 affects the peripheral nerve; lesion 2, the dorsal root; lesion 3, the ventral root; and lesion 4, the anterior horn cells.

LESIONS OF THE POSTERIOR ROOTS

• • • • • • • • •

The posterior (dorsal) roots can be damaged by local tumors, infections, or injuries (see Fig. 26, lesion 2). A frequent cause of injury to dorsal roots is herniation of the nucleus pulposus (i.e., "slipped disc"), which can protrude from between adjacent vertebral bodies and compress one or more dorsal roots. The result is pain and paresthesias (sensations of numbness and tingling) that characteristically occur in the distribution of the affected roots. Examination usually reveals loss of sensation in a dermatomal distribution (see left sides of Figs. 17 and 18 in Chap. 6) and loss of the associated muscle stretch reflexes.

LOWER MOTONEURON LESIONS: HYPOTONIC PARALYSIS OF MUSCLES

• • • • • • • • •

The term **lower motoneuron** is used to designate the anterior horn cells of the spinal cord, which innervate the skeletal muscles of the body, and the motor nerve cells of the brain stem, which innervate muscles supplied by the cranial nerves. Destruction of these neurons (Fig. 26, lesion 4), their axons in ventral nerve roots (Fig. 26, lesion 3), or motor fibers of peripheral nerves (Fig. 26, lesion 1) abolishes both the voluntary and reflex responses of muscles. In addition to paralysis, the affected muscles show hypotonia (i.e., diminished resistance to passive manipulation of the limbs) and absence of the muscle stretch reflexes. Within a few weeks of injury, the fibers of the muscles begin to show **atrophy**. The atrophy of muscle fibers deprived of their motoneurons is more profound than the atrophy that occurs in muscles that are rendered inactive. This is because the anterior horn cells exert a trophic influence on muscle fibers that is essential for maintaining their normal state. Muscles undergoing early stages of atrophy display **fibrillations** and **fasciculations**. Fibrillations are fine twitchings of single muscle fibers that generally cannot be seen on clinical examination but can be detected on electromyographic examination. Fasciculations are brief contractions of **motor units** and can be seen in skeletal muscle through the intact skin.

Lesions that damage sensory fibers in the dorsal roots (Fig. 26, lesion 2) or their cell bodies in spinal ganglia also disrupt the stretch reflex pathway (see Fig. 15 in Chap. 4) and, as a consequence, produce hypotonia and loss of the muscle stretch reflexes. In this instance, the lower motoneurons remain intact, and there is no loss of voluntary motor strength. The trophic influence of anterior horn cells is preserved, and neither muscle atrophy (except that of disuse) nor fasciculations appear. Coordinated movements are performed poorly because of the loss of sensory feedback to the nervous system.

UPPER MOTONEURON LESION: SPASTIC PARALYSIS OF MUSCLES

• • • • • • • • •

The term **upper motoneuron** is used to describe nerve cell bodies that originate in high levels of the central nervous system and send their axons into the brain stem or spinal cord, where they make contact, directly or indirectly, with motor nuclei of the cranial nerves and anterior horn cells in the spinal cord. Examples of upper motoneuron pathways include the corticospinal, corticobulbar, reticulospinal, vestibulospinal, and rubrospinal tracts.

A lesion in the **posterior limb of the internal capsule** (Fig. 27, lesion 1) disrupts the influence of the cerebral cortex on lower motoneurons on the contralateral side of the body. The corticospinal and corticobulbar tracts are not the only pathways involved in such a lesion, because the lesion also interrupts connections between the cerebral cortex and the origin of the rubrospinal and reticulospinal pathways. Immediately following such a lesion, the patient develops paralysis of the face, arm, and leg (hemiplegia) of the opposite side of the body, with hypotonia and depression of the muscle stretch reflexes. After an interval that varies from a few days to a few weeks, stretch reflexes return in these muscles and then progress to become more active than normal. Hypertonia develops, as shown by fixed posture of the limbs and increased resistance to positive manipulation of the limbs. As the examiner manipulates the limbs, the resistance is most marked in the flexor muscles of the arm and the extensor muscles of the leg. This resistance is strong at the beginning of the movement but gives way in a "clasp-knife" fashion as the movement is continued. The hypertonia is velocity dependent; the characteristic clasp-knife reaction requires rapid movement of the limb to be appreciated and may be missed with slow movement. The muscle stretch reflexes are hyperactive and occasionally may show **clonus** (i.e., a sustained series of rhythmic jerks) as a tendon is maintained in extension by the examiner. Muscles showing the clasp-knife reaction and hyperreflexia are said to be **spastic** or to show **spasticity**. Other conditions may produce hypertonic muscles, but they have distinguishing features that differentiate them from the spasticity associated with internal-capsule lesions. Some examples of these are **decerebrate rigidity**, **dystonia**, **parkinsonian rigidity**, and **myotonia**. Rigidity is not velocity dependent; even slow movements of the limbs disclose increased resistance. In addition to spastic weakness with hyperreflexia, internal-capsule lesions result in the appearance of **Babinski's sign**. This reflex response is described in the following section.

The **pyramidal tract** consists of upper motoneurons in the cerebral cortex with axons coursing through the pyramidal tract in the medulla and terminating on anterior horn cells or interneurons in the spinal cord. The pyramidal tract is also termed the **corticospinal tract**. In humans, signs of upper motoneuron disease (e.g., spastic paralysis, increased muscle stretch reflexes, clonus, Babinski's sign, clasp-knife response to passive movements, lack of muscle atrophy except for disuse atrophy) result from pyramidal (corticospinal) tract lesions. This has been verified in a small number of patients whose brains, when examined after death, showed lesions restricted to the pyramidal tract in the medulla. Experimentally placed pyramidal tract lesions in the monkey, however, do not cause spasticity; these lesions result in limb hypotonia. In most humans with spasticity, multiple upper motoneuron projections, in addition to the corticospinal tract, are affected.

There has been considerable debate about the lower motoneurons that mediate spasticity, with some experts claiming that gamma (or beta and gamma) motoneurons are responsible and others stating that alpha motoneurons are responsible. Hypersensitive gamma and beta fibers can stimulate muscle spindles to a higher rate of discharge, resulting in enhanced responses to muscle stretch. Hypersensitive alpha motoneurons can react excessively to proprioceptive input from muscle stretch receptors. Although it is not yet clear whether the responses of both gamma and alpha motoneurons are enhanced in spasticity, the bulk of evidence suggests that hyperactive alpha motoneurons account for the abnormalities.

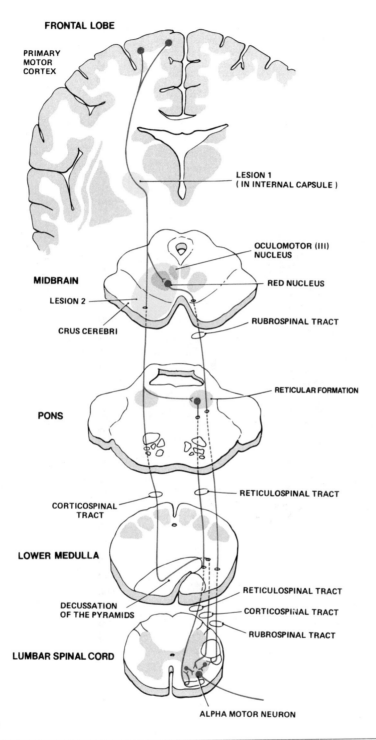

FIGURE 27

• • • • • • • • •

Several of the major motor pathways of the central nervous system. Lesion 1 affects the internal capsule and causes a contralateral hemiplegia affecting the lower portion of the face and the arm and leg; the pathways to the facial nucleus and cervical cord are not shown. Lesion 2 causes an ipsilateral cranial nerve disorder (loss of function of the third cranial nerve) and a contralateral hemiplegia affecting the lower portion of the face and the arm and leg (see Fig. 48 in Chap. 14).

The symptoms listed for corticospinal tract lesions occur because other descending upper motoneuron pathways tend to be involved as well. An important neurologic sign that clearly can be attributed selectively to lesions of the corticospinal tract is **Babinski's sign**, which is described in the following section. A corticospinal tract lesion rostral to the level of the pyramidal decussation gives rise to **contralateral** spasticity, muscle weakness, and Babinski's sign. A lesion of this tract caudal to the level of the pyramidal decussation (i.e., in the spinal cord) causes these signs on the **ipsilateral** side of the body.

The effects of lower motoneuron lesions are limited to the muscles that they innervate, but a small lesion that interrupts the corticospinal tract removes voluntary motor control from the whole sector of the body that lies downstream from the level of the injury. Thus, a lesion of the posterior limb of the internal capsule (see Fig. 27, lesion 1) causes paralysis of the contralateral face, arm, and leg. Involvement of the face is limited to the lower portion because the muscles in the upper portion are innervated by a region of the facial nucleus that receives much less input from the upper motoneurons than the region innervating muscles of the lower face, and because this input to the upper facial area comes from the cortex of both hemispheres (see Chap. 13). A lesion on one side of the brain stem commonly affects one of the cranial nerves (e.g., the third nerve in the instance of lesion 2 in Fig. 27), and thus the patient will have loss of function of a cranial nerve on the side ipsilateral to the lesion, with a hemiplegia on the contralateral side.

Paralysis affecting the arm and leg of one side of the body is termed **hemiplegia**. **Paraplegia** is paralysis of both legs, as, for example, after a transverse lesion of the spinal cord that destroys the upper motoneurons of both sides of the cord. Paralysis of a single extremity is termed **monoplegia**, and paralysis that includes all four extremities is called **quadriplegia**. Lesions that impair function but are not sufficiently severe to cause total paralysis produce weakness that is clinically designated as **paresis**.

REFLEXES ASSOCIATED WITH LESIONS OF THE MOTOR PATHWAY

• • • • • • • •

Certain reflexes that are not elicited in normal individuals may be present after injuries of the corticospinal tract. **Babinski's sign** (extensor plantar reflex) is an abnormal reflex obtained by stroking the plantar surface of the outer border of the foot with a blunt object such as a key. The normal response is plantar flexion of the great toe; however, if Babinski's sign is present, there is dorsiflexion of the great toe, at times accompanied by fanning of the other toes. When it is found, Babinski's sign is a strong indication of a disorder of the corticospinal tract. Many similar pathologic reflexes have been described. **Hoffmann's sign** is elicited by flicking the nail of the patient's middle finger. When the sign is present, there is prompt adduction of the thumb and flexion of the index finger. Hoffmann's sign is commonly associated with injury of the corticospinal tract, but it can occur in normal persons.

Superficial reflexes, which normally are obtained by stroking certain areas of the skin, may be absent if the corticospinal tract is injured. If the skin of the abdominal wall is scratched gently, the abdominal musculature contracts locally, causing the umbilicus to deviate momentarily in the direction of the stimulus. In the male, stroking the upper inner aspect of the thigh normally causes reflex contraction of the cremaster muscle, with elevation of the testicle on the stimulated side. Loss of the **abdominal** or **cremasteric** reflexes confirms the presence of a corticospinal tract lesion, but absence of these reflexes bilaterally in an otherwise normal individual may have no significance.

TRANSECTION OF THE SPINAL CORD

• • • • • • • • •

Immediately after complete transection of the spinal cord, sensation and all voluntary movement are lost below the level of the lesion. The finding of a level on the body below which sensation and motor function are lost provides strong clinical evidence of a spinal cord disorder. Control of the bladder and bowel is also lost. If the spinal cord lesion occurs between cervical levels 1 and 3, respirations stop. Following acute spinal transection, **spinal shock** appears (i.e., the paralysis is flaccid, the deep tendon reflexes are lost, and plantar stimulation gives no response). The expected signs of upper motoneuron lesions appear only after several weeks have elapsed. Eventually, extensor plantar responses (Babinski's sign) can be detected, followed by the gradual appearance of hyperactive deep tendon reflexes, clonus, and spasticity of the affected limbs. Flexor spasms of the legs appear intermittently, often triggered by local cutaneous stimulation. Bladder and bowel function usually becomes automatic, with these structures emptying in response to filling.

Partial injury to the spinal cord results in damage to some ascending and descending pathways and sparing of others. The symptoms and signs of partial spinal injury vary depending on the location of the injury.

HEMISECTION OF THE SPINAL CORD
(BROWN-SÉQUARD SYNDROME)

• • • • • • • •

Lateral hemisection of the spinal cord (e.g., from a bullet or knife wound) produces the **Brown-Séquard syndrome** (Fig. 28B). The specific effects in a patient with a chronic lesion can be understood by considering the fiber tracts and roots affected by the lesion.

1. Lateral column damage results in paralysis of muscles on the same side of the body below the injury, with spasticity, hyperactive reflexes, clonus, loss of superficial reflexes, and Babinski's sign.
2. Dorsal column damage, along with the lateral column injury, causes loss of position sense, vibratory sense, and tactile discrimination on the same side of the body below the level of the injury. Because of the paralysis, sensory ataxia, which might otherwise occur, cannot be demonstrated readily.
3. Damage to the anterolateral system involves loss of the sensations of pain and temperature **on the side opposite the lesion** beginning one or two dermatomes below the level of the injury (review Fig. 23 in Chap. 7).

Simple touch sensation may be unimpaired because the dorsal columns (carrying touch sensation from that side of the body) are intact opposite the lesion, and the anterolateral system on the opposite side of the cord, subserving the ipsilateral side of the body, is also intact.

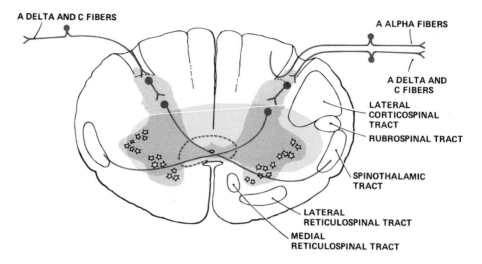

A. Syringomyelia

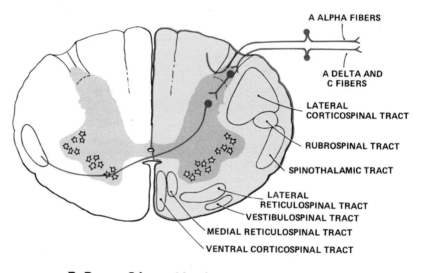

B. Brown-Séquard Lesion

FIGURE 28

• • • • • • • • •

(*A*) A cross section of the spinal cord showing the pathways interrupted by a cavitating lesion of a small syringomyelia (*dotted line*) and a larger syringomyelia (*shaded area*). (*B*) A cross section of the spinal cord showing the pathways interrupted by hemisection of the cord (Brown-Séquard lesion).

In addition to the effects produced by interrupting the long ascending and descending tracts of the spinal cord, symptoms are likely the result of damage to dorsal and ventral nerve roots at the level of the injury. These symptoms occur on the side of the lesion, and when present, they are of great value in localizing the individual cord segments involved.

1. Irritation of fibers in the dorsal root zone lead to paresthesias or radicular pain in a band over the affected dermatomes.

2. Destruction of dorsal roots results in a band of anesthesia over the dermatome(s) supplied by the involved roots.
3. Destruction of ventral roots evokes a flaccid paralysis affecting only the muscles innervated by fibers that have been destroyed.

Few lesions are precisely localized to one lateral half of the spinal cord. More often, spinal lesions involve one sector of the cord and produce a partial, or incomplete, Brown-Séquard syndrome. The particular symptoms and signs in each case are determined by the position and extent of the lesion. Brown-Séquard syndrome more often results from lesions compressing the spinal cord from the outside than it does from lesions that arise within the spinal cord.

The sensory pathways of the spinal cord show a characteristic layering, so that the sacral segments are outermost and progressively higher segments are in sequential order progressing inward. Consequently, lesions affecting the central part of the spinal cord, such as tumors or traumatic injury, can result in **sacral sparing**. With sacral sparing, sensation below the level of the lesion is lost except in the sacral dermatomes, where it is preserved.

Current evidence indicates that patients with traumatic injury to the spinal cord regain function more effectively if treated with corticosteroids soon after the injury. Therefore, the rapid diagnosis of a spinal cord disorder is critical in people who have sustained traumatic injury.

LESIONS OF THE CENTRAL GRAY MATTER

In **syringomyelia**, there is progressive cavitation around or near the central canal of the spinal cord, most commonly in the region of the cervical enlargement. A small lesion in this position interrupts the lateral spinothalamic fibers that pass through the ventral white commissure as they cross from one side to the other (Fig. 28A, lesion enclosed by dotted line). Because these fibers conduct impulses mediating pain and temperature from dermatomes on both sides of the body, the result is loss of pain and temperature sensibility, with a segmental distribution in the upper extremities on both sides. The spinothalamic tracts from the lumbosacral segments remain intact, and thus there is no sensory impairment in the lower extremities. Position, vibration, and simple touch sensations are spared in the affected dermatomes of the arms. Loss of pain and temperature sense with preservation of position, vibration, and touch sensation is termed **sensory dissociation**. In later stages of the disease, as the lesion enlarges, degeneration often extends to the anterior gray horns (see Fig. 28A, shaded area) and causes paralysis with atrophy of muscles innervated by the segments involved. Signs of upper motoneuron disease may appear in the lower extremities as a result of compression of the lateral corticospinal tracts by the cystic cavity.

LESIONS INVOLVING THE ANTERIOR HORNS AND THE CORTICOSPINAL TRACTS

Amyotrophic lateral sclerosis (**ALS**) is a progressive, fatal disease of unknown cause characterized by degeneration of neurons in the motor nuclei of the cranial nerves and in the anterior gray horns of the spinal cord, with degeneration of the pyramidal tracts bilaterally. Sensory disturbance is not part of the disorder. Weakness and atrophy are noted in some muscles, with spasticity and hyperreflexia in others. An asymmetrical distribution at the onset of the disease is the most common pattern of limb involvement. The classic form of this disease starts with weakness, atrophy, and fasciculations of the muscles of the hands and arms, followed later by spastic paralysis of the limbs. Difficulty in speaking and swallowing results from involvement of the nuclei of the lower cranial nerves.

LESIONS INVOLVING POSTERIOR AND LATERAL FUNICULI

• • • • • • • • •

Subacute degeneration of the spinal cord (combined systems disease) is most often seen in **pernicious anemia**, but it is sometimes seen with other types of anemia or nutritional disturbances. The dorsal and lateral columns of the spinal cord undergo degeneration, but the gray matter ordinarily is not affected. Degeneration of the dorsal and lateral columns results in complaints of difficulty in walking and tingling sensations in the feet. Examination reveals loss of position and vibration sense in the legs and a positive Romberg sign. Degeneration of upper motoneuron projections in the lateral columns leads to weakness in the legs, with spasticity, hyperactive muscle stretch reflexes, and bilateral Babinski's signs. Later in the course of the disease, the muscle stretch reflexes may disappear because of the development of a peripheral neuropathy.

THROMBOSIS OF THE ANTERIOR SPINAL ARTERY

• • • • • • • • •

The anterior spinal artery runs in the anterior median sulcus, sending terminal branches to supply the ventral and lateral funiculi and most of the gray matter of the spinal cord. The anterior horns, lateral spinothalamic tracts, and pyramidal tracts are included in this artery's territory, but the dorsal funiculi and posterior part of the dorsal horns are supplied independently by a pair of posterior spinal arteries (Fig. 29). Thrombosis of the anterior spinal artery in the cervical region of the cord produces bilateral atrophy, fasciculations, and flaccid paralysis at the level of the lesion because of destruction of anterior horn cells. An accompanying spastic paraplegia results from bilateral corticospinal tract involvement and, usually, loss of pain and temperature sense below the lesion because of bilateral spinothalamic tract damage. The onset of symptoms is abrupt and is often accompanied by severe pain.

TUMORS OF THE SPINAL CORD

• • • • • • • • •

Tumors that arise within the vertebral canal but outside the spinal cord (extramedullary tumors) gradually impinge on the cord as they enlarge. Compression of nerve roots often occurs first and accounts for pain distributed over the dermatomes supplied by these roots. This is followed by gradual involvement of the

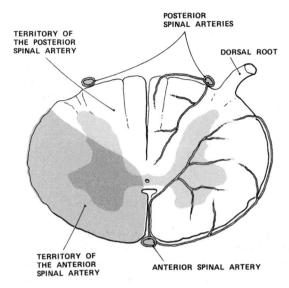

FIGURE 29

• • • • • • • • •

A cross section of the spinal cord showing the locations of the anterior and posterior spinal arteries and their branches (*right*) and the territories supplied by these arteries (*left*).

tracts within the spinal cord until a Brown-Séquard syndrome, or some modification of the syndrome, occurs. The order of appearance of symptoms may furnish a clue to the site of the tumor. For example, loss of pain and temperature sensibility involving all segments below a certain level on the left side followed by spastic paralysis on the right imply that the tumor has arisen from the ventrolateral region of the cord on the right side. Loss of proprioception on the right side followed by an extension of the proprioceptive deficit to the left side and the development of spastic paralysis on the right indicate that the tumor is compressing the spinal cord from the dorsomedial region on the right side.

4

Brain Stem
and Cerebellum

10

Anatomy of the Brain Stem: Medulla, Pons, and Midbrain

MEDULLA

The **medulla (medulla oblongata or bulb)** is the most caudal part of the brain stem. It is continuous with the spinal cord at the foramen magnum and extends rostrally for 2.5 cm to the caudal border of the pons. The central canal of the spinal cord continues through the caudal half of the medulla and then, at a point called the **obex**, flares open into the wide cavity of the fourth ventricle. The rostral part of the medulla thus occupies the floor of the fourth ventricle. The roof of the ventricle is formed by the **tela choroidea** (a thin sheet of apposed ependyma and pia mater), the **choroid plexus** (tela choroidea with blood vessels between the ependyma and pia), and the cerebellum.

External Markings of the Medulla

Figures 30, 31, and 32 represent specimens of the basal ganglia, diencephalon, and brain stem from which the overlying cerebral cortex, cerebellum, and ependymal roof of the fourth ventricle have been removed.

ANTERIOR (VENTRAL) ASPECT

The **pyramids**, which contain the **pyramidal (corticospinal) tracts**, form two longitudinal ridges on either side of the ventral median fissure (see Fig. 30). The decussation of the pyramids can be seen obliterating the fissure at the extreme caudal end of the medulla.

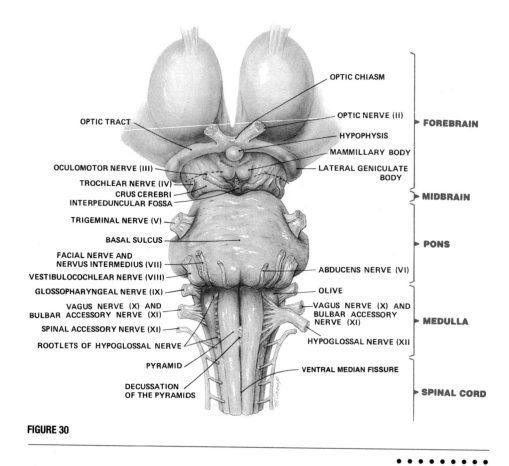

OPTIC CHIASM

OPTIC NERVE (II)

OPTIC TRACT

HYPOPHYSIS

MAMMILLARY BODY

OCULOMOTOR NERVE (III)

LATERAL GENICULATE BODY

TROCHLEAR NERVE (IV)

CRUS CEREBRI

INTERPEDUNCULAR FOSSA

TRIGEMINAL NERVE (V)

BASAL SULCUS

FACIAL NERVE AND NERVUS INTERMEDIUS (VII)

ABDUCENS NERVE (VI)

VESTIBULOCOCHLEAR NERVE (VIII)

GLOSSOPHARYNGEAL NERVE (IX)

OLIVE

VAGUS NERVE (X) AND BULBAR ACCESSORY NERVE (XI)

VAGUS NERVE (X) AND BULBAR ACCESSORY NERVE (XI)

SPINAL ACCESSORY NERVE (XI)

ROOTLETS OF HYPOGLOSSAL NERVE

HYPOGLOSSAL NERVE (XII

PYRAMID

VENTRAL MEDIAN FISSURE

DECUSSATION OF THE PYRAMIDS

FOREBRAIN

MIDBRAIN

PONS

MEDULLA

SPINAL CORD

FIGURE 30

The ventral surface of the human lentiform nucleus, head of the caudate, hypothalamus, brain stem, and upper cervical spinal cord.

LATERAL ASPECT

Two longitudinal grooves are present in the lateral aspect: the ventrolateral sulcus and the dorsolateral sulcus (see Fig. 31). The ventrolateral sulcus extends along the lateral border of the pyramid, and from this groove, the rootlets of the hypoglossal nerve (XII) exit. Radicles of the **bulbar (cranial) accessory nerve (XI)**, **vagus nerve (X)**, and **glossopharyngeal nerve (IX)** are attached in line along the dorsolateral sulcus. The **spinal portion of the accessory nerve (XI)** arises from the gray matter of spinal cord segments C2 to C5. Its rootlets exit through the lateral funiculus of the cord, join and ascend along the lateral surface of the medulla. The prominent oval swelling of the lateral area of the medulla between the ventrolateral and dorsolateral sulci is the olive (see Figs. 30 and 31). This marks the site of the inferior olivary nuclear complex inside the medulla.

POSTERIOR (DORSAL) ASPECT

In Figure 32, the fasciculus gracilis and the fasciculus cuneatus are visible as low ridges in the spinal cord. The fasciculus gracilis forms the ridge between the dorsal median and dorsal intermediate sulci. The fasciculus cuneatus lies between the dor-

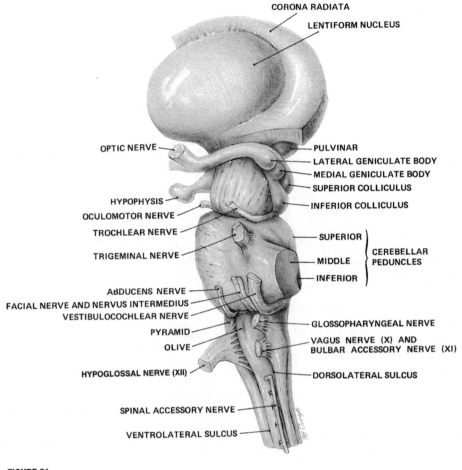

FIGURE 31

The lateral surface of the human spinal cord, brain stem, lentiform nucleus, and corona radiata.

sal intermediate and dorsolateral sulci. The sites of termination of these two tracts in the nucleus gracilis and the nucleus cuneatus are marked by small eminences named, respectively, the **clava** and the **cuneate tubercle**. The fibers from the nuclei gracilis and cuneatus extend ventrally into the tegmentum (floor) of the medulla. Thus, at the rostral end of these nuclei, the dorsal area "opens up," exposing the floor of the fourth ventricle rostral to the **obex**. Two pairs of small swellings can be seen in the floor of the ventricle. The lateral ridges constitute the **vagal trigone**; the medial ridges are the **hypoglossal trigone**. These trigones are bulges that indicate the locations of underlying nuclei, the **dorsal motor nucleus of the vagus** and the **hypoglossal nucleus**, respectively. The **striae medullares of the fourth ventricle** are ridges formed by fibers passing toward the cerebellum. Laterally, these fibers mark the location of the **lateral recesses**, leading to openings (the **foramina of Luschka)** where cerebrospinal fluid (CSF) flows from the fourth ventricle into the subarachnoid space. CSF also leaves the ventricle through a single, midline opening at the obex, the **foramen of Magendie** (see Fig. 81 in Chap. 27).

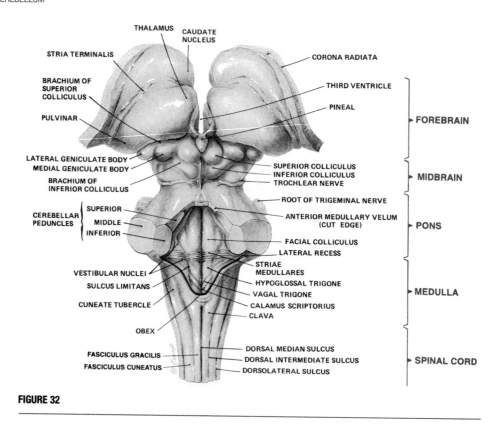

THALAMUS
CAUDATE NUCLEUS
STRIA TERMINALIS
CORONA RADIATA
BRACHIUM OF SUPERIOR COLLICULUS
THIRD VENTRICLE
PINEAL
PULVINAR
FOREBRAIN
LATERAL GENICULATE BODY
MEDIAL GENICULATE BODY
SUPERIOR COLLICULUS
INFERIOR COLLICULUS
TROCHLEAR NERVE
MIDBRAIN
BRACHIUM OF INFERIOR COLLICULUS
ROOT OF TRIGEMINAL NERVE
CEREBELLAR PEDUNCLES
SUPERIOR
MIDDLE
INFERIOR
ANTERIOR MEDULLARY VELUM (CUT EDGE)
PONS
FACIAL COLLICULUS
LATERAL RECESS
STRIAE MEDULLARES
VESTIBULAR NUCLEI
HYPOGLOSSAL TRIGONE
SULCUS LIMITANS
VAGAL TRIGONE
MEDULLA
CUNEATE TUBERCLE
CALAMUS SCRIPTORIUS
CLAVA
OBEX
DORSAL MEDIAN SULCUS
FASCICULUS GRACILIS
DORSAL INTERMEDIATE SULCUS
SPINAL CORD
FASCICULUS CUNEATUS
DORSOLATERAL SULCUS

FIGURE 32

The dorsal surface of the human spinal cord, brain stem, diencephalon, caudate nucleus, and corona radiata. The cerebellum has been removed by cutting through the peduncles. The colored line indicates the line of attachment of the tela choroidea, which forms the roof of the fourth ventricle.

Internal Structures of the Medulla

Some of the long fiber tracts of the spinal cord (e.g., spinothalamic tracts) pass directly through the medulla without any major changes in their relative positions, but both the corticospinal fibers and the dorsal columns of the spinal cord undergo shifts that radically change the arrangement of the gray and white matter in the medulla as compared with the spinal cord.

Figures 33 through 39 are drawings of histologic sections of the human brain stem. These thin slices of tissue were cut perpendicular to the long axis of the brain stem and stained with the Weigert method, in which chemicals in the stain bind to components of myelin. Thus, the dark areas on the left side of each of these cross sections represent myelinated fibers, and the light areas represent areas free of such fibers. The light areas are filled with neuron cell bodies forming the various nuclei of the brain stem.

CAUDAL HALF OF THE MEDULLA

A **central gray area** surrounds the **central canal** and merges at its perimeter with a zone containing a network of fibers and cells known as the **reticular formation**. The reticular formation extends throughout the medulla, pons, and midbrain. This is the origin of the reticulospinal tracts, which influence lower motoneurons in the

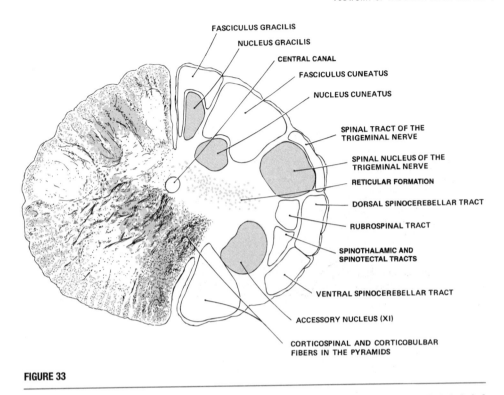

FASCICULUS GRACILIS
NUCLEUS GRACILIS
CENTRAL CANAL
FASCICULUS CUNEATUS
NUCLEUS CUNEATUS
SPINAL TRACT OF THE TRIGEMINAL NERVE
SPINAL NUCLEUS OF THE TRIGEMINAL NERVE
RETICULAR FORMATION
DORSAL SPINOCEREBELLAR TRACT
RUBROSPINAL TRACT
SPINOTHALAMIC AND SPINOTECTAL TRACTS
VENTRAL SPINOCEREBELLAR TRACT
ACCESSORY NUCLEUS (XI)
CORTICOSPINAL AND CORTICOBULBAR FIBERS IN THE PYRAMIDS

FIGURE 33

Cross section of the lowest level of the medulla, through the decussation of the pyramids. The left side represents the general appearance of this level in a myelin-stained histologic preparation. On the right, the major nuclei (*color*) and tracts (*white*) are outlined and labeled.

spinal cord. It is also an area that contains nuclear groups carrying out vital functions such as the control of blood pressure and respiration. Reticulospinal fibers to sympathetic and parasympathetic preganglionic neurons in the cord assist in these functions. Neurons of the reticular formation also project rostrally to the thalamus and hypothalamus, and some of these cell groups serve as an ascending "activating" system, which regulates general levels of activity in the brain and is important in cycles of sleep and wakefulness.

The corticospinal tracts descend through the most anterior part of the medulla in the pyramids, and at the caudal end of the medulla, most of these fibers cross in a prominent decussation (see Fig. 33) that brings them to the lateral position that they maintain in the spinal cord. On the posterior side at this level, the fasciculi gracilis and cuneatus remain present, but the nuclei in which their fibers terminate appear. Axons of the cells in these nuclei take an anterior, arched course, forming the **internal arcuate fibers** that cross the midline as the **decussation of the medial lemniscus** (see Fig. 34). Lateral to the rostral part of the cuneate nucleus, the **accessory cuneate nucleus** appears (see Fig. 34). Cells in this nucleus do not contribute axons to the medial lemniscus. Their axons ascend laterally into the inferior cerebellar peduncle as the cuneocerebellar tract (see Fig. 20 in Chap. 7). In the posterolateral region, a clear nuclear area capped by a peripheral zone of fine fibers represents the **spinal nucleus and spinal tract of the trigeminal nerve**. These two structures extend from the pontine region through the medulla to end in the second segment of the cervical spinal cord.

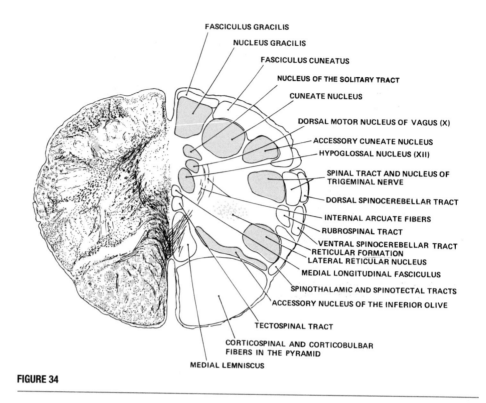

FASCICULUS GRACILIS

NUCLEUS GRACILIS

FASCICULUS CUNEATUS

NUCLEUS OF THE SOLITARY TRACT

CUNEATE NUCLEUS

DORSAL MOTOR NUCLEUS OF VAGUS (X)

ACCESSORY CUNEATE NUCLEUS

HYPOGLOSSAL NUCLEUS (XII)

SPINAL TRACT AND NUCLEUS OF TRIGEMINAL NERVE

DORSAL SPINOCEREBELLAR TRACT

INTERNAL ARCUATE FIBERS

RUBROSPINAL TRACT

VENTRAL SPINOCEREBELLAR TRACT
RETICULAR FORMATION
LATERAL RETICULAR NUCLEUS

MEDIAL LONGITUDINAL FASCICULUS

SPINOTHALAMIC AND SPINOTECTAL TRACTS

ACCESSORY NUCLEUS OF THE INFERIOR OLIVE

TECTOSPINAL TRACT

CORTICOSPINAL AND CORTICOBULBAR
FIBERS IN THE PYRAMID

MEDIAL LEMNISCUS

FIGURE 34

Cross section of the lower medulla at the level of the decussation of the internal arcuate fibers forming the medial lemniscus.

ROSTRAL HALF OF THE MEDULLA

The principal nucleus of the **inferior olivary nuclear complex**, a prominent structure in the anterolateral region, resembles a crinkled sac with an opening (hilus) directed toward the midline (see Fig. 35). Many of the complex's efferent fibers cross the midline and stream toward the posterolateral corner of the medulla to join dorsal spinocerebellar and cuneocerebellar fibers in the thick **inferior cerebellar peduncle (restiform body)**.

Several distinct, symmetrically paired cellular areas occupy the posterior part of the medulla close to the floor of the ventricle. Because these areas extend longitudinally through the upper medulla, they represent nuclear columns (see Fig. 41 in Chap. 11). The **nucleus of the hypoglossal nerve (XII)** is nearest the midline. Fibers from this nucleus pass anteriorly and emerge between the pyramid and the olive (see Fig. 35) as the rootlets of the hypoglossal nerve, which innervates the striated muscles of the tongue. The **dorsal motor nucleus of the vagus nerve (X)** lies at the side of the hypoglossal nucleus and contains neurons that form an important part of the parasympathetic division of the autonomic nervous system. The most lateral nuclear column, separated from the motor nuclei by the sulcus limitans, contains the **vestibular nuclei** (medial and inferior at this level of the medulla), which receive afferent fibers from the vestibular division of the vestibulocochlear nerve (VIII). This nerve brings information to the brain concerning position and movement of the head in space.

The **nucleus ambiguus**, seen indistinctly in Weigert-stained preparations, is located in the anterolateral part of the reticular formation. Its fibers course postero-

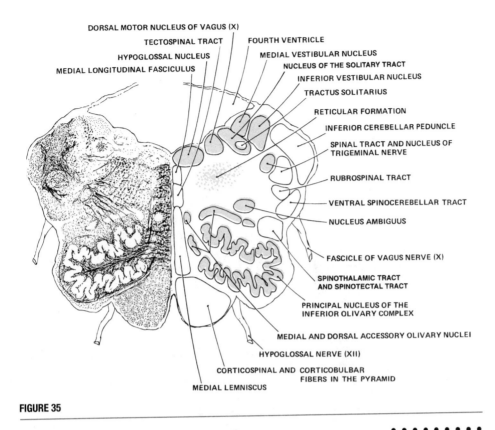

DORSAL MOTOR NUCLEUS OF VAGUS (X)
TECTOSPINAL TRACT
HYPOGLOSSAL NUCLEUS
MEDIAL LONGITUDINAL FASCICULUS
FOURTH VENTRICLE
MEDIAL VESTIBULAR NUCLEUS
NUCLEUS OF THE SOLITARY TRACT
INFERIOR VESTIBULAR NUCLEUS
TRACTUS SOLITARIUS
RETICULAR FORMATION
INFERIOR CEREBELLAR PEDUNCLE
SPINAL TRACT AND NUCLEUS OF
TRIGEMINAL NERVE
RUBROSPINAL TRACT
VENTRAL SPINOCEREBELLAR TRACT
NUCLEUS AMBIGUUS
FASCICLE OF VAGUS NERVE (X)
SPINOTHALAMIC TRACT
AND SPINOTECTAL TRACT
PRINCIPAL NUCLEUS OF THE
INFERIOR OLIVARY COMPLEX
MEDIAL AND DORSAL ACCESSORY OLIVARY NUCLEI
HYPOGLOSSAL NERVE (XII)
CORTICOSPINAL AND CORTICOBULBAR
FIBERS IN THE PYRAMID
MEDIAL LEMNISCUS

FIGURE 35

• • • • • • • •

Cross section of the upper medulla.

medially at first, but they arch back and leave the medulla anterior to the inferior cerebellar peduncle as fibers of the glossopharyngeal (IX), vagus (X), and bulbar accessory (XI) nerves (see Fig. 35 and Fig. 43 in Chap. 12). These nerve fibers control the branchiomeric muscles of the pharynx and larynx, and thus control swallowing and vocalization. An isolated bundle of longitudinal fibers accompanied by a small nucleus appears in the posterior part of the reticular formation. This bundle is known as the **solitary tract** and is composed of afferent root fibers from the facial, glossopharyngeal, and vagus nerves. The cells of the **nucleus of the solitary tract** surround the tract and receive fibers from it that carry information about taste and visceral sensations. The spinal tract and nucleus of V continue rostrally in a lateral position, somewhat ventral to the other nuclei surrounding the ventricle.

The anterolateral fiber system from the spinal cord (including the spinothalamic tract) is adjacent to the nucleus ambiguus on its anterolateral side. Two large bands of fibers lie vertically at either side of the midline. The extreme posterior portion of each band contains the **medial longitudinal fasciculus (MLF)**, a structure that extends from the upper thoracic spinal cord to the midbrain. At this level in the medulla, the MLF contains several descending pathways, including the **medial vestibulospinal**, **interstitiospinal**, and some of the **pontine reticulospinal tracts**. The **tectospinal pathway**, which descends through the brain stem anterior to the MLF, joins the fibers of this fasciculus in the caudal medulla and extends into the spinal cord as part of this tract. The **medial lemniscus** comprises the remainder and largest portion of this vertical band of fibers.

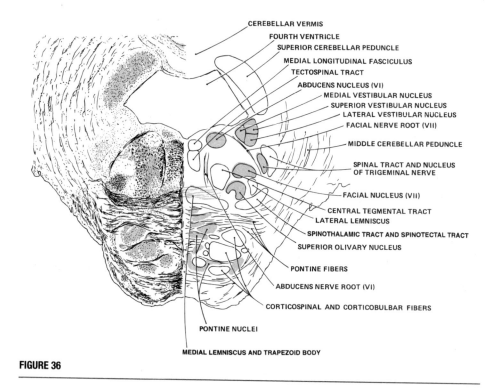

FIGURE 36

Cross section of the pons at the level of the nuclei of cranial nerves VI and VII.

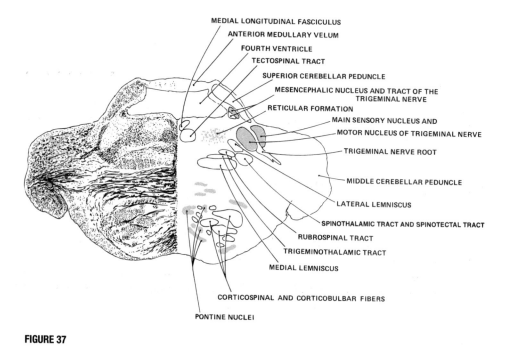

FIGURE 37

Cross section of the pons at the level of the main (principal) sensory and motor nuclei of V.

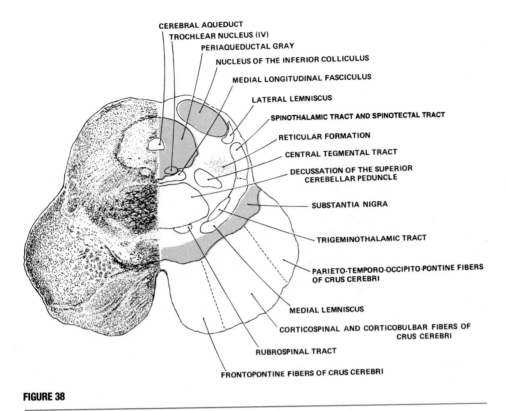

CEREBRAL AQUEDUCT
TROCHLEAR NUCLEUS (IV)
PERIAQUEDUCTAL GRAY
NUCLEUS OF THE INFERIOR COLLICULUS
MEDIAL LONGITUDINAL FASCICULUS
LATERAL LEMNISCUS
SPINOTHALAMIC TRACT AND SPINOTECTAL TRACT
RETICULAR FORMATION
CENTRAL TEGMENTAL TRACT
DECUSSATION OF THE SUPERIOR CEREBELLAR PEDUNCLE
SUBSTANTIA NIGRA
TRIGEMINOTHALAMIC TRACT
PARIETO-TEMPORO-OCCIPITO-PONTINE FIBERS OF CRUS CEREBRI
MEDIAL LEMNISCUS
CORTICOSPINAL AND CORTICOBULBAR FIBERS OF CRUS CEREBRI
RUBROSPINAL TRACT
FRONTOPONTINE FIBERS OF CRUS CEREBRI

FIGURE 38

• • • • • • • • •

Cross section of the lower midbrain at the level of the inferior colliculus and decussation of the superior cerebellar peduncles.

PONS

• • • • • • • • •

The pons is a large mass rostral to the medulla. On the ventral surface of the brain stem, the cerebral peduncles pass into the pons from above, and the pyramids emerge from its caudal margin (see Fig. 30).

External Markings of the Pons

ANTERIOR ASPECT

The anterior aspect is entirely occupied by a band of thick, transverse fibers, which constitute the pons (or "bridge") proper (see Fig. 30). A shallow furrow (i.e., the basal sulcus) extends along the midline, coinciding with the course of the basilar artery. The **abducens nerves (VI)** exit in the inferior pontine sulcus at the caudal border of the pons close to the pyramids.

LATERAL ASPECT

The transverse fibers of the pons are funneled into compact lateral bundles—the **middle cerebellar peduncles (brachia pontis)**—that attach the pons to the over-

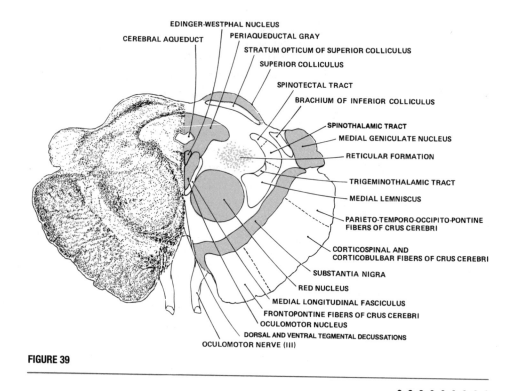

EDINGER-WESTPHAL NUCLEUS
CEREBRAL AQUEDUCT
PERIAQUEDUCTAL GRAY
STRATUM OPTICUM OF SUPERIOR COLLICULUS
SUPERIOR COLLICULUS
SPINOTECTAL TRACT
BRACHIUM OF INFERIOR COLLICULUS
SPINOTHALAMIC TRACT
MEDIAL GENICULATE NUCLEUS
RETICULAR FORMATION
TRIGEMINOTHALAMIC TRACT
MEDIAL LEMNISCUS
PARIETO-TEMPORO-OCCIPITO-PONTINE FIBERS OF CRUS CEREBRI
CORTICOSPINAL AND CORTICOBULBAR FIBERS OF CRUS CEREBRI
SUBSTANTIA NIGRA
RED NUCLEUS
MEDIAL LONGITUDINAL FASCICULUS
FRONTOPONTINE FIBERS OF CRUS CEREBRI
OCULOMOTOR NUCLEUS
DORSAL AND VENTRAL TEGMENTAL DECUSSATIONS
OCULOMOTOR NERVE (III)

FIGURE 39

● ● ● ● ● ● ● ● ●

Cross section of the upper midbrain at the level of the superior colliculus and red nucleus.

lying cerebellum (see Figs. 31 and 32). The triangular space formed between the caudal border of the middle cerebellar peduncle, the adjoining part of the cerebellum, and the upper part of the medulla constitutes the **cerebellopontine angle**. The **facial nerve (VII)** and the **vestibulocochlear nerve (VIII)** are attached to the brain stem in this niche (see Fig. 31). The **trigeminal nerve (V)**, one of the largest of the cranial nerves, penetrates the brachium pontis near the middle of the lateral surface of the pons.

POSTERIOR ASPECT

The posterior surface of the pons forms the rostral floor of the fourth ventricle (see Fig. 32). It is a triangular area with its widest point at the pontomedullary junction, where the lateral recesses of the ventricle are situated. Faint, transverse striations observed in this region are named the **striae medullares**. These striations are formed by arcuatocerebellar fibers. Rostral to the striae medullares in the floor of the ventricle is the **facial colliculus**. This colliculus (i.e., "little hill") is formed by the abducens nucleus (VI) and the fibers of the facial nerve (VII) that cross over the nucleus of VI (Fig. 36). The two fiber bands that form the walls of the fourth ventricle at this level are the **superior cerebellar peduncles (brachia conjunctiva)**. The peduncles are joined in the midline by the cerebellar vermis in the caudal pons (see Fig. 36) and rostrally by the **anterior medullary velum**, completing the roof of the ventricle (see Figs. 32 and 37).

Internal Structures of the Pons

Examination of histologic sections of the pons reveals two evident subdivisions: a posterior portion known as the **tegmentum** and an anterior part called the **basilar portion**. In this region of the brain stem the roof portion, overlying the cavity of the ventricle, is expanded and specialized to form the cerebellum.

CAUDAL PORTION

The corticospinal tracts are located centrally in the basilar portion. The gray matter that surrounds them contains the cells of the **pontine nuclei**. Transverse **pontine fibers** (i.e., the pontocerebellar tract) crossing from one side to the other, posterior and anterior to the corticospinal tracts, are the axons from cell bodies in the pontine nuclei (see Fig. 36). These fibers form the **middle cerebellar peduncle** and pass to the cortex of the cerebellum. The pontine nuclei receive input from the cerebrum, and their projections to the cerebellum constitute a major route by which the cerebral cortex communicates with the cerebellar cortex.

The **medial lemniscus** is seen as an ellipsoid bundle of fibers. In the medulla, the long axis of this ellipse is oriented in the anterior-posterior axis. In the tegmentum of the pons, these fibers shift, and the long axis of the ellipse extends transversely along the boundary with the basilar portion of the pons. The **MLF** retains its position near the midline in the floor of the fourth ventricle. At this level of the pons, the fibers in the MLF are primarily ascending. They arise from the vestibular nuclei and project to the nuclei supplying the extraocular muscles. The descending **interstitiospinal and pontine reticulospinal tracts** are partially intermingled with the MLF.

The **trapezoid body**, an auditory relay structure, is a prominent band of decussating fibers in the anterior part of the tegmentum. Its fibers interlace at right angles with the rostrocaudally oriented fibers of the medial lemniscus (see Fig. 36). The **superior olive** is a small nucleus that lies lateral and slightly posterior to the trapezoid body. It also is a structure belonging to the auditory system. The **central tegmental tract** is an isolated bundle in the anterior part of the reticular formation containing descending pathways (mainly **rubroolivary tracts)** and part of the important ascending reticular formation projections to the **thalamus** and **hypothalamus**. At this level, the central tegmental tract also carries ascending taste fibers from the solitary nucleus to the ventral posteromedial nucleus of the thalamus. The spinal nucleus and tract of the trigeminal nerve have not changed their position, but they are covered on the lateral side by the fibers of the middle cerebellar peduncle.

The **motor nucleus of the facial nerve (VII)** is immediately posterior to the superior olive and medial to the nucleus of the spinal tract of the trigeminal nerve (V). Before leaving the brain stem, the fibers of the facial nerve form an internal loop **(the internal genu of the facial nerve)**. The first segment of this loop courses posteromedially toward the floor of the fourth ventricle, passing close and just caudal and medial to the **nucleus of the abducens nerve**. The facial nerve then courses rostrally and laterally around the abducens nucleus. After completing this "hairpin" bend, the nerve takes a direct course anterolaterally and slightly caudally (see facial nerve root in Fig. 36) to its exit at the pontomedullary junction. Peripherally, its fibers innervate a thin sheet of branchiomeric muscles underneath the skin of the face. These are the muscles that control facial expression. Fibers of the abducens nerve take a straight course through the tegmentum of the pons and exit close to the lateral border of the pyramidal tract on the anterior aspect of the brain stem (see Fig. 30). These fibers innervate the lateral rectus muscle in the orbit.

The **vestibular nuclei** continue to occupy a lateral area in the floor of the fourth ventricle. The individual subnuclei at this level are the lateral, superior, and medial subnuclei (see Fig. 36). The spinal (inferior) nucleus is found in the medulla.

Paired, deep cerebellar nuclei are generally observed in sections through the cerebellum at the lower level of the pons. These nuclei are not shown in Figure 36 but are shown in Figures 54 and 55 in Chapter 17. The deep cerebellar nuclei are the source of most of the neuronal outflow from the cerebellum. They include the following structures:

1. **Nucleus fastigiatus**: located in the midline of the roof of the fourth ventricle in the region of the vermis.
2. **Nucleus globosus**: a small group of cells located just lateral to the nucleus fastigii.
3. **Nucleus emboliformis**: a slightly elongated cellular mass located between the globose and dentate nuclei.
4. **Nucleus dentatus**: the largest and most lateral of the cerebellar nuclei, it is similar in appearance to the inferior olivary nuclear complex, purselike in shape, with an anteromedial hilum.

MIDDLE PORTION

The basilar portion of the pons is widened and thickened at the level of the middle portion. The corticospinal tracts are dispersed in separate fascicles. Mingling with them are numerous other scattered longitudinal fibers. These are the **corticopontine tracts** descending from the frontal, temporal, parietal, and occipital lobes to synapse with cells of the pontine nuclei (see Fig. 37).

Two oval-shaped nuclei lie side by side in the posterolateral part of the tegmentum. The more lateral nucleus is the **main (principal) sensory nucleus of the trigeminal nerve**; the medial nucleus is the **motor nucleus of the trigeminal nerve**. Small filaments of the nerve pass posteriorly and rostrally as the **mesencephalic tract** of the trigeminal nerve. These fibers are processes of cells in the adjacent **mesencephalic nucleus**. The spinal, main sensory, and mesencephalic components of the trigeminal nerve are all sensory, conveying information from pain, temperature, touch, and muscle stretch receptors. The small motor component of the trigeminal nerve (V) arises from neurons in the motor nucleus and innervates the muscles of mastication. Trigeminal fibers emerging from the surface of the pons pass directly through the middle cerebellar peduncle (see Figs. 30 and 31).

The **superior cerebellar peduncles (brachia conjunctiva)** appear in the walls of the fourth ventricle as large, compact bands (see Figs. 36 and 37). The anterior medullary velum forms the roof of the ventricle.

MIDBRAIN

• • • • • • • • •

The **midbrain** is a short segment of brain stem between the pons and the diencephalon. It is traversed by the **cerebral aqueduct**, an extraordinarily small tubular passage connecting the third ventricle with the fourth.

External Markings of the Midbrain

ANTERIOR ASPECT

The inferior surface is formed by two ropelike bundles of fibers, the **crura cerebri**, and a deep **interpeduncular fossa** that separates them (see Fig. 30). Just before it disappears within the substance of the cerebral hemisphere above, each crus cerebri is skirted by the optic tract, a continuation of fibers in the optic nerves (II). At its caudal end, the peduncle passes directly into the basilar portion of the pons. The oculomotor nerves (III) exit from the sides of the interpeduncular fossa and emerge on the surface at the transverse groove between the pons and midbrain.

POSTERIOR ASPECT

The posterior surface (tectum) of the midbrain presents four rounded elevations— the **corpora quadrigemina** (see Fig. 32). The rostral pair of swellings constitute the **superior colliculi,** and the somewhat smaller caudal pair constitute the **inferior colliculi**. The **trochlear nerves** (IV), the smallest of the cranial nerves, emerge from the posterior surface just behind the inferior colliculi after decussating in the anterior medullary velum.

Internal Structures of the Midbrain

In cross sections of the midbrain, three zones are designated: (1) a basal portion, or crus cerebri; (2) the tegmentum, similar to the pontine **tegmentum** (the crus cerebri and the tegmentum together make up the cerebral peduncle); and (3) the tectum, or roof portion, lying above the aqueduct and forming the quadrigeminal plate.

CAUDAL HALF OF THE MIDBRAIN (LEVEL OF THE INFERIOR COLLICULUS)

Each crus cerebri appears in cross section as a prominent, crescent-shaped mass of fibers within which the corticospinal and corticobulbar tracts occupy a central position, intermingled with and flanked at either side by corticopontine fibers (see Fig. 38). The **substantia nigra** lies between the crus cerebri and the tegmentum. In the freshly sectioned brain and in some histologic preparations, the neurons of this area appear brown because of the melanin pigment contained in their cell bodies.

The central part of the tegmentum contains a massive interlacement of fibers— the **decussation of the superior cerebellar peduncle**. The **medial lemniscus** is displaced laterally and rotated slightly. Its outer border is in close relation to adjacent fibers of the anterolateral system (spinothalamic tracts). The **lateral lemniscus,** containing ascending fibers of the special sensory path of hearing, is clearly defined in the lateral part of the tegmentum posterior to the anterolateral system. Many of the fibers in the lateral lemniscus terminate dorsally in the **nucleus of the inferior colliculus**. The small, globular **nucleus of the trochlear nerve** lies near the **MLF** in the anterior part of the central gray substance **(periaqueductal gray matter)**.

ROSTRAL HALF OF THE MIDBRAIN (LEVEL OF THE SUPERIOR COLLICULUS)

The crura cerebri and the substantia nigra continue to occupy the basal portion of the midbrain. The **red nuclei** are conspicuous globular masses in the anterior portion of the tegmentum (see Fig. 39). The crossed fibers of the superior cerebellar peduncle pass into the red nucleus and around its edges. Many of these fibers terminate in the red nucleus; others pass forward to the thalamus. Together, these structures comprise an important part of the outflow from the cerebellum. The tectospinal and rubrospinal tracts arise from this part of the midbrain. Both tracts cross near their origin: the tectospinal in the **dorsal tegmental decussation** and the rubrospinal in the **ventral tegmental decussation**.

The nuclear complex of the oculomotor nerve lies in the anterior part of the central gray matter, with the **MLF** beside it. The root fibers of the oculomotor nerve stream through and around the red nucleus before converging at their exit in the interpeduncular fossa (see Fig. 48 in Chap. 14). From there, the root fibers travel to the orbit, where they innervate four of the six muscles that control eye movements and one muscle that elevates the eyelid. This nerve also contains preganglionic parasympathetic fibers, which are responsible for constriction of the pupil and for changes in the shape of the lens within the eye.

The **medial geniculate bodies** appear as projections on the lateral surfaces of the midbrain. They are auditory relay centers, properly considered to be a part of the thalamus rather than of the midbrain.

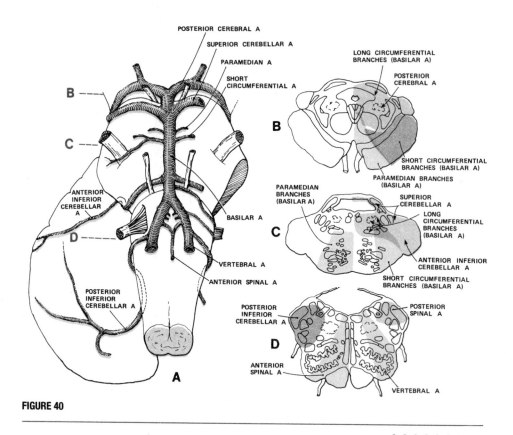

FIGURE 40

The blood supply to the brain stem, illustrated on the ventral surface of the brain stem (*A*) and on the cross sections at three levels through the brain stem (*B, C,* and *D*). In *B, C,* and *D,* the territories of individual arteries, or arterial branches, are shaded and labeled. Note that in some cases these territories overlap. Cross sections in *B, C,* and *D* correspond to Figures 39, 37, and 35 respectively.

BLOOD SUPPLY TO THE BRAIN STEM AND CEREBELLUM

• • • • • • • • •

Blood is supplied to the brain stem primarily from the **vertebral arteries**. Direct branches of the left and right vertebral arteries supply the anterolateral parts of the medulla. The anteromedial medulla receives blood from the anterior spinal artery. At the pontomedullary junction, the two vertebral arteries join to form the **basilar artery**, which supplies branches to the pons and the midbrain (Fig. 40). Branches of the vertebral and basilar arteries also wrap dorsally around the brain stem to supply the dorsal aspect of the brain stem and the entire cerebellum. These arteries include the posterior inferior cerebellar arteries, which supply the medulla as well as the cerebellum; the anterior inferior cerebellar arteries, which provide blood for the pons and the cerebellum; and the superior cerebellar arteries, which distribute to both the midbrain and the cerebellum (see Fig. 40). At the rostral end of the midbrain, the basilar artery terminates by dividing into the right and left posterior cerebral arteries, which pass superior to the tentorium cerebelli to supply the posterior and ventral surfaces of the cerebral hemispheres.

CHAPTER

11

Overview of the Cranial Nerves

The cranial nerves that have functions similar to those exhibited by spinal nerves are classified as **general**. The cranial nerves that have specialized functions, such as those supplying the eye and ear, conveying olfactory and gustatory impulses, or innervating the branchiomeric muscles, are classified as **special**. ✓

FUNCTIONAL COMPONENTS OF THE CRANIAL NERVES

General Afferent Fibers
— TOWARDS BRAIN

General afferent fibers have their cells of origin in the cranial and spinal dorsal root ganglia. **General somatic afferent (GSA)** fibers carry exteroceptive (i.e., pain, temperature, and touch) and proprioceptive impulses from sensory endings in the body wall, tendons, and joints.

General visceral afferent (GVA) fibers carry impulses from the visceral structures (i.e., hollow organs and glands) within the thoracic, abdominal, and pelvic cavities.

Special Afferent Fibers

Cells of origin of sensory fibers in this category are found only in the ganglia of certain cranial nerves. **Special somatic afferent (SSA)** nerves carry sensory impulses from the special sense organs in the eye and ear (i.e., vision, hearing, and equilibrium).

Special visceral afferent (SVA) fibers carry information from the olfactory and gustatory receptors. These fibers are designated as visceral because of the functional association of these sensations with the digestive tract.

107

↗ Away from Brain

General Efferent Fibers

General efferent fibers arise from motoneurons in the spinal cord, brain stem, and autonomic ganglia. General efferent fibers innervate all musculature of the body except the branchiomeric muscles.

General somatic efferent (GSE) fibers convey motor impulses to somatic skeletal muscles (myotomic origin). Fibers in the ventral roots of spinal nerves are of this type. In the head, the somatic musculature is that of the tongue and the extraocular muscles.

General visceral efferent (GVE) fibers are autonomic axons that control smooth muscle and cardiac muscle and regulate glandular secretion. Autonomic fibers are both preganglionic and postganglionic and are subdivided into the sympathetic and parasympathetic types. Although both are found in spinal nerves, spinal parasympathetic fibers are limited to the sacral nerves. In addition, four cranial nerves have parasympathetic components.

Special Efferent Fibers

Cranial nerves that innervate the skeletal musculature of branchiomeric origin arise from certain cranial nerve nuclei in the brain stem.

Special visceral efferent (SVE) fibers are nerve components that innervate striated skeletal muscles derived from the branchial arches. These muscles comprise the jaw muscles, the muscles of facial expression, and the muscles of the pharynx and larynx. The SVE fibers are not part of the autonomic nervous system.

There are no special somatic efferent fibers.

ANATOMIC POSITIONS OF CRANIAL NERVE NUCLEI

• • • • • • • • •

Early in development, the lateral walls of the embryonic brain and spinal cord are demarcated into an alar plate and a basal plate by the appearance of the sulcus limitans. The motor nuclei of the basal plate differentiate slightly earlier than the sensory nuclei in the alar plate. The relative mediolateral locations of the motor and sensory cranial nerve nuclei in the brain stem are shown in Figure 41. In Figure 42, which is a cross section at the level of the medulla, the nuclei at that level are shown in relation to the functional columns to which they belong. Throughout the brain stem, the basal plate cells are medial and the alar plate cells are lateral.

Most cranial nerves contain fibers of more than one functional type; thus, most cranial nerves are associated with more than one nucleus in the brain stem. For example, the vagus nerve contains motor fibers that originate within a GVE nucleus and within an SVE nucleus in the medulla, and its afferent fibers synapse on cells in the nucleus solitarius (see Fig. 42).

The **GSE** fibers of cranial nerves III, IV, VI, and XII arise from nuclei that are arranged as a discontinuous column of cells in the floor of the basal plate adjacent to the midline (see Fig. 41). These nuclei are continuous with, and homologous to, the anterior horn cells of the spinal cord. They innervate musculature derived from somatic myotomes. The **GVE** nuclei of cranial nerves VII, IX, and X occupy a posi-

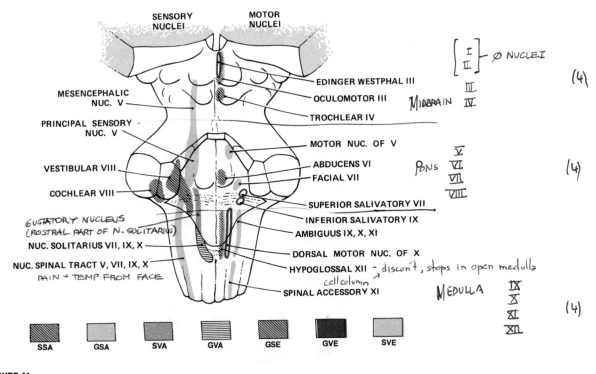

FIGURE 41

• • • • • • • • •

Dorsal surface of the brain stem showing the relative positions of the nuclear columns (functional cell columns) associated with cranial nerves III to XII. For clarity, motor nuclei are shown on the right and sensory nuclei on the left. Compare this illustration with Figure 42.

tion lateral to the somatic efferent column. Note that the GVE nucleus of III is "misplaced" medially. These are the four parasympathetic cranial nerve nuclei. The **SVE** nuclei of cranial nerves V, VII, IX, X, and XI, which provide the innervation of the branchiomeric musculature, form the most lateral discontinuous column of neurons derived from the basal plate.

The sensory fibers of cranial nerves V, VII, VIII, IX, and X arise from cell bodies in the cranial nerve ganglia. Like the central processes of cells in the dorsal root spinal ganglia, they enter the central nervous system and terminate in nuclei located in the alar plate. The **visceral afferent fibers** terminate in the **nucleus of the tractus solitarius**, a nuclear area adjacent to the visceral efferent column. The nucleus of the tractus solitarius receives **GVA fibers** in its caudal part and gustatory **(SVA)** fibers in its cephalic or rostral portion. The **GSA** column of nuclei receives fibers primarily from cranial nerve V. This column extends from the midbrain through the caudal extent of the medulla and into the cervical spinal cord. It consists of the **mesencephalic nucleus**, the **principal sensory nucleus**, and the **nucleus of the spinal tract of V**. In the spinal cord, the nucleus of the spinal tract is continuous with the **substantia gelatinosa**. The spinal cord and cranial nerve components that terminate in the substantia gelatinosa and the nucleus of the spinal tract of V, respectively, have the same functions—pain and temperature reception. Figure 42 indicates that the **SSA fibers** of nerve VIII terminate in the most dorsolateral portion of the alar plate of the brain stem.

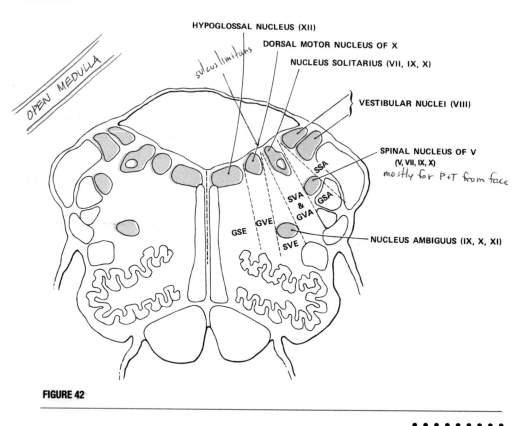

HYPOGLOSSAL NUCLEUS (XII)

DORSAL MOTOR NUCLEUS OF X

NUCLEUS SOLITARIUS (VII, IX, X)

VESTIBULAR NUCLEI (VIII)

SPINAL NUCLEUS OF V
(V, VII, IX, X)

mostly for P+T from face

NUCLEUS AMBIGUUS (IX, X, XI)

sulcus limitans

OPEN MEDULLA

SSA

SVA & GVA

GSA

GSE

GVE

SVE

FIGURE 42

Schematic cross section of the upper medulla showing the anatomic organization of the functional cell columns (*color*) that contribute motoneurons to, and receive sensory input from, the cranial nerves. GSA = general somatic afferent; GSE = general somatic efferent; GVA = general visceral afferent; GVE = general visceral efferent; SSA = special somatic afferent; SVA = special visceral afferent; SVE = special visceral efferent. Refer to Figure 35 for identification of unlabeled structures.

On entering the brain stem, the functionally distinct sensory components of individual cranial nerves subdivide into fascicles that make connections with their respective, functionally distinct nuclei. For example, the central processes of the gustatory neurons of cranial nerves VII, IX, and X synapse with neurons in the cephalic portion of the solitary complex, whereas the somatic afferent fibers from these same nerves enter the spinal tract of V and terminate in its adjacent nucleus. Similarly, the motor nuclei of the brain stem may give rise to functional components contributing to more than one cranial nerve. The nucleus ambiguus (see Figs. 41 and 42, and Fig. 43 in Chap. 12) is the origin of the SVE fibers for IX, X, and the cranial, or bulbar, portion of XI.

A SURVEY OF THE FUNCTIONAL COMPONENTS IN EACH OF THE CRANIAL NERVES

Olfactory Nerve (I)

The axons of the bipolar olfactory receptor cells are **SVA** fibers. Collectively, fascicles of these fibers constitute the olfactory nerve and terminate in the olfactory bulb.

Optic Nerve (II)

The **SSA** fibers that arise from the ganglion cells of the retina (third-order neurons) constitute the so-called optic nerve. The optic nerve is not a true peripheral nerve, but represents an evaginated fiber tract of the diencephalon. Fibers from the nasal half of each retina decussate in the optic chiasm, and beyond the chiasm, these fiber bundles are called the optic tracts.

Oculomotor Nerve (III)

Proprioceptive fibers from the extrinsic ocular muscles form the **GSA** component of the oculomotor nerve. The location of the neurons of origin of these fibers is not entirely clear. In some species, these fibers have their cell bodies of origin in the mesencephalic nucleus of V. In others, clusters of ganglion cells have been identified along the third nerve. The central processes of these cells are thought to terminate in the trigeminal nuclear complex.

The **GSE** fibers of cranial nerve III arise in the oculomotor nucleus and innervate the extrinsic muscles of the eye, except for the superior oblique and lateral rectus. These extrinsic muscles arise from preotic myotomes—thus the term "general."

The **GVE** component of cranial nerve III consists of the preganglionic parasympathetic fibers that arise in the accessory oculomotor (Edinger-Westphal) nucleus and terminate in the ciliary ganglion. Through their connections with the postganglionic neurons, they constrict the pupil and participate in the light and accommodation reflexes.

Trochlear Nerve (IV)

The cells of origin of **GSA** proprioceptive fibers from the superior oblique muscles are unknown, but may be in the mesencephalic nucleus of V.

GSE fibers arise in the trochlear nucleus and innervate the superior oblique muscle of the contralateral eye. This muscle is derived from the preotic myotomes.

Trigeminal Nerve (V)

GSA fibers of the trigeminal nerve are of two types: exteroceptive and proprioceptive. Exteroceptive fibers from the skin of the face and the anterior part of the scalp, the ectodermal mucous membranes of the head (mouth and nasal chamber), and the dura mater of most of the cranial cavity have their cells of origin in the trigeminal ganglion. Proprioceptive fibers from the muscles of mastication and the other muscles innervated by the mandibular division of V arise from cells in the mesencephalic nucleus of the trigeminal nerve.

SVE fibers from the motor nucleus of the fifth nerve contribute to the mandibular nerve and innervate the muscles of mastication, tensor veli palatini, tensor tympani, mylohyoid, and the anterior belly of the digastric muscles. These muscles arise embryologically from the first branchial arch.

Abducens Nerve (VI)

The proprioceptive **GSA** fibers from the lateral rectus muscle have unknown cells of origin, but these cells, like those contributing to the trochlear nerve, are probably located within the mesencephalic nucleus of V.

GSE fibers that arise in the abducens nucleus innervate the lateral rectus muscle of the eye, which is derived from the preotic myotomes.

Facial Nerve (VII)

Cell bodies in the geniculate ganglion give rise to **GSA** fibers conveying exteroceptive sensations (pain and temperature) from the external auditory meatus and skin of the ear. The central processes of these cells terminate in the nucleus of the spinal tract of V.

SVA cells in the geniculate ganglion have peripheral fibers that terminate in the taste buds of the anterior two thirds of the tongue. The fibers reach the tongue by way of the chorda tympani and lingual nerves. Central branches pass through the nervus intermedius and terminate in the rostral portion of the nucleus solitarius.

The preganglionic parasympathetic **GVE** fibers of cranial nerve VII arise in the poorly defined superior salivatory nucleus and pass through the nervus intermedius. Some distribute to the pterygopalatine ganglion by way of the greater superficial petrosal nerve, others by way of the chorda tympani and lingual nerves to the submandibular ganglion. Postganglionic fibers from these ganglia terminate in the lacrimal gland and in the submandibular and sublingual salivary glands, respectively.

SVE fibers arise from neurons of the motor nucleus of the facial nerve. They innervate the superficial muscles of the face and scalp (muscles of facial expression), platysma, stapedius, stylohyoid, and posterior belly of the digastric muscles. These muscles originate from the second branchial arch.

Vestibulocochlear Nerve (VIII)

The cochlear portion of nerve VIII has bipolar cells of origin in the spiral ganglion. Peripheral processes of the **SSA** fibers receive stimuli from the hair cells in the cochlear duct. The central processes terminate in the dorsal and ventral cochlear nuclei. The vestibular portion of VIII originates from **SSA** bipolar neurons in the vestibular ganglion. Peripheral processes receive stimuli from hair cells in the maculae of the utricle and saccule and from cristae in the ampullae of the semicircular canals. The central processes terminate in four vestibular nuclei in the medulla and pons.

Glossopharyngeal Nerve (IX)

GSA cell bodies located in the superior ganglion of IX have peripheral fibers conveying exteroceptive sensations (pain and temperature) from the external auditory meatus and skin of the ear. Their central processes terminate in the nucleus of the spinal tract of V.

Peripheral processes of the cell bodies located in the inferior (petrosal) ganglion of IX are **GVA** fibers that carry general sensory input from the posterior one third of the tongue and the pharynx. A special branch of their fibers innervates the carotid sinus and the carotid body. Most of the central processes terminate in the caudal part of the nucleus of the solitary tract; others may end in the spinal nucleus of V.

Other cell bodies of the inferior ganglion give rise to **SVA** fibers that carry gustatory sensations from the posterior one third of the tongue. Central processes of these cells terminate in the rostral portion of the nucleus of the solitary tract.

GVE preganglionic parasympathetic fibers from cells in the inferior salivatory nucleus synapse in the otic ganglion. Postganglionic fibers from this ganglion innervate the parotid gland.

SVE fibers originating from neurons in the nucleus ambiguus pass through branches of IX to innervate the single skeletal muscle of the third branchial arch, the stylopharyngeus.

Vagus Nerve (X)

GSA cell bodies in the superior (jugular) ganglion of X have fibers conveying exteroceptive sensations (touch, pain, and temperature) from the skin of the auricle. Central processes of these cells end in the spinal nucleus of V.

GVA cell bodies in the inferior (nodose) ganglion of X have fibers conveying general sensations from the pharynx and larynx and from the thoracic and abdominal viscera. Central processes of these neurons terminate in the caudal part of the nucleus solitarius.

SVA processes of other neurons in the inferior ganglion receive gustatory stimuli from epiglottal taste buds by way of the internal laryngeal nerve. These neurons also send their central processes into the nucleus solitarius, but to its more rostral regions.

Preganglionic parasympathetic **GVE** fibers from neurons in the dorsal motor nucleus of X terminate on postganglionic neurons in the visceral walls of the thoracic and abdominal viscera. Reports indicate that the nucleus ambiguus also gives rise to such fibers, particularly to fibers innervating the heart. Postganglionic fibers innervate glands, cardiac muscle, and smooth muscle.

SVE fibers from cells in the nucleus ambiguus innervate the skeletal musculature of the fourth branchial arch in the soft palate and pharynx.

Accessory Nerve (XI)

BULBAR (CRANIAL) PORTION

SVE fibers arising from neurons in the nucleus ambiguus accompany those of the vagus nerve and supply the muscles of the sixth branchial arch in the larynx. Evidence suggests that neurons in this group also innervate the heart.

SPINAL PORTION

SVE neurons in the spinal accessory nucleus, located in the dorsal part of the anterior horn of the upper cervical (C2 to C5) spinal cord, give rise to fibers that exit from the cord through the lateral funiculus, collect into a nerve at the lateral cord surface, pass rostrally through the foramen magnum, and then exit from the skull in association with cranial nerves IX and X (see Fig. 43 in Chap. 12). These fibers innervate the sternomastoid and trapezius muscles.

Hypoglossal Nerve (XII)

GSA proprioceptive fibers from the lingual musculature (similar to that proposed for cranial nerves III, IV, and VI) are thought to arise from scattered neurons that have been found along the hypoglossal nerve.

GSE fibers from neurons in the hypoglossal nucleus innervate the musculature of the tongue, which is derived from the three occipital myotomes.

CHAPTER

12

Cranial Nerves of the Medulla

HYPOGLOSSAL NERVE (XII)

The **hypoglossal nerve** is the motor nerve of the tongue. Its general somatic efferent fibers arise from lower motoneuron cell bodies in the **hypoglossal nucleus**. This nucleus is a column of cells that extends nearly the entire length of the medulla in a position just under the fourth ventricle close to the midline. Axons of these cells pass between the pyramid and the olive to exit as rootlets of the hypoglossal nerve. Among the muscles supplied by the hypoglossal nerve are the genioglossi, which together draw the root of the tongue forward and cause the tip of the tongue to protrude. The genioglossus muscle of each side causes the tongue, on protrusion, to deviate to the opposite side. Injury to the hypoglossal nerve on one side causes a lower motoneuron lesion, with paralysis and atrophy of the muscles on the side of the lesion. On voluntary protrusion, the tongue deviates to the paralyzed side.

ACCESSORY NERVE (XI)

The **accessory nerve** has two distinct parts. The spinal root arises from a dorsal group of anterior horn cells **(spinal accessory nucleus)** in cervical cord segments C2 through C5, exits the spinal cord through the lateral funiculus as a series of rootlets, ascends through the foramen magnum, and courses along the side of the medulla. Here it joins the cranial root of the same nerve from the medulla. After traveling together for a short distance, the two roots again separate. The cranial fibers turn away to join the vagus nerve and are distributed with the terminal branches of the vagus to the muscles of the larynx. The spinal portion of nerve XI passes through the jugular foramen and descends in the neck to end in the sternomastoid and trapezius muscles. Injury to the spinal accessory nerve results in paralysis of the sternomastoid muscle, which causes weakness in rotating the head to the opposite side. Paralysis of the upper part of the trapezius muscle results in downward and outward rotation of the upper part of the scapula, sagging of the shoulder, and weakness in attempts to shrug the shoulder.

THE VAGAL SYSTEM (IX, X, AND PORTIONS OF VII AND XI)

Four nerves of the medulla and pons are closely related in function and in the configuration of their nuclear groups: (1) the nervus intermedius, which contains the sensory and parasympathetic fibers of the facial nerve (VII); (2) the glossopharyngeal nerve (IX); (3) the vagus nerve (X); and (4) the **cranial portion of the accessory nerve** (XI). These are considered collectively as the **vagal system**.

The vagal system contains special visceral motor, preganglionic parasympathetic, and sensory fibers, but there is no separation of bundles into dorsal and ventral nerve roots as in the spinal nerves. All fibers enter and leave the medulla in a series of rootlets arranged in a longitudinal row posterior to the olive (Fig. 43).

Three nuclear columns that contribute fibers to, or receive fibers from, these four nerves are discussed. These are: (1) the special visceral motor column of the medulla, the nucleus ambiguus; (2) the preganglionic parasympathetic column, consisting of the salivatory nuclei and the dorsal motor nucleus of X; and (3) the visceral sensory column, the nucleus of the tractus solitarius, the solitary nucleus.

Motor Portion of the Vagal System

The cells of the **nucleus ambiguus** are lower motoneurons. Their axons enter the glossopharyngeal and vagus nerves and the cranial root of the accessory nerve to furnish motor innervation to the striated branchiomeric musculature of the soft palate, pharynx, and larynx. All of these fibers except the glossopharyngeal branch to the stylopharyngeus follow the peripheral branches of the vagus. The nucleus ambiguus also gives rise to fibers that follow branches of the vagus nerve to the heart, where they contribute to the cardiac slowing resulting from the carotid sinus reflex.

A unilateral lesion of the vagus nerve leads to difficulty in coughing, clearing the throat, and swallowing. Frothy mucus collects in the pharynx and overflows into the larynx. The palatal arch droops on the side of the lesion. During phonation, the soft palate is elevated on the normal side, and the uvula deviates to the normal side. Bilateral lesions of the vagus nerves result in difficulty swallowing (dysphagia), regurgitation of food into the nose on swallowing, difficulty producing certain vocal sounds (dysphonia) and the development of a nasal quality to the voice, a tendency toward mouth breathing and snoring at night, and difficulty in draining mucus from the nasal passages into the pharynx. One of the recurrent laryngeal nerves, carrying innervation to the larynx, may be injured inadvertently during operations on the thyroid gland, resulting in transient or permanent hoarseness. Paralysis of both recurrent nerves produces stridor and dyspnea, which may necessitate tracheotomy.

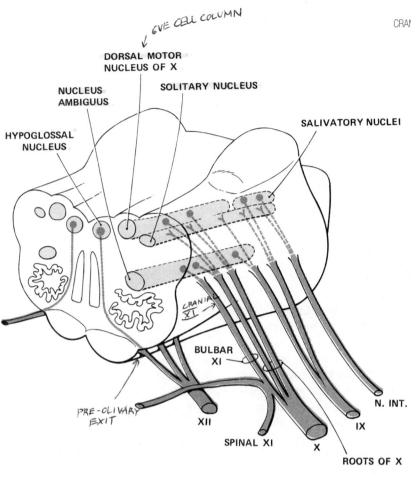

GVE CELL COLUMN

DORSAL MOTOR
NUCLEUS OF X

NUCLEUS
AMBIGUUS

SOLITARY NUCLEUS

HYPOGLOSSAL
NUCLEUS

SALIVATORY NUCLEI

CRANIAL
XI

BULBAR
XI

PRE-OLIVARY
EXIT

XII

SPINAL XI

X

ROOTS OF X

IX

N. INT.

FIGURE 43

• • • • • • • • •

The major nuclei of the vagal system and their connections with the four nerves of that system. The hypoglossal nucleus and nerve root are also shown. N. INT. = nervus intermedius.

Parasympathetic Portion of the Vagal System

The **dorsal motor nucleus of the vagus nerve** consists of nerve cell bodies whose axons leave the medulla and project to parasympathetic ganglia located in the head, neck, thorax, and abdomen. The ganglia are located near or within the viscera that they innervate and send short fibers directly to the smooth muscle, cardiac muscle, and gland cells of these organs. The fibers that arise in the dorsal motor nucleus are preganglionic fibers; those proceeding from the ganglia to muscle and gland cells are postganglionic. Stimulation of vagal parasympathetic fibers slows the heart rate, constricts the smooth muscle of the bronchial tree, stimulates the glands of the bronchial mucosa, promotes peristalsis in the gastrointestinal tract, relaxes the pyloric and ileocolic sphincters, and stimulates the secretion of gastric and pancreatic juices.

At the rostral end of the dorsal motor nuclear column is a group of neurons belonging to the **salivatory nuclei**; activity of these cells stimulates secretion by the salivary glands. The cells in the superior salivatory nucleus send their preganglionic fibers to the nervus intermedius; those in the inferior nucleus send preganglionic fibers to the glossopharyngeal nerve (see Fig. 43). The nervus intermedius is a root-let of the facial nerve (VII); it contains the preganglionic parasympathetic and sensory fibers that belong to this cranial nerve, whereas the larger motor root of VII contains only branchiomotor fibers to the muscles of facial expression. Some of the preganglionic fibers entering the nervus intermedius terminate in the pterygopalatine ganglion. This parasympathetic ganglion sends postganglionic fibers to the lacrimal gland and to the mucosal glands of the palate, pharynx, and posterior nasal chambers. Other preganglionic fibers of the nervus intermedius end in the submandibular ganglion, which innervates the submandibular and sublingual salivary glands. Preganglionic fibers of the glossopharyngeal nerve end in the otic ganglion, the parasympathetic ganglion that innervates the parotid gland.

Sensory Portion of the Vagal System, Including Taste

The sensory fibers of the vagus and glossopharyngeal nerves have their cell bodies in the **superior** and **inferior sensory ganglia** of each nerve. These ganglia are found near the base of the skull. The **geniculate ganglion**, located at the external genu of the facial nerve, contains the cell bodies of the sensory fibers of the nervus intermedius. After entering the medulla in the dorsolateral sulcus, most of the sensory fibers of the vagal system pass directly into the **solitary tract**. From this tract, they distribute branches to the nucleus of the solitary tract.

The sense of taste, initiated by chemical stimulation of special receptor cells in the taste buds of the tongue, is carried from ganglion cells subserving taste to the rostral (gustatory) portion of the solitary tract by sensory fibers of the nervus intermedius and the glossopharyngeal nerves. Ganglion cells subserving taste in the geniculate ganglion of the facial nerve have peripheral processes in the chorda tympani nerve and central processes in the nervus intermedius. The peripheral processes of these cells receive input from taste buds on the anterior two thirds of the tongue. The taste buds on the caudal one third of the tongue are innervated by peripheral processes of cells in the inferior ganglion of the glossopharyngeal nerve. In addition, a small number of taste buds located on the epiglottis receive innervation from neurons in the inferior ganglion of the vagus. This small component of the taste system is not shown entering the gustatory portion of the nucleus solitarius in Figure 43.

Secondary fibers (the ascending gustatory tract) from the cells of the rostral portion of the nucleus of the solitary tract ascend ipsilaterally through the brain stem in the central tegmental tract to the region of the ventral posteromedial nucleus (VPM) of the thalamus. In many mammals, but apparently not in primates, these ascending solitarius fibers synapse in the parabrachial nucleus (or pontine taste area), which projects to the VPM. From the VPM, thalamocortical fibers go to cerebral cortical area 43, a taste recognition area located in the opercular cortex at the ventral end of the central sulcus, where the precentral and postcentral gyri meet. This area is adjacent to, but separate from, the lingual somesthetic area (see Fig. 67 in Chap. 24).

The glossopharyngeal and vagus nerves supply the afferent fibers of touch and pain senses to the mucosa of the posterior part of the soft palate, middle ear cavity, auditory tube, pharynx, larynx, and trachea. These fibers, whose nerve cell bodies are in the inferior ganglia of nerves IX and X, enter the solitary tract along with the special sensory fibers of taste, but they terminate in the caudal portion of the nucleus of the solitary tract.

The vagus nerve also conducts sensory stimuli from the heart, bronchi, esophagus, stomach, small intestine, and ascending colon. Vagal stimulation may be responsible for the sensation of nausea, but otherwise, afferent impulses from viscera are not recognized consciously when they are conducted by the vagal route. Visceral pain is transmitted by the anterolateral system of the spinal cord, which receives its input from visceral afferents accompanying the sympathetic nerves. The chief function of the nontaste afferent fibers of the vagal system concerns the operation of visceral reflexes.

Somatic sensation (pain, touch, temperature) from the skin of the posterior part of the auricle and the external auditory meatus is transmitted to the brain stem over fibers whose cell bodies are in the superior ganglia of IX and X and the geniculate ganglion of VII. Upon entering the brain stem, the central processes of these cells are believed to enter the spinal tract of V and to terminate, along with the other fibers in that tract, on cells in the adjacent nucleus of the spinal tract. This functional component of the vagal system is not illustrated in Figure 43.

Course and Distribution of Nerves of the Vagal System

NERVUS INTERMEDIUS

The **nervus intermedius**, the smaller of the two divisions of the facial nerve root, exits from the brain stem at the junction of the medulla and pons. It enters the internal acoustic meatus and proceeds laterally in the facial canal toward the medial wall of the middle ear cavity. The sensory ganglion (**geniculate ganglion**) is located on the external genu of the facial nerve, at the angle of a sharp bend in the facial canal. The cell bodies of the taste fibers of nervus intermedius are located here. The preganglionic parasympathetic fibers are simply passing through this sensory ganglion on their way to synapses in the more peripheral autonomic ganglia. From the external genu, some peripheral fibers continue as the **greater superficial petrosal nerve** to the **pterygopalatine ganglion**. The rest of the taste and parasympathetic fibers pass downward in the facial canal but leave it abruptly and cross the tympanic cavity as the **chorda tympani nerve**. Leaving the middle ear at the medial end of the **petrotympanic fissure**, the chorda tympani descends between the pterygoid muscles to join the lingual branch of the mandibular division of the trigeminal nerve. Some fibers of the chorda tympani are given off to the submandibular ganglion, and the rest are distributed to taste receptors in the anterior two thirds of the tongue.

GLOSSOPHARYNGEAL NERVE (IX)

The **glossopharyngeal nerve** leaves the skull through the **jugular foramen**, where its two sensory ganglia, superior and inferior, are located. The nerve passes downward and forward to be distributed to the stylopharyngeus muscle and the mucosa of the palatine tonsil, the fauces, and the posterior one third of the tongue.

The glossopharyngeal nerve has five branches:

1. The **tympanic branch** enters the tympanic plexus, provides sensory innervation to the membranes of the tympanic cavity, proceeds from the plexus as the **lesser superficial petrosal nerve**, and terminates in the otic ganglion.

2. The **carotid branch** descends along the internal carotid artery to the carotid sinus and the carotid body.
3. The **pharyngeal branch** enters the pharyngeal plexus with the vagus nerve and supplies the mucous membrane of the pharynx with sensory branches.
4. The **stylopharyngeal branch** consists of motor fibers to the stylopharyngeus muscle.
5. The **lingual branch** sends taste and general sensory fibers to the posterior third of the tongue.

VAGUS NERVE (X)

The two **sensory ganglia** of the vagus nerve, the **superior (jugular)** and **inferior (nodose)**, are located near the jugular foramen through which the nerve passes. The nerve courses down the neck within the carotid sheath and enters the thorax, passing anterior to the subclavian artery on the right and anterior to the aortic arch on the left. Both nerves pass behind the roots of the lungs. The left nerve continues on the anterior side and the right nerve on the posterior side of the esophagus to reach the gastric plexus. Fibers diverge from this plexus to the duodenum, liver, biliary ducts, spleen, kidneys, and to the small and large intestine as far as the splenic flexure.

The vagus nerve has several branches:

1. The **auricular branch** extends to skin in the external auditory canal and a small sector of the auricle. The central connections of this branch are to the nucleus of the spinal tract of V.
2. The **pharyngeal branch** extends to the pharyngeal plexus, along with the glossopharyngeal nerve. It is the chief motor nerve of the pharynx and soft palate.
3. The **superior laryngeal internal branch** is sensory to mucosa of the upper part of the larynx and epiglottis; its external branch innervates inferior pharyngeal constrictor and cricothyroid muscles.
4. The **recurrent laryngeal branch**, on the left side, loops around the aortic arch from anterior to posterior; on the right side, it takes a similar course around the subclavian artery. Both nerves ascend in the laryngotracheal grooves and supply motor fibers to the intrinsic muscles of the larynx and sensory fibers to the mucosa below the vocal cords.
5. The **cardiac (superior and inferior cervical cardiac rami and thoracic) branches** enter the cardiac plexus on the wall of the heart with cardiac nerves from the sympathetic trunks. They terminate in the ganglia of the plexus near the sinoatrial and atrioventricular nodes.
6. The **pericardial, bronchial, esophageal, and other branches** divide to enter the pulmonary, celiac, superior mesenteric, and other plexi to the thoracic and abdominal viscera.

CRANIAL ACCESSORY NERVE

The cranial accessory nerve joins the vagus nerve and contributes to the laryngeal branches of that nerve, particularly the recurrent laryngeal.

Reflexes of the Vagal System

SALIVARY-TASTE REFLEX

The secretory function of the vagal system is illustrated by the salivary taste reflex. When a gustatory stimulus, such as a drop of lemon juice, is placed on the anterior two thirds of the tongue, the salivary glands increase their output of saliva. The afferent stimulus is carried by taste fibers in the facial nerve to the nucleus of the solitary tract. Connecting fibers from this nucleus project through interneurons in the adjacent reticular formation to parasympathetic neurons in the superior and inferior salivatory nuclei. Parasympathetic preganglionic neurons in the superior salivatory nuclei project through the facial nerve to the submandibular ganglion, where a synapse occurs and postganglionic fibers connect with the submandibular and sublingual salivary glands. Parasympathetic preganglionic neurons in the inferior salivatory nuclei project through the glossopharyngeal nerve to the otic ganglion, where a synapse occurs and postganglionic fibers connect with the parotid salivary glands. The reflex pathway for gustatory stimuli on the posterior one third of the tongue is similar to that described above, except the afferent stimulus is carried by the glossopharyngeal nerve.

CAROTID SINUS REFLEX

Increased blood pressure stimulates special **baroreceptors** in the wall of the **carotid sinus** and sends impulses over afferent fibers of the glossopharyngeal nerve to the nucleus of the solitary tract. Second-order neurons in this nucleus project through reticular formation interneurons to the dorsal motor nucleus of x. Parasympathetic fibers from this nucleus project through the vagus nerve to the sinoatrial and atrioventricular nodes, as well as to atrial muscle itself. The result of activating this reflex is slowing of the heart rate. Simultaneously, other reflex connections are made to neurons in the rostral ventrolateral medulla that descend to sympathetic neurons of the spinal cord. Activation of this reflex pathway evokes dilation of peripheral blood vessels and further reduces blood pressure. Some individuals with hypersensitive carotid sinus reflexes are subject to attacks of syncope brought on by light external pressure over the sinus.

CAROTID BODY REFLEX

The **carotid body** contains special chemoreceptors that respond to changes in the carbon dioxide and oxygen content of the circulating blood. Activation of these chemoreceptors sends impulses through the glossopharyngeal nerve to the nucleus of the solitary tract. Fibers from the solitary nucleus then go to the "respiratory center" of the medulla, where they influence the rate of respiration. The respiratory center consists of diffusely arranged cells of the reticular formation with reticulospinal fibers descending to the lower motoneurons of the phrenic and intercostal nerves.

Propagation of nerve impulses over the **reticulospinal fibers** from the respiratory center produces inspiration. As the lungs become inflated, stretch receptors in the walls of bronchioles discharge impulses that ascend to the medulla through the vagus nerve. Connecting neurons reach the respiratory center and, by inhibition, temporarily arrest the inspiratory phase of respiration. The respiratory center depends on impulses descending from the pons for maintenance of the rhythm. The activity of neurons in the respiratory center can be controlled voluntarily for acts such as singing and talking.

COUGH REFLEX

Coughing is usually a response to irritation of the larynx, trachea, or bronchial tree, but at times it may also be produced by stimulation of vagus nerve fibers in other locations, including the external auditory canal or the tympanic membrane. Afferent impulses reach the solitary nucleus and tract by way of the vagus nerve. Connections are made to the respiratory center to bring about forced expiration. At the same time, fibers going to the nucleus ambiguus cause efferent impulses to descend to the muscles of the larynx and pharynx for their participation in coughing.

GAG REFLEX

Touching the posterior wall of the pharynx results in contraction of the muscles in the soft palate and pharynx. The afferent fibers for this reflex are sensory fibers of the glossopharyngeal nerve. After entering the solitary tract, they make synaptic connections with the nucleus ambiguus, which sends efferent fibers through the vagus nerve to the striated muscles of the pharynx.

VOMITING REFLEX

Forceful emptying of the stomach is brought about by relaxation of the gastroesophageal sphincter and contraction of the muscles of the anterior abdominal wall, which expels the gastric contents. At the same time, inspiration is avoided by closure of the glottis. The stimulus, which may arise in any part of the gut innervated by the vagus nerve, evokes impulses sent to the nucleus of the solitary tract by sensory fibers of the vagus nerve. From here, impulses go to the nucleus ambiguus to close the glottis, and to neurons of the medullary reticular formation. Impulses in the reticular formation are transmitted over the reticulospinal pathways into the spinal cord and activate the appropriate lower motoneurons to cause contraction of the diaphragm and abdominal muscles.

A general elevation of intracranial pressure can cause vomiting. This probably results from transmission of the increased pressure onto the floor of the fourth ventricle. Vomiting can also occur if there is localized pressure on the medulla from a pathologic process such as a local tumor or hemorrhage.

Initiation of vomiting has also been attributed to the **area postrema**, which is immediately rostral to the obex, on the floor of the fourth ventricle. This area is thought to be a chemoreceptor region with connections to the nucleus solitarius, through which it can elicit vomiting in response to drugs or other emetic agents in the cerebrospinal fluid.

CHAPTER

13

Cranial Nerves of the Pons and Midbrain

ABDUCENS NERVE (VI)

The abducens nerve, arising from its nucleus beneath the fourth ventricle in the pons, supplies the motor fibers of the **lateral rectus** muscle of the eye. Leaving the brain stem anteriorly at the junction of the medulla and pons, the nerve passes along the floor of the posterior fossa of the skull between two layers of dura mater. It then enters the **cavernous sinus**, passes through the sinus, and enters the orbit through the **superior orbital fissure**. The abducens nerve has the longest intracranial course of the cranial nerves and can be damaged in the brain stem or, more often, in its intracranial course. In addition, prolonged elevation of intracranial pressure from any cause may damage the abducens nerve. Complete loss of function of the nerve makes it impossible for the patient to turn the eye outward beyond the midline. The unopposed pull of the medial rectus muscle causes the eye to turn inward (adduct), thereby producing an **internal strabismus**. **Strabismus**, or **squint**, is an abnormality of eye movement in which the axes of the eyes are not parallel. When strabismus occurs from a nerve VI lesion, visual images do not fall on corresponding points of the left and right retinas, and as a result, the images cannot be fused properly. The result is **diplopia (double vision)**, which worsens when the patient attempts to gaze to the side of the lesion. The two images are seen side by side; therefore; the disorder is termed **horizontal diplopia**. The patient usually attempts to minimize the diplopia by rotating the head so that the chin turns toward the side of the lesion. With bilateral abducens nerve paralysis, both eyes are turned inward and neither eye can be moved in a lateral direction past the midposition.

TROCHLEAR NERVE (IV)

• • • • • • • • •

The nucleus of the trochlear nerve is located anterior to the periaqueductal gray area in the midbrain, in the region of the inferior colliculus. The fibers of the trochlear nerve travel caudally a short distance, then curve posteriorly around the central gray area. The fibers decussate in the anterior medullary velum and exit from the posterior surface of the tectum caudal to the inferior colliculus. The trochlear nerve is the only cranial nerve with fibers emerging from the posterior aspect of the brain stem. The trochlear nerve then passes around the outside of the brain stem to its ventral surface, courses through a sheath in the lateral wall of the cavernous sinus, and enters the orbit through the superior orbital fissure. The trochlear nerve innervates the superior oblique muscle on the side opposite to its nucleus of origin. The muscle depresses the eye, especially when it is adducted (turned medially). Thus, an isolated lesion of the trochlear nerve results in loss of downward ocular movement when the eye is turned toward the nose. The patient with an isolated trochlear nerve lesion complains of vertical diplopia and tilts his or her head to align the eyes and thereby eliminate the diplopia. Lesions limited to the trochlear nerve are rare.

OCULOMOTOR NERVE (III)

• • • • • • • • •

The nucleus of the oculomotor nerve is located anterior to the periaqueductal gray area in the midbrain, in the region of the superior colliculus. The fibers course ventrally, and some penetrate the medial portions of the red nucleus and the cerebral peduncle. The oculomotor nerve exits from the brain stem at the interpeduncular fossa, passes along the brain stem, courses through a sheath in the lateral wall of the cavernous sinus, and enters the orbit through the superior orbital fissure. Shortly after its exit from the brain stem, the nerve passes close to the circle of Willis, which is an anastomotic group of arteries at the base of the brain. An aneurysm (saccular dilatation) in one of the arteries in this region may compress the oculomotor nerve. Tumor or hemorrhage above the tentorium cerebelli may push the inferior margin of the temporal lobe under the edge of the tentorium and exert pressure on the oculomotor nerve as it crosses the tentorium. Mass lesions in the cavernous sinus or superior orbital fissure may also compress the nerve.

The oculomotor nerve innervates the **medial, superior**, and **inferior recti**, the **inferior oblique**, and the **levator palpebrae superioris** muscles. Each of these muscles is innervated by fibers from its own subgroup of neurons in the oculomotor nuclear complex. The medial rectus, inferior rectus, and inferior oblique muscles receive input only from neurons on the same side of the brain stem; the superior rectus muscle is innervated by neurons on the contralateral side; and each levator palpebrae muscle is innervated by axons of cells in both the right and left nuclei. A special subgroup of cells in this complex, the **Edinger-Westphal nucleus**, contributes **preganglionic parasympathetic fibers** to the **ciliary ganglion**, whose postganglionic fibers innervate the **ciliary muscle** for accommodation and the **sphincter muscle of the iris** for constriction of the pupil.

Lesions of the oculomotor nerve cause an ipsilateral lower motoneuron paralysis of the muscles supplied by the nerve. This results in (1) outward deviation (abduction) of the eye **(external strabismus)**, because of the unopposed action of the lateral rectus muscle and inability to turn the eye vertically or inward; (2) **ptosis**, or drooping of the upper eyelid, with inability to raise the lid voluntarily; and (3) dilation of the pupil **(mydriasis)** because of the unopposed action of the radial muscle fibers of the iris, which are supplied by the sympathetic system. The patient with a lesion of the oculomotor nerve complains of a drooping lid and double vision. Incomplete lesions produce partial effects. There may be some weakness of all functions, or one symptom may appear without the others (e.g., dilation of the pupil without paralysis of eye movements). Patients with diabetes mellitus are prone to develop vascular lesions of the oculomotor nerve with loss of all functions except for pupillary responses.

The pathways mediating conjugate ocular movement are described in Chapter 20.

FACIAL NERVE (VII)

The seventh cranial nerve consists of motor, sensory, and parasympathetic divisions. The motor division innervates the **muscles of facial expression** (mimetic muscles). The sensory and parasympathetic divisions are parts of the **nervus intermedius**. These components of the nerve convey parasympathetic secretory fibers to the salivary and lacrimal glands and to the mucous membranes of the oral and nasal cavities, taste sensation from the anterior two thirds of the tongue, and general somatic sensation from the auricle and external auditory meatus. The course and distribution of the nervus intermedius are described in Chapter 12.

The motor division arises from nerve cell bodies in the facial nucleus of the pontine tegmentum (see Fig. 36 in Chap. 10). The neuronal cell groups in this nucleus are subdivided according to the particular muscles that they innervate. The fibers emerging from these neurons pass dorsally, encircling the nucleus of the abducens nerve, and emerge at the lateral aspect of the caudal border of the pons in the angle formed by the junction of the cerebellum and the pons (i.e., the **cerebellopontine angle)**. The nerve enters the **internal auditory canal** and then the **facial canal**, leaves the skull by way of the **stylomastoid foramen**, and courses through the substance of the parotid gland behind the ramus of the mandible. The fibers then divide into branches that fan out to the face and scalp. The fibers also supply the stapedius, the posterior belly of the digastric, and the stylohyoid muscles. The nervus intermedius courses together with the facial nerve from the brain stem to the internal auditory meatus and then into the facial canal. The fibers of the nervus intermedius leave the facial nerve during its course through the facial canal.

Loss of function of the facial nerve from a lesion at the stylomastoid foramen causes total paralysis of the muscles of facial expression on that side. The muscles of the affected side of the face sag, and the normal lines around the lips, nose, and forehead appear "ironed out." When the patient attempts to smile, the corner of the mouth on the paralyzed side does not move, and saliva may ooze from between the lips on the paralyzed side. The cheek may puff out during expiration because the buccinator muscle is paralyzed. Although corneal sensation persists, the corneal reflex is lost on the side of the lesion because the motor fibers to the orbicularis oculi do not function. The patient's inability to close the eye on the side of the paralysis leads to irritation of the cornea and a predisposition to infection; thus, the patient must use protective eyedrops and wear a bandage over the eye. It is not uncommon for the facial nerve to lose function overnight without any known cause except for marked swelling with compression of the nerve in the distal part of the bony facial canal, a condition known as Bell's palsy. Fortunately, most patients with Bell's palsy recover spontaneously in 1 or 2 months.

If a lesion affects the facial nerve in the cerebellopontine angle, within the internal auditory canal, or in the proximal parts of the facial canal, the facial nerve fibers to the stapedius muscle and the fibers of the nervus intermedius are involved. Consequently, in addition to paralysis of facial muscles, these patients have (1) hyperacusis (increased sensitivity to sounds because of paralysis of the stapedius muscle); (2) absent taste sensation on the anterior two thirds of the tongue ipsilaterally (from injury to the nervus intermedius); and (3) disturbed secretion of tears and saliva ipsilaterally (from injury to the nervus intermedius).

In contrast to lower motoneuron or peripheral nerve lesions, which usually cause paralysis of muscles in both the upper and lower parts of the ipsilateral face, upper motoneuron lesions in the sensorimotor cortex or in the course of the corticobulbar fibers cause weakness only of the muscles innervating the lower parts of the face on the contralateral side. The muscles of the brow usually are spared. The brow appears unaffected relative to the lower face, because the cerebral cortex provides a small but equal amount of direct bilateral input to the lower motoneurons of both facial nerve nuclei that control the forehead muscles. In contrast, the cerebral cortex densely innervates the lower motoneurons projecting to the contralateral lower facial muscles but provides only modest input to these lower motoneurons ipsilaterally. This explanation for the sparing of upper facial muscles is relatively new and is based on experimental work in the nonhuman primate. The older explanation is that the upper facial muscles receive supranuclear innervation from both cerebral hemispheres, whereas the lower facial muscles receive supranuclear innervation only from the contralateral hemisphere.

When paralysis results from injury to upper motoneurons rather than to the facial nerve itself or its nucleus, involuntary contraction of the muscles of facial expression remains possible. In response to an emotional stimulus, the muscles of the lower face will contract symmetrically when the patient smiles or laughs. This is presumably because the neural mechanism for emotional facial expression is separate from that for voluntary facial movement. The anatomic pathways mediating emotional facial expression are unknown.

TRIGEMINAL NERVE (V)

• • • • • • • • •

The fifth cranial nerve is termed the trigeminal nerve because it divides into three major peripheral nerves: the **ophthalmic**, the **maxillary**, and the **mandibular**. The trigeminal nerve is a mixed nerve with a large motor root supplying the muscles of mastication and an even larger sensory root distributed to the face, mouth, nasal cavity, orbit, anterior half of the scalp, and dura mater. Sensory branches of the ophthalmic nerve innervate the skin of the forehead and nose; the branches of the maxillary nerve innervate the cheeks and upper lip; and the branches of the mandibular nerve innervate the lateral side of the face and the lower jaw (see Fig. 17 in Chap. 6).

Motor Division of Nerve V

Fibers from the motor nucleus of nerve V in the lateral tegmentum of the rostral pons enter the mandibular branch of the fifth nerve and innervate the **muscles of**

mastication (i.e., the temporalis, masseter, and medial and lateral pterygoid muscles) and several other smaller muscles (the tensor tympani, tensor veli palatini, mylohyoid, and anterior belly of the digastric muscles). Peripheral lesions of this portion of the fifth nerve cause atrophy and weakness, which can be recognized by feeling the size and tautness of the masseter muscles as the jaws are clenched. Fasciculations may be seen in the denervated muscle fibers. Because of the action of the pterygoid muscles, which draws the mandible forward and toward the midline, the chin deviates in the direction of the paralyzed side when the jaw opens. The motor nucleus of each side of the brain stem receives input from upper motoneurons originating in both the left and right motor areas of the cerebral cortex, and supranuclear lesions confined to one side do not produce any marked effects. The motor nucleus also receives monosynaptic inputs from the muscle spindle afferents in the muscles of mastication. These afferents arise from the cells of the mesencephalic nucleus of V (Fig. 44). These cells form the afferent side of the reflex arc that mediates the jaw jerk. The **jaw jerk** is a stretch reflex obtained by placing the examiner's index finger over the middle of the patient's chin with the patient's mouth slightly open, and tapping the finger gently with a reflex hammer. The normal response is a slight contraction of the masseter and temporalis muscles bilaterally, causing the jaw to close slightly. This response can become exaggerated by upper motoneuron lesions rostral to the level of the pons and is decreased or absent with lesions that interrupt the reflex arc.

Sensory Division of Nerve V

The **trigeminal (semilunar, gasserian) ganglion** contains cell bodies of the afferent fibers of the fifth nerve, with the exception of the proprioceptive fibers from muscle spindles located in muscles of the head. These proprioceptive fibers are peripheral processes of neurons in the **mesencephalic nucleus**, which is located in the dorsolateral part of the tegmentum of the pons and the lateral periaqueductal gray area of the midbrain (see Fig. 37 in Chap. 10 and Fig. 44). The unipolar nerve cell bodies of this nucleus are essentially displaced ganglion cells and are unique in that they are located within the central nervous system.

Fibers of trigeminal ganglion cells mediating the sensations of pain, temperature, and touch turn caudally after entering the pons and form the **spinal tract of the trigeminal nerve**, giving off terminal branches to the **nucleus of the spinal tract of V** as they descend through the pons and medulla into the upper cervical segments of the spinal cord. Fibers arising from cells of the nucleus of the spinal tract cross to the opposite side of the brain stem and ascend with the spinothalamic tract through the pons and midbrain to the medial part of the **ventral posteromedial nucleus (VPM)** of the thalamus, from which thalamocortical fibers project to the postcentral gyrus (see Fig. 44 and Fig. 19 in Chap. 6). In the medulla, these fibers ascend as they cross; therefore, in the lower medulla, they are near the medial lemniscus, but they gradually shift laterally to join the spinothalamic tract.

Trigeminal nerve fibers mediating tactile discrimination project to the principal sensory nucleus (see Fig. 44 and Fig. 37 in Chap. 10) and the rostral part of the nucleus of the spinal tract. These nuclei send crossed fibers to accompany the contralateral medial lemniscus. These crossed fibers terminate in the VPM with fibers from the nucleus of the spinal tract of V. In addition, the dorsal portion of the principal sensory nucleus gives off uncrossed fibers that ascend to the ipsilateral VPM as part of the central tegmental tract (see Fig. 44). These fibers have traditionally

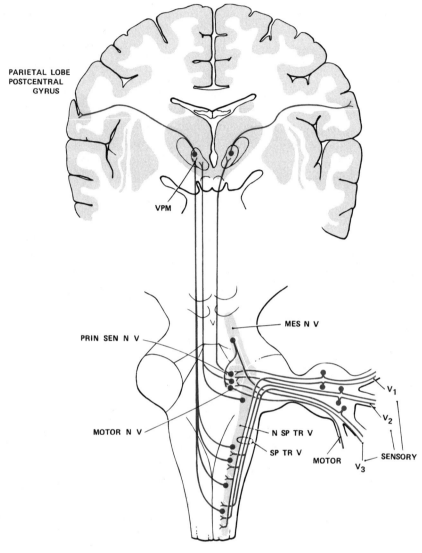

FIGURE 44

• • • • • • • • •

Dorsal view of the brain stem showing the connections of the afferent and efferent fibers of the trigeminal nerve. MES N V = mesencephalic nucleus of V; N SP TR V = nucleus of the spinal tract of V; PRIN SEN N V = principal sensory nucleus of V; SP TR V = spinal tract of V; V$_1$ = ophthalmic nerve; V$_2$ = maxillary nerve; V$_3$ = mandibular nerve; VPM = ventral posteromedial nucleus of the thalamus.

been referred to as the **dorsal trigeminothalamic tract** (see Fig. 44). The name **trigeminal lemniscus** is sometimes applied to all of the trigeminothalamic fibers, although they are never gathered into a single distinct separate bundle.

Lesions in the lateral part of the medulla or lower pons that damage the spinal tract of the trigeminal nerve are likely to include the spinothalamic tract as well. This causes loss of pain and temperature sense on the same side of the face as the lesion and loss of pain and temperature sense on the opposite side of the body beginning at the neck. In the upper pons and midbrain, the fibers crossed mediating pain, temperature, touch, joint position sense, and vibration sense are all close together; in these regions, one lesion produces anesthesia of the opposite side of the body, including the face.

When a foreign body such as a wisp of cotton touches the cornea, the **corneal reflex** produces prompt closing of the eyelids. Sensory fibers entering the upper part of the spinal tract of V synapse with cells of the nucleus of the spinal tract, which send axons to the nucleus of the facial nerve. Motor fibers of the facial nerve then activate the orbicularis oculi muscle to close the eye on the side that had been touched. Connecting fibers from the nucleus of the spinal tract go to the facial nucleus of the opposite side to close the eye on that side as well. The response on the side that is stimulated is the **direct corneal reflex**; that in the other eye is the **consensual corneal reflex**. Interrupting the trigeminal nerve on one side abolishes both responses. On the other hand, if the facial nerve is destroyed on one side, a direct response is not observed after stimulation of the cornea on that side, but a consensual reflex is obtained. Touching the cornea also activates reflex connections with autonomic neurons in the superior salivatory nucleus to produce increased lacrimation. These reflex pathways are not illustrated in Figure 44.

Tic douloureux, or **trigeminal neuralgia**, is a disorder characterized by attacks of unbearably severe pain lasting only for seconds at a time over the distribution of one or more branches of the trigeminal nerve. A small **trigger zone** may be present, and its stimulation by light touch, temperature changes, or facial movement may set off a painful paroxysm. No cause for this disorder has been discovered, but medical therapy can relieve symptoms in most patients.

CHAPTER

14

Lesions of the Brain Stem

Because the brain stem contains a compact arrangement of diverse structures, a single lesion commonly damages several of them simultaneously. The structures frequently injured are (1) the afferent or efferent components of the cranial nerve nuclei, most of which innervate structures on the ipsilateral side of the body, and (2) the long descending motor and long ascending sensory pathways, both of which innervate structures on the contralateral side of the body. As a consequence of this anatomic arrangement, a unilateral lesion of the brain stem often causes loss of function of one or more cranial nerves on the ipsilateral side and a hemiplegia with a hemisensory loss on the contralateral side.

The location of the lesion, whether in the mesencephalon, pons, or medulla, frequently can be determined by the cranial nerve affected. For example, lesions of the mesencephalon affect cranial nerve III, lesions of the pons affect cranial nerve V, and lesions of the medulla affect cranial nerve XII.

The corticospinal tract and the medial lemniscus remain in relatively consistent positions through the medulla and pons, close to the midline and near the base. Consequently, unilateral, medial lesions in these regions of the brain stem generally cause a contralateral hemiplegia with loss of the sensations of position and vibration. In contrast, laterally placed lesions usually spare the corticospinal tract and medial lemniscus but often involve the (1) spinothalamic tract, (2) descending sympathetic fibers, (3) spinal nucleus and tract of V, (4) vestibular nuclei, and (5) cerebellar connections. Thus, lateral lesions do not cause contralateral hemiplegia or loss of position and vibration sense, but they do cause (1) loss of pain and temperature sense contralaterally on the body, (2) ipsilateral **Horner's syndrome** (small pupil, ptosis of the eyelid, decreased sweating on the face, and enophthalmos), (3) loss of pain and temperature sensation on the face, (4) nystagmus, and (5) ataxia of the limbs ipsilaterally. Additional cranial nerve nuclei and fibers are affected by lateral lesions; the specific nuclei affected depend on the location of the lesion.

In addition to the cranial nerves and the long pathways, the brain stem contains the **reticular formation**, which includes autonomic components important in the control of respiration, blood pressure, and gastrointestinal functions. The reticular formation is also important in arousal, wakefulness, and sleep. Brain stem lesions can interfere with each of these functions, and large brain stem lesions such as medullary hemorrhage (which occurs usually in people with chronic, uncontrolled high blood pressure) can cause sudden death.

Brain stem lesions result from diverse types of pathology, including hemorrhages, vascular occlusions, tumors, and lesions of multiple sclerosis. Many of the resulting clinical disorders have been given eponyms, but because there is considerable lack of uniformity in their usage, only the more familiar ones are presented.

LESIONS OF THE MEDULLA

The Medial Sector

Several of the individual cranial nerves pass close to the pyramidal tract before they emerge from the brain stem. A single lesion that includes the nerve and the tract at this point produces loss of function of the cranial nerve on the side of the lesion and a contralateral hemiplegia. For example, a lesion of the right hypoglossal nerve and the right pyramid results in paralysis of the muscles of the right half of the tongue, and left hemiplegia (Fig. 45, lesion 1). The paralysis of the arm and leg is on the side opposite the lesion because the pyramidal tract crosses to the left after it has passed caudal to the site of the lesion, at the junction of the medulla and the cervical spinal cord. The muscles of the face are not involved because the lesion is caudal to the connections of the corticobulbar fibers with the facial nerve nucleus. If the lesion occurs acutely, as with a vascular occlusion, the arm and leg show a hypotonic paralysis, with weakness, diminished resistance to passive manipulation, decreased muscle stretch (deep tendon) reflexes, loss of superficial reflexes, and absence of the response to plantar stimulation. Within 1 month to 6 weeks after an acute lesion, or with a chronic lesion, the arm and leg develop a spastic paralysis, with weakness, "clasp-knife" resistance to passive manipulation, hyperreflexia, loss of superficial reflexes, and an extensor plantar (Babinski's) response. The tongue deviates to the right side when protruded, and the right half of the tongue becomes progressively atrophic.

An extension of this lesion across the midline may damage the left pyramid and produce additional signs of upper motoneuron involvement in the right extremities (see Fig. 45, lesion 1a). In some patients, disease of the anterior spinal artery, the vascular supply to this area of the medulla, results in recurring symptoms with recovery of function between attacks (see Fig. 40 in Chap. 10). If lesions 1 and 1a in Figure 45 occur temporarily at different times, the result is an **alternating hemiplegia**. If the same lesion is enlarged in the dorsal direction, it affects the right medial lemniscus and defects occur in position sense, vibration sense, and tactile discrimination (see Fig. 45, lesion 1b). Because the fibers of the medial lemniscus cross in the lower part of the medulla caudal to this level, the sensory signs appear on the left side of the body.

The Lateral Sector

A small lesion in the lateral part of the reticular formation of the medulla may include the nucleus ambiguus and the lateral spinothalamic tract simultaneously (see

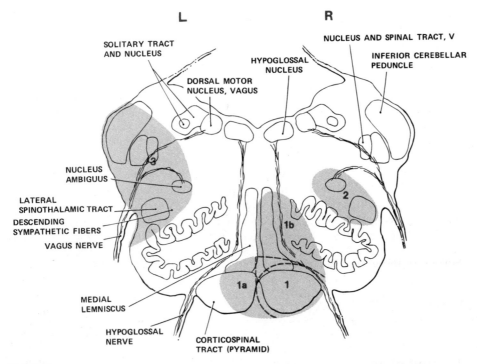

FIGURE 45

A cross section of the medulla. The shaded areas indicate the positions of lesions. (*1*) A lesion of the right hypoglossal nerve and right pyramid. (*1a*) An extension of the lesion involving the medial lemniscus on the right. (*2*) A lesion of the nucleus ambiguus and spinothalamic tract. (*3*) A lesion affecting the dorsolateral portion of the medulla, involving the inferior cerebellar peduncle, the spinal tract and nucleus of the trigeminal nerve, the spinothalamic tract. the nucleus ambiguus, the vestibular nuclei (not shown), the decending sympathetic pathways, and the emerging fibers of the vagus nerve.

Fig. 45, lesion 2). When the lesion is on the right side, it causes a loss of pain and temperature sense on the left side of the body, except for the face. The sensory effects are contralateral because fibers of the lateral spinothalamic tract are crossed near their origin. Destruction of the nucleus ambiguus paralyzes the voluntary muscles in the pharynx and larynx supplied by the right glossopharyngeal, vagus, and bulbar accessory nerves. Failure of the right side of the soft palate to contract causes difficulty in swallowing, and on phonation, the palate and uvula are drawn to the nonparalyzed left side. Loss of function of the right vocal cord results in dysphonia (i.e., hoarseness of the voice).

The Dorsolateral Sector of the Upper Medulla (Wallenberg's Syndrome)

The posterior inferior cerebellar artery, a branch of the vertebral artery, supplies the dorsolateral portion of the medulla and the inferior surface of the cerebellar vermis (see Fig. 40 in Chap. 10). A lesion in these regions commonly results from arterial occlusion by thrombosis of the posterior inferior cerebellar artery or the vertebral artery. The damage involves the inferior cerebellar peduncle, spinal tract and nucleus of the trigeminal nerve, lateral spinothalamic tract, nucleus ambiguus, descending sympathetic pathways, and emerging fibers of the vagus nerve (see Fig. 45, lesion 3). The vestibular nuclei often are affected as well. Loss of function of the spinocerebellar fibers in the inferior cerebellar peduncle results in cerebellar ataxia and hypotonia (i.e., diminished resistance to passive manipulation of the limbs) on the side of the lesion. Injury to the spinal tract of the trigeminal nerve causes loss of pain and temperature sensation on the ipsilateral side of the face and loss of the ipsilateral corneal reflex, whereas damage to the lateral spinothalamic tract results in loss of pain and temperature sensation in the limbs and trunk of the side opposite from the lesion. Damage to the vestibular nuclei causes nystagmus. Injury to the descending sympathetic pathways leads to an ipsilateral Horner's syndrome, with pupillary constriction, ptosis (i.e., partial closure of the upper eyelid), enophthalmos, and loss of sweating in half of the face. Loss of function of the nucleus ambiguus or the peripheral fibers in IX, X, and bulbar XI leads to ipsilateral paralysis of the soft palate, pharynx, and larynx, with dysphagia (i.e., difficulty swallowing) and dysphonia.

LESIONS OF THE PONS

● ● ● ● ● ● ● ● ●

The Medial Sector of the Caudal Part

A lesion that includes the right corticospinal tract and the emerging fibers of the right abducens nerve results in an ipsilateral abducens palsy (i.e., internal deviation of the right eye caused by paralysis of the lateral rectus and the unopposed pull of the medial rectus muscle) and a contralateral hemiplegia (Fig. 46, lesion 1). In the patient with a chronic lesion, an upper motoneuron type of paralysis of the left arm and leg are observed.

Lesions of this part of the brain stem often extend far enough laterally to include fibers of the facial nerve, and thus also produce a peripheral type of facial paralysis. When unilateral loss of function of the abducens and facial nerves is accompanied by contralateral hemiplegia, the condition is called the **Millard-Gubler syndrome** (see Fig. 46, lesion 1a).

A similar lesion with considerable dorsal expansion into the pontine tegmentum involves the right medial lemniscus, the paramedian pontine reticular formation, and the right medial longitudinal fasciculus (see Fig. 46, lesion 1b). The effect of interrupting fibers of the medial lemniscus is loss of position sense, vibration sense, and tactile discrimination on the left side of the body. Damage to the neurons responsible for conjugate lateral gaze in the paramedian pontine reticular formation abolishes the ability to turn the eyes voluntarily to the right, resulting in paralysis of right lateral gaze. The eyes may be drawn to the left by the predominating influence of the unaffected (left) side of the paramedian pontine reticular formation, but such an effect is temporary. Pathways controlling eye movements are described in Chapter 20. The combination of symptoms produced by this lesion is known as **Foville's syndrome**.

Damage to the medial longitudinal fasciculus bilaterally results in **internuclear ophthalmoplegia**, a disorder commonly found in multiple sclerosis. With attempted gaze to one side, the adducting eye (i.e., the eye moving toward the nose) fails to

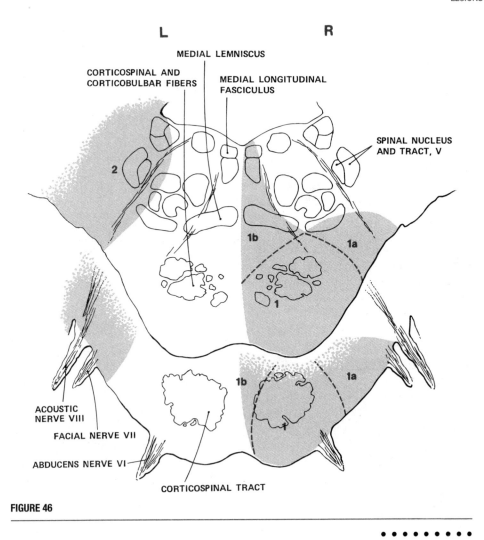

L   **R**

MEDIAL LEMNISCUS

CORTICOSPINAL AND
CORTICOBULBAR FIBERS

MEDIAL LONGITUDINAL
FASCICULUS

SPINAL NUCLEUS
AND TRACT, V

ACOUSTIC
NERVE VIII

FACIAL NERVE VII

ABDUCENS NERVE VI

CORTICOSPINAL TRACT

FIGURE 46

• • • • • • • • •

A cross section of the caudal portion of the pons. The shaded areas indicate the positions of lesions. (*1*) A lesion of the right corticospinal tract and the emerging fibers of the right abducens nerve. (*1a*) An extension of the lesion to include the facial nerve. (*1b*) An extension of this lesion into the pontine tegmentum, involving the right medial lemniscus and right medial longitudinal fasciculus. (*2*) The region affected by a cerebellopontine angle tumor. (For unidentified structures, see Fig. 36 in Chap. 10.)

move beyond the midline, and coarse nystagmus develops in the abducting eye (i.e., the eye moving away from the nose). The same abnormality develops with gaze to the opposite side. Despite loss of adduction on attempted lateral gaze, convergence often is preserved. Damage to the medial longitudinal fasciculus unilaterally causes loss of adduction of the eye on the side of the lesion and nystagmus of the abducting eye. The eye that fails to adduct with gaze to one side can adduct with convergence, demonstrating that the loss of adduction is a supranuclear abnormality (i.e., an abnormality of structures at a higher level than that of the neurons directly causing eye movement). Unilateral internuclear ophthalmoplegia occurs usually with vascular disease of the brain stem, but it can also result from multiple sclerosis or, rarely, a tumor (glioma).

The Cerebellopontine Angle

An acoustic neuroma is a slow-growing tumor that arises from Schwann cells in the sheath of nerve VIII close to the attachment of the nerve to the brain stem. The tumor exerts pressure on the lateral region of the caudal part of the pons near the cerebellopontine angle (see Fig. 46, lesion 2). Initially, the symptoms are those of eighth nerve damage. Progressive deafness is noted, as well as spontaneous horizontal nystagmus and, if the patient is tested, absence of normal labyrinthine (vestibular) responses. (Labyrinthine responses are tested by placing cold or warm water in the ear and observing the patient for nystagmus. These responses can be tested also by rotating the patient in a special chair and observing for nystagmus). Later in the course of the disease, cerebellar ataxia appears on the side of the lesion as a result of compression of the cerebellar peduncles. If the tumor becomes extremely large, damage to the spinal tract and nucleus of nerve V can occur, abolishing the corneal reflex and causing diminished pain and temperature sensibility in the face on the side of the injury. A peripheral type of facial paralysis, also occurring on the side of the lesion, can result from damage to the fibers of nerve VII. If they are detected in time, cerebellopontine angle tumors usually can be removed surgically and neurologic function fully restored.

The Middle Region

A large lesion in the basal part of the right side of the middle pons can affect the right corticospinal tract and the emerging fibers of the right trigeminal nerve to produce an ipsilateral fifth nerve palsy and a contralateral hemiplegia (Fig. 47, lesion 1). Involvement of the motor fibers of nerve V leads to paralysis of the muscles of the right side of the jaw, causing the jaw to deviate to the right when the mouth is opened. Damage to the sensory fibers of nerve V causes anesthesia of the right side of the face and mouth, with loss of the right corneal reflex. In the patient with a chronic lesion, there is an upper motoneuron paralysis of the left arm and leg.

A lesion in the same region that extends farther dorsally enters the tegmentum of the pons and destroys the medial lemniscus. This results in loss of position sense, vibration sense, and tactile discrimination on the left side of the body. Extension of the lesion to the spinothalamic tract causes loss of pain and temperature on the contralateral side of the body. A lesion in this location also interrupts the small number of aberrant **uncrossed** fibers of the corticobulbar and corticotectal tracts that have separated from the corticospinal tracts and in this region lie near the medial lemniscus (see Fig. 47, lesion 1a). In addition to a left hemiplegia, the patient exhibits paralysis of the superficial muscles of the lower part of the left side of the face. Lesions of the middle part of the pons also destroy the tectal projections to the paramedian pontine reticular formation before they cross, interrupting the pathway from the right frontal lobe that produces voluntary turning of the eyes to the left. This results in paralysis of left lateral gaze and deviation of the eyes tonically to the right. If the neurons of the paramedian pontine reticular formation are damaged directly, there is paralysis of conjugate ocular deviation to the side of the lesion and tonic deviation of the eyes to the opposite side. If there is an associated hemiplegia, the limb paralysis is on the side opposite the lesion. Thus, the patient will "look toward the hemiplegia."

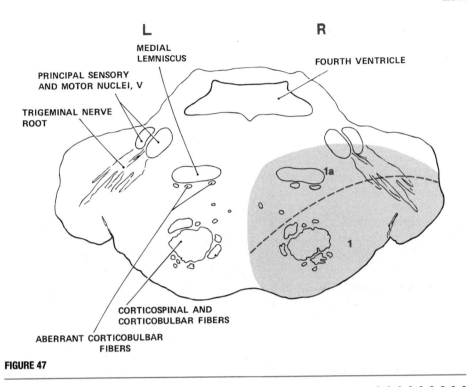

L   R

MEDIAL
LEMNISCUS   FOURTH VENTRICLE

PRINCIPAL SENSORY
AND MOTOR NUCLEI, V

TRIGEMINAL NERVE
ROOT

1a

1

CORTICOSPINAL AND
CORTICOBULBAR FIBERS

ABERRANT CORTICOBULBAR
FIBERS

FIGURE 47

A cross section of the middle region of the pons. The shaded areas indicate the positions of the lesions. (*1*) A lesion affecting the right corticospinal tract and the emerging fibers of the right trigeminal nerve. (*1a*) An extension of this lesion to involve the medial lemniscus and the aberrant corticobulbar tract.

LESIONS OF THE MIDBRAIN

The Medial Basal Part (Weber's Syndrome)

A lesion of the right crus cerebri and the right oculomotor nerve usually produces left hemiplegia with involvement of the face, arm, and leg combined with external strabismus of the right eye as a result of action of nerve VI, closure (i.e., ptosis) of the right upper eyelid, loss of the ability to raise the right upper eyelid, dilation of the right pupil, loss of adduction of the eye beyond the midline, and loss of upward and downward movement of the eye (Fig. 48, lesion 1). The right pupil is dilated because of interruption of the parasympathetic fibers in nerve III. The combination of unilateral oculomotor palsy and contralateral hemiplegia is termed **Weber's syndrome**. In some cases the corticobulbar tract may not be affected because many of its fibers diverge from the corticospinal tract at this level and shift to a more dorsal position as they continue downward. If the lesion extends dorsally, however, it may include most of these fibers and cause weakness of the face.

The Tegmentum (Benedikt's Syndrome)

A lesion of the tegmentum of the midbrain affects the fibers of the oculomotor nerve, medial lemniscus, red nucleus, and fibers of the superior cerebellar pedun-

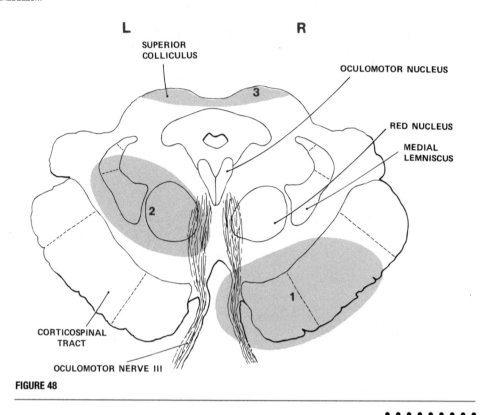

FIGURE 48

• • • • • • • • •

A cross section of the midbrain. The shaded areas indicate the positions of lesions. (*1*) A lesion of the right crus cerebri and oculomotor nerve. Dorsal extension of this lesion will involve the aberrant corticobulbar pathway. (*2*) A lesion of the tegmentum of the midbrain, affecting the oculomotor nerve, medial lemniscus, red nucleus, and fibers of the superior cerebellar peduncle. (*3*) A lesion involving the superior colliculi.

cle, which pass around the red nucleus in this area (see Fig. 48, lesion 2). If the lesion is located on the left side, loss of function of the left oculomotor nerve results in paralysis of movement of the left eye and ptosis and dilation of the pupil. An external strabismus is noted; the eye can be adducted only to the midposition, and up-and-down movements are lost. The right side of the body, including the face, shows a loss of tactile, muscle, joint, vibratory, pain, and temperature sensation from injury to the ascending sensory tracts; the left medial lemniscus at this level has joined the spinothalamic tracts. Involvement of the red nucleus and the superior cerebellar peduncle, which contains efferent fibers from the right cerebellar hemisphere, produces ataxia and involuntary (i.e., choreic) movements of the right arm and leg. Because the corticobulbar and corticospinal tracts are spared, the patient does not become hemiplegic. The combination of third nerve palsy with contralateral loss of sensation, ataxia, and involuntary movements is termed **Benedikt's syndrome**.

The Mesencephalic Tectum
(Parinaud's Syndrome)

Injury in the vicinity of the superior colliculi (see Fig. 48, lesion 3) causes paralysis of conjugate upward gaze, a disorder termed **Parinaud's syndrome**. The loss of upward gaze may be accompanied by pupillary abnormalities. The pupils may be fixed and unreactive to any stimulus, or they may react in the near-point reaction but not to light. Paralysis of convergence can occur as well. This disorder often results from tumors of the pineal gland that compress the tectal and pretectal regions of the mesencephalon.

BRAIN STEM LESIONS CAUSING COMA AND "LOCKED-IN" SYNDROME

• • • • • • • • •

Bilateral lesions that damage substantial amounts of reticular formation in the upper pons and midbrain lead to **coma**, which is a state of unresponsiveness. Bilateral lesions of the ventral pons, usually caused by occlusion of the basilar artery, may completely interrupt the corticobulbar and corticospinal tracts. As a result, the patient becomes essentially totally paralyzed and unable to speak, but is fully awake. Usually, the patient can open the eyelids and make slight vertical movements of the eyes. These movements are retained because of sparing of the dorsal parts of the midbrain, including the rostral interstitial nucleus of the medial longitudinal fasciculus and its projections to the posterior commissure and the interstitial nucleus of Cajal. Communication can be established by asking the patient to move the eyes in response to a command. This establishes that the patient is completely immobile, or "**locked in**," but is not in a coma.

CHAPTER

15

Hearing

AUDITORY APPARATUS

The eighth cranial nerve has two divisions: vestibular and cochlear. Each is so distinct in its function and anatomic relations that they can be considered as separate cranial nerves. The vestibular division is discussed in Chapter 16.

Sound consists of sinusoidal waves—alternating condensations and rarefactions—of air molecules. The frequency of the waves, measured in **hertz (Hz)**, determines the **pitch** of the sound. The amplitude of each wave is related to loudness and is measured in **decibels (dB)**. The human ear can detect sound frequencies from about 20 to 20,000 Hz and loudness from about 1 to 120 dB.

The auditory apparatus consists of three components: the external, middle, and internal ear. There are three spaces in the skull that are separated from one another solely by membranes (Fig. 49A). The external ear, or **external auditory meatus**, is separated from the cavity of the middle ear by the **tympanic membrane**, which receives airborne vibrations. A chain of three ossicles, the **malleus**, the **incus**, and the **stapes**, spans the middle ear (Fig. 49B). The first of the ossicles, the malleus, is attached to the tympanic membrane. The last of the ossicles, the stapes, has a footplate that fits into the **oval window** between the middle and inner ear cavities. The stapes is secured to the margin of the oval window by a ligamentous membrane that seals this window and separates the air-filled middle ear from the fluid-filled inner ear.

Sound mediated by air strikes the tympanic membrane and induces motions in this membrane that are conveyed to the oval window by the ossicles. The chain of three ossicles in the middle ear serves as an amplifier as well as an impedance-matching device that decreases the amount of energy lost by the sound waves in going from the air to the fluid **(perilymph)** behind the oval window. The oval window is an opening into the **vestibule** portion of the inner ear (Fig. 49C). Continuous with the perilymph-filled vestibule is the **cochlea**, a tube resembling a snail shell about 3.5 cm long and exhibiting 2.5 turns. The vestibule and cochlea constitute two of

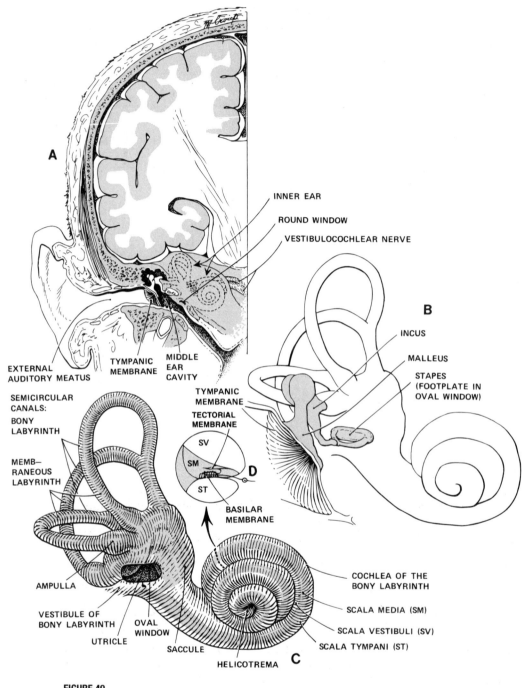

FIGURE 49

The ear. (*A*) The location of the three parts of the ear (external, middle, and inner) in relation to the skull and the brain. (*B*) The relationships among the eardrum (tympanic membrane) and the three bones (ossicles) in the middle ear that connect the eardrum to the inner ear. (*C*) The bony labyrinth, and the membranous labyrinth (color) within it, form the inner ear. (*D*) A cross section through the bony and membranous labyrinths of the cochlea shows the location of the basilar membrane and tectorial membrane the three chambers of the inner ear. The third is the set of **semicircular canals**, which are discussed further in Chapter 16. These three connected chambers within the temporal bone of the skull make up the **bony labyrinth**. Within this perilymph-filled bony cavity lies a **membranous labyrinth**, which is similar in shape to the bony labyrinth (except in the vestibule) and is filled with another fluid, the **endolymph**.

In the cochlear part of the bony labyrinth, the central bony core, or **modiolus**, is the axis around which the turns of the cochlea are wrapped. The modiolus provides support for the bony **spiral lamina**, which partially divides the cavity of the cochlea into two perilymphatic chambers: the **scala vestibuli** and the **scala tympani**. The membranous labyrinth within the cochlea is called the **scala media**, or **cochlear duct**. Stretching across the cochlea from the spiral lamina to the opposite wall of the cochlea, the cochlear duct completes the separation of the scala vestibuli and scala tympani. The **organ of Corti**, which contains the sensory epithelium, or hair cells, stretches along the length of the cochlear duct, resting on the **basilar membrane** (Fig. 49D) as it spirals around the turns of the cochlea.

The piston action of the stapes produces an instantaneous pressure wave in the perilymph of the **scala vestibuli** that travels to the **helicotrema** (i.e., the apical connection between the scala vestibuli and tympani) within microseconds. A traveling wave is set up on the basilar membrane as a result of the pressure wave in the perilymph of the scala vestibuli. The basilar membrane is narrower at the base of the cochlea (near the vestibule) than at the apex (near the helicotrema); thus, the mechanical properties of the basilar membrane, on which the organ of Corti is located, vary gradually from base to apex. As a result, the pressure wave produced by a sound of a specific frequency (i.e., pitch) causes the basilar membrane to vibrate maximally at a particular point along its length.

The hair cells of the organ of Corti are the auditory receptor cells. The base of each hair cell is indirectly attached to the basilar membrane. The apex of each cell bears stereocilia, which extend above the surface of the cell. The tips of the stereocilia are embedded in the **tectorial membrane**, which is attached to the wall of the cochlear duct separately from the attachment of the basilar membrane to the bony spiral lamina. When sound waves enter the cochlea, the basilar and tectorial membranes move independently of each other, and the stereocilia are subjected to shearing forces. The resultant bending of the stereocilia opens ionic channels and produces potential changes in the hair cell membrane. Synapses at the base of each hair cell activate the closely applied dendritic processes of the spiral ganglion cells. The **spiral ganglion**, located in the modiolus of the cochlea, contains the bipolar cells of the cochlear division of the eighth nerve.

The organ of Corti contains two types of hair cells. The **outer hair cells** are more numerous, and each spiral ganglion cell innervates as many as 50 of these cells. These cells have contractile properties and are thought to control the sensitivity of the organ of Corti by regulating the apposition of the tectorial membrane to the inner hair cells. It is the **inner hair cells** that are the primary auditory receptor cells. Each inner hair cell receives dendritic innervation from as many as 10 spiral ganglion cells, and each of these ganglion cells innervates only one inner hair cell. Thus, the activity of 30 to 50 outer hair cells converges onto a single spiral ganglion cell, whereas the activity of each inner hair cell diverges and singly controls the activity of as many as 10 spiral ganglion cells.

The organ of Corti serves as an audiofrequency analyzer. It is tonotopically organized so that the highest tones (in pitch and frequency) maximally stimulate the hair cells in the most basal portion of the cochlea, where the basilar membrane is nar-

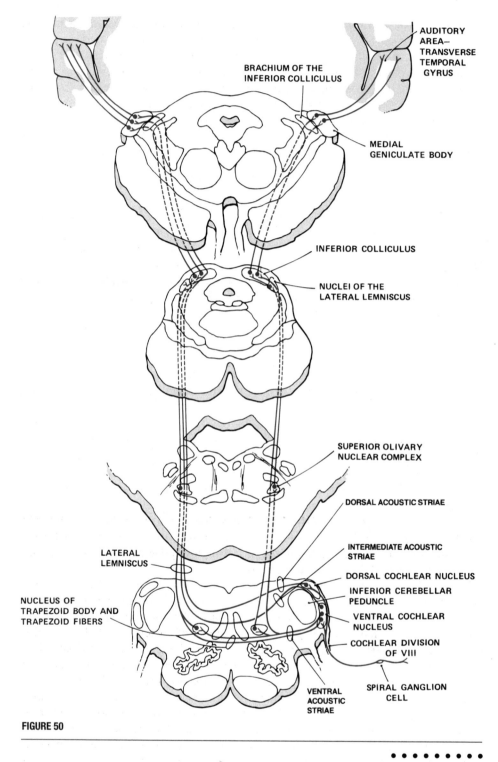

AUDITORY
AREA—
TRANSVERSE
TEMPORAL
GYRUS

BRACHIUM OF THE
INFERIOR COLLICULUS

MEDIAL
GENICULATE BODY

INFERIOR COLLICULUS

NUCLEI OF THE
LATERAL LEMNISCUS

SUPERIOR OLIVARY
NUCLEAR COMPLEX

DORSAL ACOUSTIC STRIAE

INTERMEDIATE ACOUSTIC
STRIAE

DORSAL COCHLEAR NUCLEUS

INFERIOR CEREBELLAR
PEDUNCLE

VENTRAL COCHLEAR
NUCLEUS

COCHLEAR DIVISION
OF VIII

SPIRAL GANGLION
CELL

VENTRAL
ACOUSTIC
STRIAE

LATERAL
LEMNISCUS

NUCLEUS OF
TRAPEZOID BODY AND
TRAPEZOID FIBERS

FIGURE 50

The auditory pathways. Axons of neurons in the cochlear nuclei actually cross the midline as they ascend, so that they enter the lateral lemniscus at the level of the pontomedullary junction. For diagrammatic convenience, they are shown crossing completely in the medulla.

row. The tones of lowest pitch maximally stimulate the most apical hair cells. Tones or sounds of intermediate pitch stimulate the hair cells in the intermediate portion of the basilar membrane. The inner hair cells and the spiral ganglion cells to which they are attached show frequency-dependent responses to sound, and each ganglion cell has a characteristic **tuning curve**; that is, each shows a characteristic relation between the amplitude of sound needed to induce a barely detectable neuronal discharge and the frequency of the sound stimulus. The pressure waves, after traversing the scala media, cross the basilar membrane, pass through the scala tympani, and are damped at the **round window** (see Fig. 49A, not in view on 49C).

AUDITORY PATHWAY

• • • • • • • • •

The cochlear nerve enters the brain stem at the junction of the medulla and pons. As it attaches to the brain stem, the nerve clings to the lateral side of the inferior cerebellar peduncle and enters the **posterior (dorsal) and anterior (ventral) cochlear nuclei**. Each entering nerve fiber bifurcates and makes synaptic connections with neurons in both cochlear nuclei. The neurons that make up these two nuclei are tonotopically organized. Three projections, the acoustic striae, arise from the cochlear nuclei to relay the information centrally and rostrally. The **dorsal acoustic stria** originates in the dorsal cochlear nucleus, passes over the inferior cerebellar peduncle, and crosses to join the contralateral **lateral lemniscus** (Fig. 50). The two other striae arise from the ventral cochlear nucleus. The **intermediate acoustic stria** takes a course that is similar to that of the dorsal stria. The **ventral acoustic stria** takes a different route and passes anterior to the inferior cerebellar peduncle to terminate in the **ipsilateral and contralateral nuclei** of the **trapezoid body** and **superior olivary nuclei** (see Fig. 36 in Chap. 10). These nuclei project fibers into the ipsilateral and contralateral lateral lemnisci. Fibers in the lateral lemniscus ascend through the brain stem to terminate in the **nucleus of the inferior colliculus** and the medial geniculate nucleus. In addition, some of these fibers terminate in small nuclear groups, the **nuclei of the lateral lemniscus**, which are intermingled with the lateral lemniscus. The fibers of the lateral lemniscus terminate in the **nucleus of the inferior colliculus**, which sends axons to the **medial geniculate body** through the **brachium of the inferior colliculus**.

The medial geniculate bodies are special sensory nuclei of the thalamus and serve as the final sensory relay stations of the hearing path. The efferent connection of the medial geniculate body to the temporal lobe forms the **auditory radiation**, which projects to the **transverse temporal gyrus, gyrus of Heschl**, located on the dorsal surface of the superior temporal convolution and partly buried in the lateral fissure. This relatively small cortical region, Brodmann's area 41, is the primary auditory receptive area. When auditory impulses arrive at area 41, a sound is heard. The neuronal processing that occurs in area 41 and the immediately surrounding cortex (areas 42 and 22) appears to be essential for discriminations requiring a response to changes in the temporal patterning of sounds and for recognition of the location or direction of a sound. The processing of information about the location of a sound may occur initially in the part of the pathway including the superior olive and inferior colliculus. Evaluation of meaningful combinations of different frequencies in a temporal sequence may begin in the cochlear nuclei, inferior colliculus, and medial geniculate nucleus. A tonotopic organization has been demonstrated for all of these central auditory nuclei, but as indicated previously, this information may be used for analysis of a variety of significant properties of sound in addition to recognition of tones. Although some mammals can make discriminations of differing frequencies and intensities without an intact auditory cortex, reviews of the rare cases of bilateral auditory cortex lesions in humans indicate that this area is critical for perception of speech and that such lesions can result in profound deafness.

Descending efferent fibers have been found in all parts of the auditory pathway. It is believed that they function as feedback loops. In the region of the superior olive, there are neurons projecting into the **olivocochlear bundle**, which travels by way of the eighth nerve and terminates either directly on hair cells of the organ of Corti or on afferent fibers of the spiral ganglion. The olivocochlear bundle has an inhibitory action on impulses originating in the cochlea. The efferent fibers of the auditory pathway, including the olivocochlear bundle, may be responsible for the phenomenon of selective auditory attention.

Bilateral Representation of the Ears in Each Temporal Lobe

As illustrated in Figure 50, above the level at which the cochlear nerve enters the brain stem, the hearing pathway is composed of crossed and uncrossed fibers, the majority of which are crossed. Opportunity for auditory information to be redistributed in both crossed and uncrossed fashions exists at many levels of the brain stem. Fibers cross from one side to the other between the superior olivary nuclei, the nuclei of the trapezoid body, the nuclei of the lateral lemnisci, and the nuclei of the inferior colliculi. (These commissural connections are not illustrated in Fig. 50.) Each lateral lemniscus, therefore, conducts stimuli from both ears. A lesion of the right lateral lemniscus, or of the right anterior transverse temporal gyrus, stops some impulses from both ears but does not interfere with other impulses from both ears going to the cortex of the left hemisphere. Therefore, deafness in one ear usually signifies damage to the acoustic (cochlear) nerve, the cochlea, or the sound-conducting apparatus of the middle ear on that side. The eighth nerve can be damaged bilaterally by toxic effects of some drugs, the most notorious of which are streptomycin, quinine, and aspirin.

HEARING DEFECTS FROM NERVE DAMAGE AND FROM CONDUCTION DEFECTS

• • • • • • • • •

Sound can be conveyed by **air conduction** or **bone conduction**. Sound is mediated by air conduction when the source of the sound is at some distance from the ear and sound waves are transmitted through air to the tympanic membrane. Sound is mediated by bone conduction when the source of the sound, a vibrating body, is in contact with the skull or bones of the body and waves are transmitted through the cranial bones. Injury to fibers of the eighth nerve commonly produces **hearing loss (sensorineural deafness)** and **tinnitus** (i.e., ringing or roaring in the ear). These disturbances may also be caused by lesions involving the auditory conducting mechanisms in the middle ear, a condition termed **conduction deafness**.

Examination with a tuning fork is helpful for distinguishing sensorineural deafness from conduction deafness. A 256-Hz tuning fork should be used. In **Weber's test**, the base of a vibrating fork is applied to the forehead in the midline, and the patient is asked whether the sound is heard in the midline or is localized in one ear. In normal individuals, the sound appears to be in the midline. In a patient with conduction deafness in one ear, the sound seems louder in the affected ear, and in a patient with sensorineural deafness in one ear, it seems louder in the other (normal) ear. This occurs because in conduction deafness, air conduction is reduced but bone conduction is relatively enhanced. By contrast, in sensorineural deafness, bone conduction of sound is as ineffective in stimulating the damaged nerve as air conduction.

Rinne's test compares the patient's ability to hear a vibrating tuning fork by bone conduction and by air conduction. The base of a vibrating 256-Hz tuning fork is placed over the mastoid process of the skull. When it can no longer be heard, it is removed, and the tines are held in front of the ear. A person with normal hearing continues to hear by air conduction after bone conduction ceases. In conduction deafness, bone conduction is better than air conduction. In sensorineural deafness, both are diminished, but air conduction remains better than bone conduction.

Audiometers provide refined testing of hearing, because pure tones can be used at controlled intensities. Receivers for both air and bone conduction are available, and it is possible to graph the results of these tests in each ear for both air and bone conduction. Conduction deafness generally is indicated by an impairment in reception of the lower frequencies of pure tones in the air conduction test. In sensorineural deafness tested in the same manner, the threshold deficit occurs in the reception of tones in the higher frequencies.

Auditory evoked potentials, also known as **brain stem auditory evoked potentials**, can be recorded from electrodes applied to the scalp. The stimulus is a recurrent series of clicks, and the potentials are amplified and then summated by a computer. The individual components of the auditory evoked potential are generated by a succession of structures in the auditory pathway from the auditory nerve to the auditory cortex. Auditory evoked potentials assist the clinician in determining the site of a disease process in the auditory pathway. Brain tumors, stroke, and multiple sclerosis are among the diseases that can alter the auditory evoked potential.

Sensorineural deafness commonly occurs with Ménière's disease, trauma, drug damage, infection, aging, and occlusion of the internal auditory artery. Conduction deafness may result from wax in the external auditory canal, otitis media, and diseases that impair the capacity of the ossicles to function properly, such as otosclerosis.

AUDITORY REFLEXES

• • • • • • • • •

Auditory reflexes consist of involuntary responses to sound and are mediated by branches from the main auditory pathway. **Audiomotor reflexes** are contractions of the tensor tympani and stapedius muscles. These muscles are innervated by the trigeminal and facial nerves, respectively, and their contraction diminishes vibrations of the middle ear ossicles, thus protecting the inner ear from damaging sound intensities. Other reflex pathways synapse in the reticular formation to evoke autonomic responses. Among several pathways mediating auditory reflexes, fibers projecting from the inferior colliculus to the superior colliculus and fibers projecting from this site downward provide auditory input to the spinal cord by way of the **tectospinal tract**. These fibers terminate on lower motoneurons in the cervical spinal cord supplying the muscles of the head and neck that respond to sound. The **gen-**

eral acoustic muscle reflex is a generalized jerking of the body in response to a loud, sudden sound. The **auditory-palpebral reflex** consists of a blink of the eyelids in response to a loud noise. The **auditory-oculogyric reflex** involves deviation of the eyes in the direction of a sound. The **cochleopupillary reflex** is dilation of the pupils (or constriction followed by dilation) in response to a loud noise.

CHAPTER

16

The Vestibular System

The **vestibular system** consists of receptors located in the inner ear on both sides of the head, peripheral nerve fibers of the eighth cranial nerve that transmit information from the receptors to the central nervous system, and central connections that analyze information about the position and movement of the head in space. The vestibular system maintains body balance; coordinates eye, head, and body movements; and permits the eyes to remain fixed on a point in space as the head moves.

VESTIBULAR RECEPTORS

The inner ear, or labyrinth, consists of two parts: a **bony labyrinth** and a **membranous labyrinth**. The bony labyrinth consists of a series of cavities in the petrous portion of the temporal bone. Inside the bony labyrinth is the membranous labyrinth, consisting of tubes of fine membranes. A fluid called **perilymph** fills the space between the bony labyrinth and the membranous labyrinth. A fluid called **endolymph** fills the membranous labyrinth. The peripheral receptors of the vestibular system, the **vestibular hair cells**, are also located inside the membranous labyrinth. The perilymphatic space of the vestibular portion of the bony labyrinth is continuous with the perilymphatic spaces of the cochlea: the scala vestibuli and scala tympani. Similarly, the endolymph within the vestibular portion of the membranous labyrinth communicates with the endolymph of the cochlear duct.

The vestibular membranous labyrinth consists of two swellings within the vestibule, the **utricle** and **saccule**, and three **semicircular canals**, the **anterior, lateral (horizontal)**, and **posterior semicircular canals**. The semicircular canals are arranged in roughly three planes at right angles to each other (see Fig. 49 in Chap. 15).

The floor of the utricle contains a specialized region, the **macula**, which is the receptor region of the utricle. The macula contains hair cells that synapse on the distal branches of vestibular ganglion cells. The apical surface of each hair cell bears stereocilia and a single kinocilium. These "hairs" extend upward into an overlying gelatinous substance containing **otoconia**, which are crystals of calcium carbonate. The macula of the utricle lies in the horizontal plane when the head is held erect, so that the otoconia rest directly on the hair cells. If the head is tilted or accelerated linearly, the gravitational pull on the otoconia moves the gelatinous matrix and bends the hairs of the receptor cells. This movement induces changes in the membrane potential of the receptor cells that elicit action potentials in the peripheral processes of the vestibular ganglion cells. The utricle responds to **gravitational forces** and to **linear acceleration**, chiefly in the horizontal plane. The saccule contains a similar receptor organ, or macula, but the function of the saccule is less well understood.

Each semicircular canal has an enlarged end called the **ampulla** (see Fig. 49 in Chap. 15). Within the ampulla is the **ampullary crest**, a ridge that bears hair cells like those of the maculae. The ampullary crest is covered with a gelatinous capsule termed the **cupula**, which extends upward almost to the roof of the ampulla. When the head undergoes angular acceleration, the viscous endolymph in the semicircular ducts lags behind as a result of inertia and pushes on the cupula. Distortion of the cupula evokes a receptor potential in the hair cells of the ampullary crest, and this alters the level of activity in the peripheral fibers of the eighth nerve innervating the hair cells. The vestibular nerve fibers to each duct respond with an increase in impulse frequency to rotation in one direction and with a decrease in impulse frequency to rotation in the opposite direction. These increases and decreases modify a baseline, tonic level of vestibular activity that provides balanced input from the two ears. Damage to the inner ear or vestibular nerve on one side causes an imbalance that can produce nausea, vertigo, postural imbalance, and abnormal eye movements.

As a broad generality, the vestibular labyrinth has two separate functions, dynamic and static. The **dynamic functions**, mediated largely by the semicircular canals, can detect motion of the head in space. The **static functions**, mediated mostly by the utricle, allow detection of the position of the head (and body) in space and are important in the control of posture.

THE VESTIBULAR NERVE AND ITS CENTRAL CONNECTIONS

• • • • • • • • •

The afferent fibers of the vestibular nerve have their cell bodies in the **vestibular ganglion of Scarpa**. Axons of bipolar cells of the vestibular ganglion pass through the internal auditory canal and reach the upper medulla in company with the cochlear nerve. The fibers of the vestibular nerve bifurcate into ascending and descending branches and terminate in the vestibular nuclei, which are clustered in the lateral part of the floor of the fourth ventricle (Fig. 51): the **lateral vestibular nucleus (of Deiters)**, the **medial vestibular nucleus (of Schwalbe)**, the **superior vestibular nucleus (of Bechterew)**, and the **inferior vestibular nucleus** (descending spinal). Despite clear, cytoarchitectural boundaries between the nuclei, there is no conclusive evidence that afferents from the vestibule and the semicircular canals are segregated in their distribution to these four cell groups.

The major efferent connections of the vestibular nuclei are to the cerebellum, spinal cord, and nuclei of the extraocular nerves (i.e., the oculomotor, trochlear, and abducens). A projection to the thalamus has also been described. The thala-

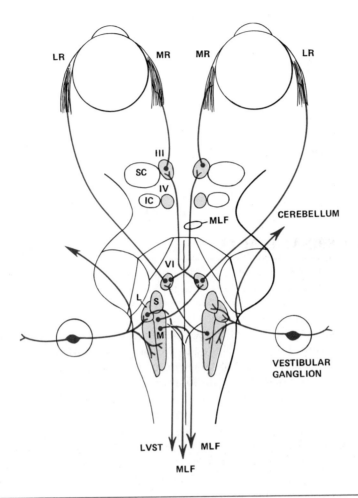

FIGURE 51

Connections of the vestibular system. The origins of the descending pathways arising from the lateral and medial nuclei are illustrated only on the left. On both sides are shown the ascending pathways that control the horizontal vestibuloocular reflex through projections to the abducens and oculomotor nuclei. I = inferior vestibular nucleus; IC = inferior colliculus; L = lateral vestibular nucleus; LR = Lateral rectus muscle; LVST = lateral vestibulospinal tract; M = medial vestibular nucleus; MLF = medial longitudinal fasciculus; MR = medial rectus muscle; S = superior vestibular nucleus; SC = superior colliculus; III = oculomotor nucleus; IV = trochlear nucleus; VI = abducens nucleus.

mic projection is the least studied of the vestibular system pathways. It is thought to arise in the medial and inferior (spinal) nuclei and to terminate ipislaterally at the rostral edge of the **ventral posterolateral nucleus** of the thalamus. The cortical projections of this area are not entirely clear. Some evidence suggests that the **frontal lobe** receives vestibular sensory projections, whereas other data indicate projections to a small region of the parietal lobe at the **anterior end** of the **intraparietal sulcus**, where the intraparietal sulcus intersects with the postcentral sulcus.

Some primary fibers of the vestibular nerve pass directly to the cerebellum, ending in the cortex of the flocculonodular lobe. Other vestibular fibers to the flocculonodular lobe cortex arise from the superior, medial, and inferior nuclei. These projections also reach the vermis of the anterior lobe of the cerebellum. From the cortex of the vermis, Purkinje cell axons project to the inferior and lateral vestibular nuclei. Neurons of the lateral vestibular nucleus are inhibited monosynaptically by the Purkinje cells. In addition, the cerebellar cortex sends information to the fastigial nucleus, which gives rise to the **fastigiobulbar tract (tract of Russell)**. The fibers of this tract are crossed and uncrossed and terminate in all of the vestibular nuclei and in the reticular formation of the pons and medulla. As they pass from the cerebellum, some of these fibers loop around the superior cerebellar peduncle to form the **uncinate fasciculus (hook bundle)**. Other fastigiobulbar fibers, which are uncrossed, pass from the cerebellum on the medial side of the inferior peduncle and constitute a portion of the peduncle sometimes referred to as the **juxtarestiform body**. The fibers of the juxtarestiform body terminate in the vestibular nuclei and in the reticular formation.

VESTIBULOSPINAL TRACTS

• • • • • • • • •

Two major projections into the spinal cord arise from the vestibular nuclei. The lateral tract, which is uncrossed, comes from the lateral vestibular nucleus. The medial tract, which is both crossed and uncrossed, comes chiefly from the medial vestibular nucleus, with some fibers contributed by the inferior (spinal) nucleus. The **lateral vestibulospinal tract** extends ipsilaterally from the cervical to the lumbosacral level of the spinal cord. The **medial vestibulospinal tract** in the descending portion of the medial longitudinal fasciculus extends bilaterally through the cervical level of the spinal cord. Both tracts terminate along their course almost exclusively on interneurons in laminae VII and VIII, which in turn synapse on alpha and gamma lower motoneurons in lamina IX (see Chap. 8). Both vestibulospinal tracts have strong facilitating effects on motoneurons innervating antigravity muscles. These effects assist the local myotatic (muscle stretch) reflexes and reinforce the tonus of the extensor muscles of the trunk and limbs, producing enough extra force to support the body against gravity and maintain an upright posture.

An animal whose brain stem has been transected at the midbrain level develops a condition known as **decerebrate rigidity**. This condition is characterized by marked rigidity of the extensor muscles of all of the limbs as well as the trunk and neck. In humans, decerebrate rigidity is characterized by extension of all the limbs, with the arms adducted and internally rotated at the shoulders. Decerebrate rigidity results from a marked tonic enhancement of activity descending from the brain stem through the vestibulospinal and reticulospinal tracts, which exert a strong excitatory influence on muscle tone, particularly in extensor muscles. Normally, muscle tone is maintained by a balance of inhibiting and facilitating activity descending from the cerebral hemispheres to the level of the spinal cord. Removal of the influence of the cerebral hemispheres by transection at the upper levels of the brain stem allows excessive activity in the vestibulospinal and reticulospinal tracts to occur without control. Decerebrate rigidity results from a marked tonic facilitation of gamma motoneuron activity in the spinal cord. This increases the rate of firing of muscle spindle afferents and thereby increases the firing of alpha motoneurons to extensor muscles. Decerebrate rigidity is abolished by transection of the dorsal roots, because this interrupts the gamma motoneuron–spindle afferent reflex arc. Decerebrate rigidity is also abolished by lesions of the central nervous system that interrupt the descending vestibular and reticular pathways.

VESTIBULOOCULAR PATHWAYS

• • • • • • • • •

The vestibular system is extremely important in controlling **conjugate eye movements** reflexly in response to head movement and to the position of the head in space. Fibers from the superior, medial, and, to a lesser extent, the lateral and inferior vestibular nuclei project rostrally in the **medial longitudinal fasciculus (MLF)**. The projections from the superior nucleus are uncrossed in the MLF until they reach the oculomotor complex, where some terminate in the opposite nucleus. Fibers from the other vestibular nuclei are both crossed and uncrossed in the MLF, but those from the medial and inferior nuclei are predominantly crossed. The fibers synapse on the somatic motor nuclei of the cranial nerves (abducens, VI; trochlear, IV; and oculomotor, III) that supply the extraocular muscles. Other fibers from the MLF, which may indirectly influence eye movements, project to several small nuclear groups located in the vicinity of the oculomotor nuclear complex and the pretectal area. These include the interstitial nucleus of Cajal, the nucleus of Darkschewitsch, and the nucleus of the posterior commissure. The interstitial nucleus of Cajal, in turn, gives rise to descending fibers that travel the length of the MLF and project to the vestibular nuclei and the spinal cord.

The labyrinth on each side of the body provides a baseline tonic discharge that constantly influences the vestibuloocular and vestibulospinal pathways. The tonic discharge can be altered by activation of the labyrinthine receptors.

Vestibular reflexes, in cooperation with certain reflexes of the optic system, enable the eyes to remain fixed on stationary objects while the head and body are moving. Turning the head slightly to the right causes a slight flow of endolymph in the horizontal semicircular canals. The flow is directed to the left because the fluid's inertia causes it to lag behind the movement of the head. This flow of endolymph causes increased neural activity in the ampulla of the right horizontal canal and decreased activity in the left. This excites the vestibular nuclei on the right through the vestibular ganglion cells. From the right vestibular nuclei, the activity passes through the MLF to excite the left abducens nucleus to innervate the left lateral rectus muscle and the right oculomotor nucleus to innervate the right medial rectus muscle (see Fig. 51). Simultaneously, activity in the MLF inhibits the innervation of the left medial rectus and the right lateral rectus muscles. As a result, the eyes are turned the proper distance to the left to keep the fields of vision unchanged.

TESTS OF VESTIBULAR FUNCTION

• • • • • • • • •

If stimulation of hair cells in the ampulla of a semicircular canal is persistent, the eyes draw slowly to one side until they reach a limit and then jerk quickly to the opposite side. These movements are repeated in rapid succession, producing tremor-like oscillations of the eyes known as **nystagmus**. The **direction of nystagmus** is designated according to the direction of the **fast component**, although this is opposite to the movement induced by stimulation from the semicircular canal. The fact that vestibular stimulation evokes nystagmus provides a basis for clinical tests of vestibular function.

A **rotation test** of vestibular function can be performed by turning the patient in a revolving chair with the head tilted forward 30 degrees to bring the horizontal canals parallel with the floor. Movement is stopped abruptly after 10 or 12 turns. Momentum causes the endolymph to continue to flow in the direction in which the head had been turning, even though the head is now stationary. The induced nystagmus, called **afternystagmus** or **postrotatory nystagmus**, lasts about 30 seconds in normal individuals. If rotation was to the left, endolymph flows to the left, and the slow component of the nystagmus is to the left. Because the quick component is to the right, it is called "nystagmus to the right." With a special chair designed to rotate the patient's head in any plane, it is possible to test each of the three pairs of semicircular canals individually. The orientation of the canals is such that the two horizontal canals are one pair; the right anterior and left posterior canals are in the same plane and constitute the second pair; and the right posterior and left anterior canals are the third pair.

Caloric, or **thermal, tests** of nystagmus permit the vestibular system of each side to be tested separately. Usually, the patient is either lying down with the head tilted forward about 30 degrees or seated with the head tilted backward about 60 degrees. Either of these positions brings the horizontal semicircular canal into a vertical plane. The external auditory canal is then irrigated with either cold or warm water. This lowers or raises the temperature of the endolymph on the side of the semicircular canal closest to the middle ear and causes a convection current in the endolymph. Stimulation of hair cells by the current flowing past the ampulla produces nystagmus. With warm water in the right ear and the head tilted backward, the current going up produces a flow equivalent to flow to the left in the horizontal position. Thus, the nystagmus has its slow component to the left and its quick component to the right. If cold water is used, the current is reversed and the nystagmus has its slow component to the right and its quick component to the left. The caloric tests of nystagmus can be recorded graphically by placing recording electrodes on the patient's face near the eyes.

Loss of the tonic labyrinthine discharge on one side by destruction of the vestibule, section of the vestibular nerve, or damage to the vestibular nuclei unbalances the stream of impulses from each side and leads to spontaneous nystagmus and vertigo. Tonic deviation of the eyes to one side, along with nystagmus and vertigo, occurs after unilateral damage to the vestibular nuclei or their connections, but tonic ocular deviation does not occur after destruction of the vestibule or section of the vestibular nerve. For example, if the right vestibular nerve is severed, the influence of the remaining left vestibular apparatus is unbalanced, causing nystagmus with the slow component to the right. In a few weeks, this effect is overcome by the compensatory influence of voluntary and visual reflex circuits.

Although **horizontal nystagmus** is the most common type, vertical or rotatory forms of nystagmus also occur. Nystagmus results from lesions of the vestibular system, including its peripheral and central connections, and also from lesions of the brain stem and cerebellum. Nystagmus can result from chronic visual impairment and from a number of toxic substances.

SENSORY ASPECTS OF VESTIBULAR STIMULATION

Stimulation of the vestibular apparatus by motion of the body or by artificial means produces a sense of motion. **Vertigo** is a sense of whirling. The individual may feel that his or her body is rotating, or it may seem that external objects are spinning around the individual. Motion sickness during travel by air or sea is a familiar manifestation of prolonged and excessive stimulation of the vestibular apparatus. Feelings of giddiness, faintness, and lightheadedness may be vaguely described in somewhat similar terms, but they should not be mistaken for true vertigo. **Ménière's disease** is a condition characterized by sudden attacks of severe vertigo, usually associated with nausea, vomiting, and prostration and accompanied by progressive unilateral deafness and tinnitus. Accumulation of fluid in the labyrinth **("hydrops")** is thought to be responsible for this condition.

CHAPTER

17

The Cerebellum

The cerebellum, along with other central nervous system structures, participates in the execution of a wide variety of movements. It is needed to maintain the proper posture and balance for walking and running; to execute sequential movements for eating, dressing, and writing; to participate in rapidly alternating repetitive movements and smooth pursuit movements; and to control certain properties of movements, including trajectory, velocity, and acceleration. Voluntary movements can proceed without assistance from the cerebellum, but such movements are slow, clumsy, and disorganized. Lack of motor skill as a result of cerebellar dysfunction is called **dyssynergia** (also **asynergia** or **cerebellar ataxia)**. Although the cerebellum receives large numbers of afferent fibers, conscious perception does not occur in the cerebellum, and its efferent fibers do not contribute to conscious sensations elsewhere in the brain. Nevertheless, evidence is mounting that the cerebellum is involved in certain aspects of cognition, particularly the mental processes needed for planning the execution of complex movements.

The cerebellum is a bilaterally symmetrical structure situated in the posterior cranial fossa. It is attached to the medulla, pons, and midbrain by the **cerebellar peduncles,** which lie at the sides of the fourth ventricle on the ventral aspect of the cerebellum. The **tentorium cerebelli,** a transverse fold of the dura mater, stretches horizontally over the superior surface of the cerebellum and separates it from the overlying occipital lobes of the cerebrum. The surface of the cerebellum is corrugated by numerous parallel folds known as **folia**. A layer of gray matter, the **cerebellar cortex,** covers the surface and encloses an internal core of white matter. Four pairs of **deep cerebellar nuclei** are buried within the cerebellum. From medial to lateral, these consist of the **fastigial, globose, emboliform**, and **dentate nuclei.** The globose and emboliform nuclei commonly are grouped together and termed the **interposed nuclei**.

PRIMARY SUBDIVISIONS OF THE CEREBELLUM

• • • • • • • • •

The cerebellum consists of a midline structure called the **vermis** and two large lateral masses known as the **cerebellar hemispheres** (Fig. 52). The cerebellum is composed of three major anatomic components:

1. The **flocculonodular lobe** consists of the paired flocculi, which are small appendages in the posterior inferior region, and the nodulus, which is the inferior part of the vermis (see Fig. 52B). The posterolateral fissure separates the flocculonodular lobe from the posterior lobe. The flocculonodular lobe is also termed the **archicerebellum**, because phylogenetically, it is the oldest part of the structure.
2. The **anterior lobe**, which is of modest size, is the portion of the cerebellum that lies anterior to the **primary fissure** (see Fig. 52A). This lobe corresponds approximately to the **paleocerebellum**, which is the second oldest part of the cerebellum phylogenetically.
3. The **posterior lobe** is the largest part of the cerebellum and is located between the other two lobes. It contains the major portions of the cerebellar hemispheres and is known as the **neocerebellum**.

The flocculonodular lobe receives many projections from the vestibular nuclei. The anterior lobe, particularly its vermal portion, receives input from the spinocerebellar pathways. The flocculonodular and anterior lobes are the predominant regions of the cerebellum in phylogenetically older vertebrates. The posterior lobe receives projections from the cerebral hemispheres and is greatly expanded in mammals that have developed an extensive cerebral cortex.

The foregoing description presents the **transverse divisions** of the cerebellum. These divisions are based on the embryonic development of 10 rostrocaudally arranged lobules (numbered I to X on the vermis in Fig. 52C). A more clinically useful method of describing the cerebellum is based on **longitudinal sagittal zonal patterns**. This classification subdivides each half of the cerebellum into three, mediolaterally arranged longitudinal strips that include the cerebellar cortex, underlying white matter, and deep cerebellar nuclei: (1) the vermal region with the fastigial nuclei, (2) the paravermal region or the intermediate zone of the hemisphere with the interposed nuclei, and (3) the lateral hemisphere region with the dentate nuclei (see Fig. 52A and B; for locations of the deep cerebellar nuclei, see Figs. 54 and 55).

THE CEREBELLAR CORTEX

• • • • • • • • •

The cerebellar cortex consists of three layers (Fig. 53):

1. The outermost is the **molecular layer**, which contains two types of neurons, the **stellate** and **basket cells**; dendrites of Purkinje and Golgi type II cells; and axons (T-shaped parallel fibers) of the granule cells.
2. The middle is the **Purkinje cell layer**, which contains the cell bodies of Purkinje cells. These are very large, flasklike neurons that have enormous dendritic arborizations extending up into the molecular layer. This dendritic arborization is

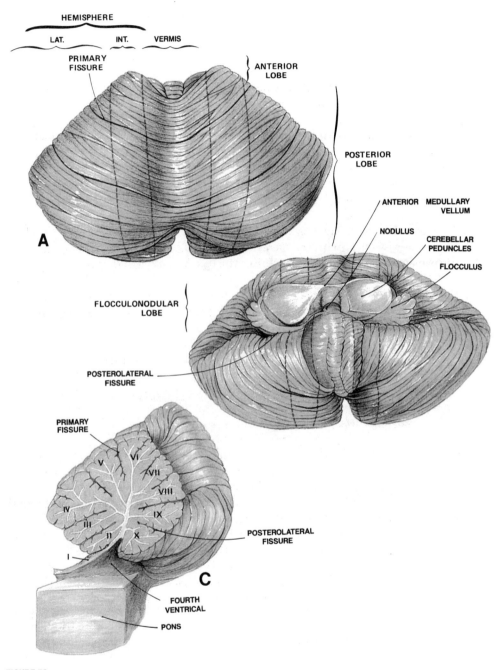

FIGURE 52

The human cerebellum seen from the dorsal (*A*) and ventral (*B*) surfaces and from the medial surface after a midline section through the vermis (*C*). The primary fissure divides the anterior and posterior lobes. The posterolateral fissure divides the posterior lobe from the flocculonodular lobe. The vermal structures are identified by Roman numerals.

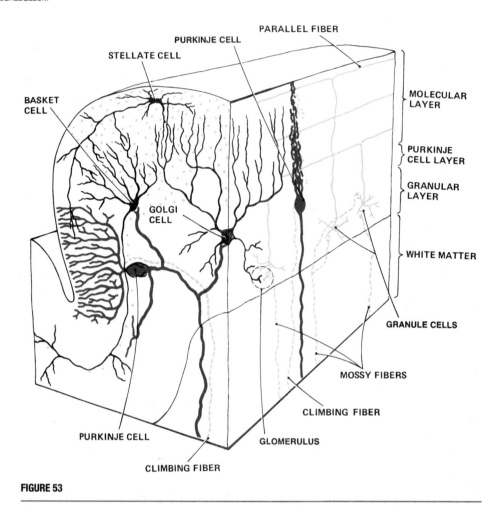

FIGURE 53

• • • • • • • • •

The smaller cut surface (*left*) represents the sagittal plane of the cerebellum, perpendicular to the length of the folium. This is the plane in which Purkinje cell dendrites arborize. At right angles to this surface, the larger cut surface (*right*) represents the mediolateral plane of the cerebellum along the length of one folium.

unusual in that it is confined to one plane—the sagittal plane of the cerebellum. The result of this arrangement of the cells is that the Purkinje cell dendrites spread out in a plane perpendicular to the course of the millions of parallel fibers, which run along the length of the folium and make thousands of synaptic contacts with the dendrites of each Purkinje cell (see Fig. 53). The Purkinje cells are the projection neurons of the cerebellar cortex. Their long axons synapse either on deep cerebellar nuclei or vestibular nuclei. Collaterals of Purkinje cell axons make synaptic contact with Golgi cells, other Purkinje cells, basket cells, and stellate cells.

3. The innermost is the **granular layer**, which contains numerous **granule** cells (neurons), **Golgi type II cells** (neurons), and **glomeruli** (synaptic complexes that contain axons of incoming mossy fibers, axons and dendrites of Golgi type II cells, and dendrites of granule cells). Each glomerulus is encased in glial cell processes.

The cerebellar cortex has a simple synaptic organization. There are two sets of excitatory inputs and two sets of inhibitory inputs; three types of interneurons, all of which are inhibitory (the exception to this is the granule cell, which is excitatory); and one output, which is inhibitory.

Most afferents to the cerebellar cortex send collateral projections to the deep cerebellar nuclei. Some afferents, notably those in the dorsal spinocerebellar and cuneocerebellar pathways, project mainly or exclusively to the cerebellar cortex. The afferents to the cerebellar cortex terminate either in the granule cell layer (in the glomeruli) as **mossy fibers** or, in the molecular layer, on the dendrites of Purkinje cells as **climbing fibers**. Mossy fiber afferents are derived from the spinal cord, pontine nuclei, vestibular ganglia and nuclei, trigeminal nuclei, reticular formation nuclei, and deep cerebellar nuclei. Climbing fiber afferents are derived exclusively from the inferior olive. Several amino acids have been identified as possible neurotransmitters in the cerebellum. The mossy fibers and the granule cells probably use glutamate as a neurotransmitter, and the climbing fibers probably use aspartate. Golgi cells, basket cells, and Purkinje cells use gamma-aminobutyric acid (GABA). The stellate cells may use taurine. The neurotransmitter of the deep cerebellar nuclei has not been established, but the projections to the inferior olive may utilize GABA, whereas the projections to the red nucleus and thalamus may utilize glutamate.

Both mossy fiber and climbing fiber inputs are excitatory to both the deep cerebellar nuclei and the cortex. Mossy fiber input excites Purkinje cells indirectly by activating granule cells and their axons, the parallel fibers. Mossy fiber excitation of Purkinje cells evokes **simple spikes**, which consist of a single action potential. Climbing fiber input excites Purkinje cells directly, evoking **complex spikes**, which consist of an action potential followed by a long-lasting depolarization with multiple small wavelets. Granule cells, through their axonal processes (parallel fibers), excite Purkinje cells, basket cells, stellate cells, and Golgi type II cells. In turn, basket cells and stellate cells inhibit Purkinje and Golgi type II cells. The Golgi type II cells inhibit granule cells. Finally, Purkinje cells, the only route for all information exiting from the cerebellar cortex, are inhibitory to the deep cerebellar and vestibular nuclei. Consequently, of all the neurons whose cells reside within the cerebellar cortex, the granule cell is the only excitatory one.

In addition to the mossy fiber and climbing fiber inputs, there are **aminergic afferent projections** to all three layers of the cerebellar cortex. These projections are thought to be inhibitory. The **locus ceruleus** gives rise to **noradrenergic fibers** that enter the cerebellum through the superior cerebellar peduncle and terminate in all parts of the cerebellar cortex. These fibers make synaptic contact with Purkinje cell dendrites and with granule cell dendrites. **Dopaminergic fibers** originating in the **ventral mesencephalic tegmentum** ascend to the interposed and dentate nuclei and to the Purkinje cell and granule cell layers of the cerebellar cortex. **Serotonergic fibers** from the **raphe nuclei** of the brain stem project to essentially all lobules of the cerebellum, terminating in both the granule cell and molecular layers.

THE PEDUNCLES OF THE CEREBELLUM

The three paired cerebellar peduncles are composed of large numbers of fibers entering and leaving the cerebellum to connect it with other parts of the nervous system.

The **inferior cerebellar peduncle (restiform body)** consists chiefly of afferent fibers. This peduncle contains a single efferent pathway, the **fastigiobulbar tract** (also called the **juxtarestiform body**; see Chap. 16), which projects to the vestibular nuclei and completes a vestibular circuit through the cerebellum. Efferents from the fastigial nucleus also reach alpha motoneurons in the cervical spinal cord. Afferent fibers enter the inferior cerebellar peduncle from at least six sources: (1) fibers from the vestibular nerve and nuclei, (2) olivocerebellar fibers from the inferior olivary nuclei, (3) the dorsal spinocerebellar tract, (4) some of the fibers from the rostral spinocerebellar tract, (5) the cuneocerebellar tract from the accessory cuneate nuclei in the medulla, and (6) reticulocerebellar fibers. The first three of these are illustrated in Figure 54.

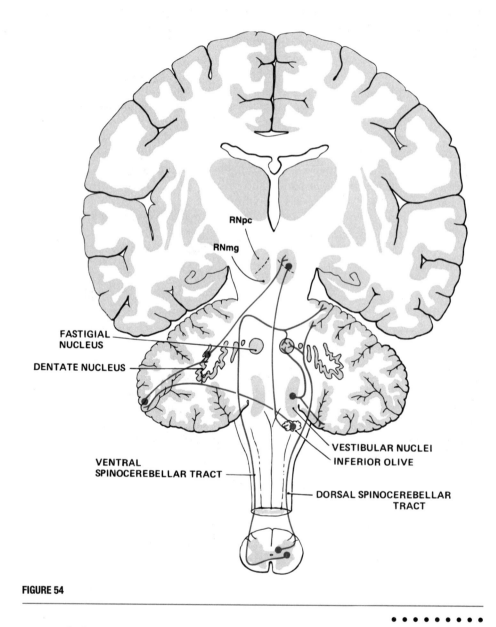

FIGURE 54

Inputs to the fastigial nucleus and cerebellar cortex from the spinal cord and vestibular nuclei. Inputs to the dentate nucleus and cerebellar cortex from the inferior olive.

The **middle cerebellar peduncle** (brachium pontis) consists almost entirely of crossed afferent fibers from the pontine nuclei in the gray substance of the basal part of the pons (pontocerebellar or transverse pontine fibers). The major projections to the pontine nuclei originate within the cerebral cortex (Fig. 55).

The **superior cerebellar peduncle** (brachium conjunctivum) consists principally of efferent projections from the cerebellum. Rubral, thalamic, and reticular projections arise from the dentate and interposed (globose and emboliform) nuclei (see Fig. 55). Some of the fastigiobulbar tract fibers also run with the superior peduncle for a short distance before they enter the inferior cerebellar peduncle. The superior cerebellar peduncle also contains afferent projections from the ventral spinocerebellar tract (see Fig. 54), a portion of the rostral spinocerebellar tract, and trigeminocerebellar projections.

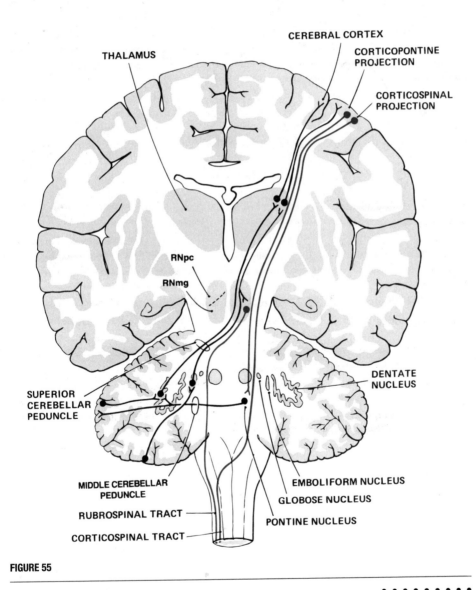

FIGURE 55

Connections of the dentate nucleus and interposed (emboliform and globose) nuclei.

AFFERENT AND EFFERENT PATHWAYS OF THE CEREBELLUM

• • • • • • • • •

The cortex of the cerebellum and the deep cerebellar nuclei are furnished with a constant account of the progress of motor activity by signals from many sources. First, they are informed of the commands being issued from the cerebral cortex by a flow of neuronal impulses through three cerebrocerebellar projection pathways. The largest of these is the corticopontocerebellar pathway, which is a crossed path connecting most of the cortex of one cerebral hemisphere with the cerebellar hemisphere on the opposite side by way of the **corticopontine tract and the ponto-cerebellar** projections. These pontocerebellar fibers ascend through the **middle cerebellar peduncle** (see Fig. 55). The other cerebrocerebellar pathways originate primarily in the motor areas of the cerebral cortex and include the **cerebroolivo-cerebellar** and **cerebroreticulocerebellar** pathways. Additional communication received by the cerebellar cortex consists of a stream of information from the skin, joints, and muscles of the limbs and trunk of the body mediated by the three spinocerebellar tracts (dorsal, ventral, and rostral) and the cuneocerebellar tract. Most other sensory modalities, including the auditory, vestibular, and visual senses, also reach the cerebellum. Finally, the cerebellum receives direct connections from neurons in the hypothalamus. All of this information enters a vast pool of cerebellar cortical neurons, where integration takes place.

In general, the vermal and intermediate zones of the anterior lobe and the caudal part of the posterior lobe receive afferent input primarily from the spinal cord; the flocculonodular lobe receives a major projection from the vestibular system; and the cerebellar hemispheres receive their major input from the cerebral cortex. This distribution is also reflected in a general functional pattern. The vermal and intermediate zones of the anterior and caudal posterior lobes are primarily concerned with posture and locomotion, the flocculonodular lobe is important in vestibular function (balance, posture, and eye movements), and the lateral zones of the cerebellar hemispheres are involved in control of finely coordinated movements of the extremities.

Afferent input from essentially all sources reaches both the deep cerebellar nuclei and the cerebellar cortex. The result is an increase in excitability of the deep nuclei and the Purkinje cells of the cerebellar cortex. The Purkinje cells provide strong inhibitory control over neurons of the deep nuclei. The inhibitory control of Purkinje cells over the excitability of the deep cerebellar nuclei is a key aspect of cerebellar function. Through information received from afferents and interactions between the cerebellar cortex and the deep nuclei, the cerebellum is able to monitor ongoing movements and trigger new or modified movements. The cerebellum can ensure that the speed and accuracy of movements is adequate for each task undertaken by the motor system.

The efferent pathways by which the cerebellum is able to influence movement are best understood by examining the projections of the deep cerebellar nuclei. The fastigial nucleus, which belongs to the vermal zone, sends projections to the reticular and vestibular nuclei of the brain stem. These nuclei send projections into the spinal cord and are concerned with posture and balance. The interposed nuclei of each side of the cerebellum send projections through the superior cerebellar peduncle to the red nucleus of the contralateral side. The magnocellular division of the red nucleus gives rise to axons of the rubrospinal tract (see Fig. 55). This projection crosses the midline and descends into the spinal cord. Thus, the origin of this pathway in the interposed nuclei and its terminations in the spinal cord are on the same side of the body.

Projections from both the dentate and the interposed nuclei exit through the superior cerebellar peduncle to the contralateral **ventral lateral nucleus** of the thalamus. Thalamocortical fibers from the ventral lateral nucleus relay impulses to the motor regions of the ipsilateral frontal lobe. Through this pathway, these thalamocortical projections make synaptic contact with cortical efferent fibers that pass through the pyramidal tract and project to the contralateral side of the spinal cord through the corticospinal pathway. Thus, the origin of this pathway in the dentate and interposed nuclei and its termination in the spinal cord are both on the same side of the body (see Fig. 55). Through its influence on the corticospinal pathway, this part of the cerebellar circuitry has its important influence on coordinated movements of the distal limb musculature.

AFFERENT–EFFERENT CIRCUITS THROUGH THE CEREBELLUM

• • • • • • • •

The general scheme of operation of the cerebellum allows neuronal impulses to be returned to the same region from which they originated. Briefly, the following are important afferent–efferent circuits involving the cerebellum:

1. The cortex of the vermal region receives information from the spinal cord and sends back information indirectly by the fastigial nucleus through the reticular formation (reticulospinal tracts) and vestibular nuclei (vestibulospinal tracts) to the spinal cord.
2. The flocculonodular lobe cortex receives information from the vestibular system and returns information through direct corticovestibular projections and through fastigioreticulovestibular pathways to the vestibular nuclei in the brain stem, where vestibulospinal pathways arise.
3. The lateral (hemisphere) cortex receives information from the cerebral cortex and sends information back through the dentatothalamocortical path to exert an influence on the cerebrum and, through the corticospinal tract, to influence the spinal cord.

FUNCTIONS OF THE CEREBELLUM

• • • • • • • •

During ongoing motor tasks, the mossy fiber inputs furnish an excitatory "mainline" pathway providing drive for neurons in the deep cerebellar nuclei. The mossy fiber input to the cerebellar cortex constitutes a "side path" consisting of a mossy fiber–granule cell–parallel fiber–Purkinje cell circuit with related interneurons. The inhibitory cerebellar cortical side loop controls the discharge of neurons in the deep cerebellar nuclei.

The climbing fiber input to the cerebellar cortex has a conditioning effect on the activity of Purkinje cells. Climbing fiber activity can adjust the flow of information through Purkinje cells by strengthening or weakening the influence of various synapses in the cerebellar cortical pathways converging on the Purkinje cells.

Moreover, climbing fiber activity is thought to influence motor learning by inducing plastic changes in the synaptic activity of Purkinje cells.

The intent to perform a movement originates in the cerebral cortical association areas, including the supplementary motor cortex. These areas act in cooperation with the lateral portions of the cerebellar hemispheres and dentate nuclei during the early phases of movement planning. The result is a command to move, which involves the dentate nuclei, followed by neurons in area 4 of the cerebral cortex. The intermediate parts of the cerebellar hemispheres, including the interpositus nuclei, are kept informed of the progress of the ongoing movement by inputs from collaterals of pyramidal tract fibers mediated by way of the pontine nuclei and also from peripheral receptors in the body parts being moved.

Studies suggest that the cerebellum participates in cognitive processing. The evidence is chiefly anatomic and is based on the demonstration of connections from the dentate nucleus to the thalamus and then to the prefrontal areas of the cerebral cortex. It is presumed that these connections are used in some kinds of thinking, such as planning ahead. The cerebellum may learn a motor program and quickly link elements within the program to a new situation so that these elements can be used quickly and automatically.

CLINICAL SIGNS OF CEREBELLAR DYSFUNCTION

• • • • • • • • •

From the clinical perspective, the cerebellum is organized into a series of sagittal zones. The clinical signs of cerebellar dysfunction can be separated into those resulting from disease of the midline zone of the cerebellum and those resulting from disease of the lateral portions.

Disease of the Midline Zone of the Cerebellum

The midline zone of the cerebellum consists of the anterior and posterior parts of the vermis, the flocculonodular lobe, and the fastigial nuclei. Disease of these regions produces the following signs and symptoms:

1. **Disorders of stance and gait**. The stance is usually on a broad base, with the feet several inches apart. There may be a severe truncal tremor. It is difficult for the patient to walk in tandem, placing the heel of one foot directly in front of the toes of the other foot. With disease of the midline zone, the gait disturbance usually occurs without ataxia of the movements of individual limbs.
2. **Titubation**. This is a rhythmic tremor of the body or head occurring several times per second.
3. **Rotated or tilted postures of the head**. The head may be maintained rotated or tilted to the left or right. The side of the deviation does not usually indicate the site of the cerebellar disease.
4. **Ocular motor disorders**. A number of disturbances of ocular function result from cerebellar disease, the most prominent of which is spontaneous **nystagmus** (i.e., not resulting from physiologic vestibular stimulation). This consists of rhythmical oscillatory movements of one or both eyes occurring with the eyes gazing straight ahead or with ocular deviation.

Disease of the Lateral (Hemispheric) Zone of the Cerebellum

For clinical purposes, the lateral cerebellar zone consists of the cerebellar hemisphere and the dentate and interposed nuclei of each side. Disease of this region produces the following signs and symptoms:

1. **Decomposition of movement**. The various components of a motor act are performed in a jerky and irregular rather than in a smooth sequence. Evidence indicates that decomposition of movement is a voluntary, adopted strategy that compensates for the inability to make complex movements accurately. The person with a cerebellar disorder learns to make movements more accurate by moving one joint at a time in a serial manner.

2. **Disturbances of stance and gait**. The stance is on a broad base, and the gait is unsteady, with a tendency to fall to the side, forward, or backward. The gait disorder is accompanied by ataxia of individual movements of the limbs.

3. **Hypotonia**. This is a decrease in the resistance to passive manipulation of the limbs, appearing in one or several limbs at the time of cerebellar injury. Hypotonia often decreases with time. It is detected clinically by manipulating the limbs about the joints and not by palpating the muscles.

4. **Dysarthria**. In cerebellar disease, speech may be slow, slurred, and labored, but comprehension remains intact and grammar does not suffer.

5. **Dysmetria**. This is a disturbance of the trajectory or placement of a body part during active movements. The limb may fall short of its goal in hypometria, or it may extend beyond its goal in hypermetria.

6. **Dysdiadochokinesis and dysrhythmokinesis**. Dysdiadochokinesis is a manifestation of the decomposition of movements in cerebellar disease, demonstrated by testing alternating or fine repetitive movements. Dysrhythmokinesis is a disorder of the rhythm of rapidly alternating movements. It can be evoked by asking the patient to tap out a rhythm such as three rapid beats followed by one delayed beat. In cerebellar disease, the rhythm of the movements is disturbed.

7. **Ataxia**. This term comprehensively describes the various problems with movement resulting chiefly from the combined effects of dysmetria and decomposition of movement. There are errors in the sequence and speed of the components of each movement. A patient with an ataxia of gait veers from side to side, having difficulty walking in a straight line.

8. **Tremor**. Cerebellar disease results in **static** and **kinetic tremors**. Static tremor is demonstrated by asking the patient to extend the arms parallel to the floor with the hands open. A rhythmic oscillation generated at the shoulder is seen. A kinetic tremor can be produced by having the patient alternately touch his or her nose and then touch the examiner's finger, which is held at a full arm's length away from the patient. Kinetic tremor can also be tested by asking the patient to place the heel of one foot on the knee of the opposite leg and run the heel down the shin. These movements result in a side-to-side coarse tremor that is generated at the proximal joints (shoulder and hip).

9. **Impaired check and rebound**. These are related signs of cerebellar dysfunction. The patient is asked to maintain the arms extended forward while the examiner taps the patient's wrist enough to displace the arm. Normally, the arm returns rapidly to the resting position, but with cerebellar disease, the limb is markedly displaced and repeatedly overshoots when returning to the original position.

10. **Ocular motor disorders**. A number of disorders of eye movement result from injury to the cerebellar hemispheres. The most common disorder is nystagmus.

Cerebellar defects gradually improve with time after sudden lesions such as traumatic injury or loss of blood supply (stroke). Improvement of motor function over time occurs partially because the patient learns compensatory strategies and partially because of the **plasticity** of the central nervous system (the capacity to form new connections or to use existing connections differently).

Somatotopic localization of separate body regions in the cerebellar cortex has been demonstrated in experimental animals. These studies have revealed an extremely complex representation of body parts. Despite the complexity of the organization of the cerebellum, however, it is clear that the right side of the body is under the influence of the right cerebellar hemisphere and that any symptoms occurring unilaterally are found on the same side as the lesion in the cerebellum. This contrasts strikingly with cerebral lesions, which produce contralateral effects.

Many neurologic diseases affect the cerebellum. **Olivopontocerebellar atrophy** is a progressive degenerative disease occurring either sporadically or genetically, usually with autosomal dominant transmission but occasionally with autosomal recessive transmission. The disease results in degeneration of the inferior olives, pons, and cerebellar cortex, causing ataxia of gait, dysarthria, cerebellar tremors of the trunk and limbs, and incoordination of movements of all limbs. **Friedreich's ataxia** is a hereditary disorder transmitted as an autosomal recessive trait that results in degeneration of the peripheral nerves, spinocerebellar pathways, dorsal columns, and corticospinal tracts in the spinal cord. The disease begins in childhood or early adolescence with ataxia of limb movements and gait, accompanied by the appearance of extensor plantar responses. As the disease progresses, patients develop scoliosis, pes cavus (high arches), limb weakness, and ataxia. The disease progresses to include paraparesis (i.e., severe weakness of the legs), with loss of the muscle stretch reflexes and position and vibration sense in the limbs. **Alcoholic cerebellar degeneration** is a disease associated with severe chronic alcoholism with malnutrition. Degenerative changes appearing in the anterior and superior parts of the cerebellar vermis are associated with ataxia of gait but with preservation of speech and coordinated movements of the upper extremities.

5

Higher Levels of the Nervous System

18

The Basal Ganglia

The cerebral cortex influences motor function directly through the corticospinal and corticobulbar pathways, whereas the cerebellum and basal ganglia influence lower motoneurons both through descending pathways and through their modulation of the cerebral cortex. The cerebral cortical modulation is accomplished through recurrent circuits that form cortical–brain stem–cerebellar–thalamic–cortical and cortical–basal ganglia–thalamic–cortical loops. Although these systems are thus tightly integrated, the differing functions of the cerebellar and basal ganglia loops produce distinctive neurologic deficits when these circuits are damaged by disease. Clinicians divide the motor system into two groups of circuits, the **pyramidal system** and the **extrapyramidal system**. The pyramidal system consists of the corticobulbar and corticospinal pathways. The extrapyramidal system is composed of all other projection pathways that influence motor control, including the basal ganglia and the projection pathways from the brain stem to the spinal cord (e.g., the rubrospinal, reticulospinal, vestibulospinal, and tectospinal tracts). The neuronal circuits of the extrapyramidal system are closely connected with those of the pyramidal system; separating these connections into two systems is artificial. Nevertheless, the term extrapyramidal system is frequently used clinically to denote the components of the basal ganglia and related subcortical nuclei that influence motor activity, and disease of the extrapyramidal system results in neurologic symptoms that are different from those occurring with disease of the pyramidal system.

STRUCTURES IN THE BASAL GANGLIA

Structures in the basal ganglia have numerous interconnections, and the terminology used in describing these structures can be confusing. A thorough understanding of the terminology is an essential prerequisite for understanding the interrelations of this system.

• • • • • • • • •

TABLE 2

BASAL GANGLIA NOMENCLATURE

Term	Descriptive Terms		Synonym	Components
	Prefix	*Suffix*		
Striatum	Strio-	-striate	Neostriatum	Caudate nucleus and putamen
Pallidum	Pallido-	-pallidal	Paleostriatum	Globus pallidus
Lenticular nucleus				Putamen and globus pallidus
Corpus striatum				Caudate nucleus, putamen, and globus pallidus
Subthalamic nucleus	Subthalamo-	-subthalamic		
Substantia nigra	Nigro-	-nigral		Pars compacta and pars reticularis

The major components of the basal ganglia include the **caudate nucleus, putamen**, and **globus pallidus**. Two other subcortical nuclei, the **subthalamic nucleus** and the **substantia nigra**, are not part of the telencephalic basal ganglia, but are interconnected anatomically and functionally with the caudate, putamen, and globus pallidus. Table 2 provides a guide to the terminology associated with the basal ganglia. Reference to Table 2 should make it apparent that "nigrostriatal" indicates a pathway that arises in the substantia nigra and terminates in the putamen, the caudate nucleus, or both. Similarly, "pallidosubthalamic" indicates a pathway that arises in the globus pallidus and projects to the subthalamic nucleus. Note that "corpus striatum" and "striatum" are not synonymous terms. They are frequently mistaken as being equivalent.

The **caudate nucleus** occupies a position in the floor of the lateral ventricle, dorsolateral to the thalamus (Figs. 56B, 57, and 58). The bulge at the cephalic end of the caudate nucleus is known as the **head** (Fig. 56A). The **body** passes backward at the side of the thalamus and tapers gradually to form the **tail**, which curves ventrally and follows the inferior horn of the lateral ventricle into the temporal lobe, ending near the amygdala.

The putamen and globus pallidus together form the **lenticular**, or **lentiform, nucleus** (see Fig. 56B), a thumb-sized mass wedged against the lateral side of the internal capsule. The lenticular nucleus is separated from the caudate nucleus by fibers of the internal capsule, except in the cephalic part, where the caudate nucleus and putamen are fused by cell bridges through the anterior limb of the internal capsule. The putamen is the lateral portion of the lenticular nucleus and has the same histologic appearance as the caudate nucleus, with numerous, densely packed, small neurons. The globus pallidus, in the medial region of the lenticular nucleus, contains sparsely distributed large cells and is traversed by many myelinated fibers. These fiber bundles account for the pale appearance of the globus pallidus in the fresh state, from which its name is derived. The globus pallidus is separated from the putamen by a cell-sparse lamina, and a similar lamina separates the globus pallidus itself into two parts, the **external globus pallidus** and the **internal globus pallidus**. The internal segment is developmentally affiliated with the diencephalon and thus with the adjacent subthalamus, from which it is separated by the fibers of the internal capsule.

The **subthalamus** is closely related to the basal ganglia anatomically and functionally. It contains the **zona incerta**, located between the lenticular fasciculus and

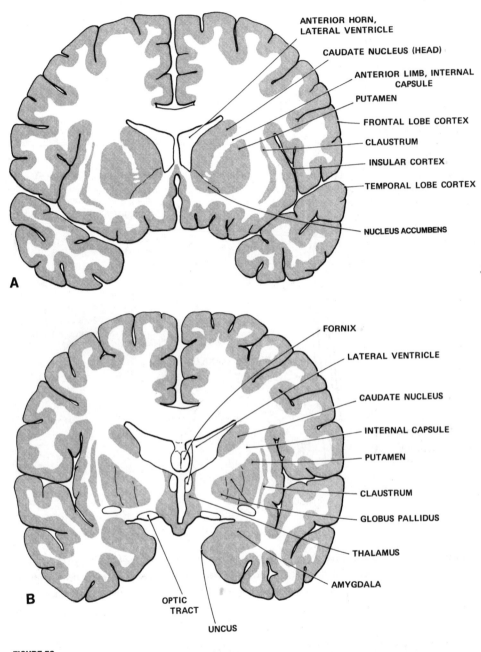

FIGURE 56

• • • • • • • • •

Two coronal sections through the cerebral hemispheres. (*A*) Section through the rostral part of the frontal lobe shows the relation of the basal ganglia to the surrounding telencephalic structures. (*B*) Section through the caudal part of the frontal lobe shows the location of the basal ganglia lateral to the diencephalon.

the thalamic fasciculus; **Forel's tegmental field H**, which includes the **prerubral field**; and the **subthalamic nucleus of Luys** (see Fig. 58). The zona incerta and the scattered cells in the prerubral field are considered by some to be a rostral continuation of the midbrain reticular formation. The rostral portions of the **substantia**

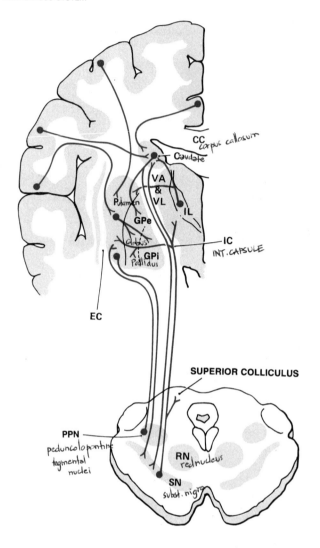

FIGURE 57

• • • • • • • • •

The afferent and efferent connections of the caudate nucleus and putamen. C = caudate nucleus; CC = corpus callosum; EC = external capsule; GPe - globus pallidus, external; GPi = globus pallidus, internal; IC = internal capsule; IL = intralaminar nuclei of the thalamus; P = putamen; PPN = pedunculopontine tegmental nucleus; RN = red nucleus; SN = substantia nigra; VA = ventral anterior nucleus of the thalamus; VL = ventral lateral nucleus of the thalamus.

nigra and the **red nucleus** extend into this region of the caudal diencephalon from the midbrain. The caudal part of the **subthalamic nucleus**, lens-shaped and lying along the medial border of the internal capsule, is adjacent to the rostral part of the substantia nigra.

CONNECTIONS OF THE BASAL GANGLIA

• • • • • • • • •

As with most regions of the brain, the nuclei of the basal ganglia contain two general types of neurons: interneurons and projection neurons. The major inputs to the corpus striatum are from the cerebral cortex, thalamus, and substantia nigra, and the major output is to the thalamus. From neurons in all areas of the neocortex, but particularly from the frontal and parietal lobes, axons project to the striatum (see Fig. 57). The primary motor (area 4), premotor (lateral area 6), supplementary motor (medial area 6) and somatosensory (areas 3, 1, and 2) cortices project preferentially to the putamen, whereas the frontal eye fields (area 8) and association areas of the

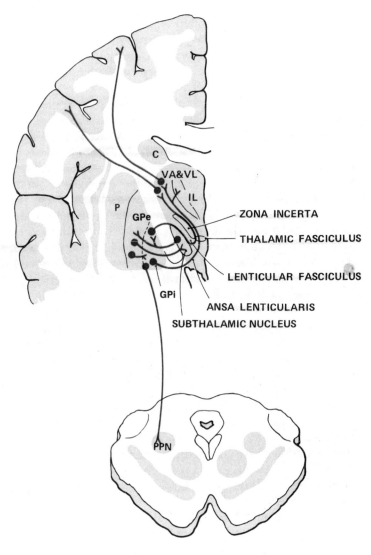

FIGURE 58

• • • • • • • • •

The efferent connections of the globus pallidus. C = caudate nucleus; GPe = globus pallidus, external; GPi = globus pallidus, internal; IL = intralaminar nuclei of the thalamus; P = putamen; PPN = pedunculopontine tegmental nucleus; VA = ventral anterior nucleus of the thalamus; VL = ventral lateral nucleus of the thalamus.

frontal and parietal lobes project heavily onto the caudate nucleus. The neurons projecting from the cerebral cortex to the striatum are strongly excitatory and use glutamate as their neurotransmitter. Stimulation of cerebral cortical neurons evokes excitatory postsynaptic potential–inhibitory postsynaptic potential (EPSP–IPSP) sequences in striatal neurons. The EPSPs result from the actions of excitatory glutamatergic cortical efferents, and the IPSPs result from feedback inhibition as a result of the recurrent collaterals of GABAergic neurons in the striatum. The striatum also receives input from the intralaminar nuclei of the thalamus, the substantia nigra and the **pedunculopontine tegmental nucleus** of the midbrain (see Fig. 57).

Neurons in the striatum project to the substantia nigra pars reticulata and both the external and internal segments of the globus pallidus (see Fig. 57). The projections are organized topographically, with faithful representation of body parts, from the cerebral cortex to the neostriatum, pallidum, and thalamus. Projections from the neostriatum to the pallidum are inhibitory and use the neurotransmitter gamma-aminobutyric acid (GABA). Many of the interneurons within the striatum are excitatory and use the neurotransmitter acetylcholine.

The major outflow of efferent fibers from the basal ganglia comes from the internal segment of the globus pallidus (see Fig. 58). Some of these fibers stream directly across the posterior limb of the internal capsule. On entering the subthalamic region, they form a bundle known as the **lenticular fasciculus** (Forel's field H$_2$), located immediately ventral to the zona incerta. Another bundle of fibers from the globus pallidus (internal segment) passes around the ventral aspect of the posterior limb of the internal capsule to form a loop, the **ansa lenticularis**. Both bundles merge on the medial aspect of the zona incerta in the prerubral field, where cerebellothalamic fibers join them. These bundles then curve dorsally and pass laterally just dorsal to the zona incerta to form a discrete bundle called the **thalamic fasciculus** (Forel's field H$_1$). The fibers in these systems synapse in the intralaminar (including the **centromedian**), **ventral lateral**, and **ventral anterior** nuclei of the thalamus. A second projection of efferents, the **pallidosubthalamic fibers**, arises from the external segment of the globus pallidus, crosses the posterior limb of the internal capsule, and synapses in the subthalamic nucleus. The cells of this nucleus project back to both parts of the globus pallidus, but primarily to the internal segment. Another important projection of the globus pallidus descends as **pallidotegmental fibers** to terminate in the pedunculopontine tegmental nucleus. The latter bundle and a pathway from the substantia nigra pars reticulata to the superior colliculus are the only pathways arising from the basal ganglia that descend caudal to the level of the substantia nigra. The projections from the globus pallidus are primarily inhibitory and use GABA as a neurotransmitter. These pallidal neurons also contain neuropeptides such as substance P and enkephalin, which are selectively distributed in specific pallidal projection pathways.

The **substantia nigra** is a subcortical nucleus that is closely related to the basal ganglia (see Fig. 57). It is reciprocally connected with the striatum and sends efferents to the **ventral anterior** and **dorsomedial**, and to some extent, to the **ventral lateral** thalamic nuclei. As mentioned previously, the substantia nigra pars reticulata also projects to the superior colliculus. Neurons that originate in the striatum and project to the substantia nigra are inhibitory and use the neurotransmitters GABA and substance P. Fibers that arise in the **pars compacta** of the substantia nigra use the neurotransmitter dopamine and synapse in the striatum, whereas GABAergic cells in the **pars reticulata** receive striatal input and project to the thalamus.

There are many circuits and feedback loops within and between the structures related to the basal ganglia. One important circuit is: cerebral cortex → striatum → internal segment of globus pallidus → thalamus → cerebral cortex. A second circuit is: cortex → subthalamic nucleus → internal and external segments of globus pallidus → thalamus → cortex. Another loop is: cortex → striatum → substantia nigra → thalamus → cortex. Many smaller circuits exist between structures that have reciprocal connections, for example, substantia nigra ⇌ striatum, and subthalamic nucleus ⇌ pallidum.

As described previously and in Chapter 17, the basal ganglia and the cerebellum interact with the cerebral cortex through a series of feedback circuits. The dentate and interposed nuclei of the cerebellum project to the ventral lateral nucleus of the thalamus, which also receives projections from the globus pallidus and the substantia nigra. Evidence indicates that none of these projections overlap in the ventral lateral nucleus. The ventral lateral nucleus projects to the primary motor and supplementary motor areas of the cerebral cortex. In turn, the motor cortex and other regions of the cerebrum project to the striatum to enter the basal ganglia circuit. Moreover, the motor cortex projects to the pons to enter the cerebellar circuit, including the corticopontocerebellar pathway, Purkinje cells, interposed and dentate nuclei, and the cerebellothalamic tract. Consequently, both the basal ganglia and the cerebellum are influenced by, and return influence to, the part of the cerebral cortex that gives rise to the descending motor pathways, which affect the activity of the lower motoneurons.

THE VENTRAL STRIATUM

• • • • • • • • •

The basal ganglia circuitry described above involves primarily the motor and sensory areas of the frontal and parietal lobes. Other areas of cortex, in the temporal and limbic lobes as well as the orbitofrontal region of the frontal lobe, project to the **nucleus accumbens** (see Fig. 56A) and the **olfactory tubercle**. These latter two structures constitute the **ventral striatum**. Like the dorsal striatum (caudate and putamen), the ventral striatum receives afferents from the intralaminar nuclei of the thalamus as well as the cerebral cortex and projects to the pallidum. These dorsal and ventral circuits are largely in parallel, however, rather than overlapping. The ventral striatum receives input from limbic and other allocortical areas that do not project to the dorsal striatum, and it projects to the **ventral pallidum**, an area adjacent to the globus pallidus. The ventral pallidum, in turn, projects to the dorsomedial nucleus of the thalamus and to the subthalamic nucleus and pedunculopontine tegmental nucleus. It also projects to the habenula.

The ventral circuitry parallels the dorsal system in that the ventral striatum is reciprocally connected with a dopaminergic cell group in the midbrain, but in this case it is the **ventral tegmental area**, a nuclear area medial to the substantia nigra.

Although little is known about the functions of the ventral striatum and pallidum, it appears that they are important in motivation, especially in behaviors that are guided by the limbic system. Experimental studies also demonstrate that these structures influence behaviors associated with addiction to a variety of abused substances.

FUNCTIONAL CONSIDERATIONS

• • • • • • • • •

Recordings from neurons in the basal ganglia of experimental animals during various motor tasks reveal that the discharge of single cells in the neostriatum shows a direct correlation with movements of the contralateral arm or leg. Neuronal activity related to movement usually occurs at the same time as the movement or even slightly after movement has occurred. Neuronal activity is also related to learned cues and to behavioral context and motivation. These findings suggest that the basal ganglia monitor the progress of movements, and are particularly concerned with the automatic execution of learned motor plans.

Lesions of the basal ganglia resulting from disease in humans cause (1) disorders of the initiation of movement (i.e., akinesia), (2) difficulty continuing or stopping an ongoing movement, (3) abnormalities of muscle tone (rigidity), and (4) the development of involuntary movements (tremor or chorea). The movements influenced by the basal ganglia include those related to posture, automatic movements (e.g., swinging the arms while walking), and skilled volitional movements, including eye movements. The basal ganglia are also important in cognition, a function that may be mediated through the circuits connecting these nuclei with the prefrontal cortex.

Many of the symptoms of basal ganglia disease reflect disorders in the function of neurotransmitter systems. Parkinson's disease is a state characterized pharmacologically by decreased dopaminergic activity and relatively increased cholinergic activity in the basal ganglia that occur because of degeneration of nigrostriatal dopaminergic projections and preservation of striatal cholinergic interneurons. A prominent symptom is akinesia. Huntington's disease is a state characterized pharmacologically by degeneration of GABA and cholinergic neurons in the striatum, with relative preservation of dopaminergic connections. A prominent symptom is chorea, which is described later in this section. Parkinson's disease and Huntington's disease represent opposite extremes of basal ganglia dysfunctional states.

Parkinson's disease, or paralysis agitans, is a common condition associated with degenerative changes (neuronal degeneration and depigmentation) in the substantia nigra and locus ceruleus. The pathologic changes in the substantia nigra involve dopaminergic neurons that project to the striatum and thus lead to the depletion of dopamine in the caudate nucleus and putamen. The depletion of dopamine leads to complex changes in the activity of striatal projection neurons. Striatal projections to the internal segment of the globus pallidus and the substantia nigra pars reticulata become less active in Parkinson's disease whereas projections to the external segment of the globus pallidus become more active. The result is loss of inhibition (disinhibition) of the output neurons of the basal ganglia, which are inhibitory, and consequently, *increased* inhibition of thalamocortical neurons.

Patients with Parkinson's disease develop akinesia, rigidity, and tremor. The akinesia is manifested as difficulty in initiating and performing volitional movements of the most common type, including standing, walking, eating, and writing. The lines of the patient's face are smooth, the expression is fixed (the so-called "masked face"), and there is little overt evidence of spontaneous emotional responses. The patient stands with the head and shoulders stooped and walks with short, shuffling steps. The arms are held at the sides and do not automatically swing in rhythm with the legs as they should. Although patients have difficulty in starting to take their first steps, once under way, the pace becomes more and more rapid, and patients have trouble in stopping the progress on reaching their goal. This abnormality of walking is termed a **festinating gait**. Rigidity of the limbs (i.e., increased resistance to passive movement) is present in most patients with Parkinson's disease and often consists of cogwheel rigidity. When the examiner passively flexes or extends one of the patient's extremities, an increased resistance occurs that suddenly gives way and then returns sequentially as the movement continues, in the manner of a cogwheel. The muscle stretch (deep tendon) reflexes usually are normal. The tremor of Parkinson's disease typically occurs when the patient is at rest and consists of 4- to 6-cycle-per-second flexion–extension movements of the fingers and wrists, at times in the form of a "pill-rolling" movement. Treatment of Parkinson's disease consists of the administration of medications that enhance the dopaminergic activity of the basal ganglia. Surgical therapy, consisting of the placement of a lesion in the ventrolateral nucleus of the thalamus, was used extensively in the past in the treatment of Parkinson's disease. A resurgence of interest in surgical treatment has resulted from the finding that patients become less responsive to medications over time. Currently, surgical therapy is directed at the globus pallidus rather than the thalamus.

A severe form of parkinsonism has been described in young adults who have taken intravenous recreational drugs. Improper synthesis of a synthetic heroinlike compound results in the production of 1-methyl-4-phenyl-1,2,3,6-tetrahydropyridine (MPTP). This drug causes severe degeneration of the dopaminergic neurons of the substantia nigra.

Basal ganglia diseases result not only in **hypokinetic movement** disorders such as Parkinson's disease, but also in **hyperkinetic movement** disorders such as **chorea, athetosis**, and **hemiballismus**. The hyperkinetic movement disorders are thought to share a pathophysiologic mechanism consisting of decreased activity of the subthalamic nucleus. Decreased subthalamic nucleus function can result from destruction of the structure (as in hemiballismus) or from dysfunction of a selective group of subthalamic neurons projecting to the external segment of the globus pallidus. The ultimate effect is loss of excitatory activity of the subthalamic nucleus on neurons of the internal segment of the globus pallidus and substantia nigra pars reticulata, and consequent **disinhibition** of thalamocortical neurons.

Chorea is a movement disorder that can result from disease of the basal striatum. Choreiform movements consist of a rapid, irregular flow of motions, including "piano-playing" flexion–extension movements of the fingers, elevation and depression of the shoulders and hips, crossing and uncrossing of the legs, and grimacing movements of the face. **Sydenham's chorea** occurs in children as a complication of rheumatic fever, but the disease is self-limited and recovery is complete. **Huntington's disease** is a disorder inherited as an autosomal dominant trait characterized by progressive dementia and choreiform movements, usually beginning in adult life. The approximate site of the genetic locus responsible for this disease has been found. There are marked degenerative changes in the basal ganglia, particularly in the caudate nucleus and putamen. There is profound destruction of striatonigral GABAergic neurons. The choreic movements are thought to result from relatively excessive activity of the preserved nigrostriatal dopaminergic neurons, with decreased activity of GABAergic neurons. This idea is compatible with the observations that L-dopa worsens the chorea in Huntington's disease and that excessive L-dopa given to parkinsonian patients can induce choreic movements. **Hemichorea** consists of choreiform movements limited to one side of the body, usually resulting from a vascular lesion of the contralateral basal ganglia. The disorder usually occurs abruptly in middle age and often is accompanied by weakness of the affected limbs.

Athetosis is a movement disorder characterized by slow, writhing movements of a wormlike character involving the extremities, trunk, and neck. Athetosis often occurs in association with **dystonia**, which is the abnormal persistence of limb and trunk postures. Athetosis is frequently seen in patients with cerebral palsy and results from brain damage that occurred at birth as a result of hypoxia and ischemia. The pathologic changes involve the cerebral cortex and the basal ganglia.

Hemiballismus is a movement disorder characterized by the onset of continuous, wild, flinging motions of the arm and leg on one side of the body. The onset is often sudden and results most often from a vascular lesion of the contralateral subthalamic nucleus.

CHAPTER

19

Vision

For vision to occur, reflected rays of light from an object must strike the eye, be refracted by the **cornea** and **lens**, and form an image on the retina. The optical properties of the lens invert and reverse the projection of the visual field on the retina; the image that is formed is upside-down (inverted) and turned left-for-right (reversed). Thus, the superior half of the visual field is projected on the inferior half of the retina, and the inferior half of the visual field is projected on the superior half of the retina. The left half of the visual field is projected on the right (nasal) half of the left retina and right (temporal) half of the right retina (see Fig. 60, colored lines), and this information is conveyed to the right cerebral hemisphere. The reverse is true for the right half of the visual field. The entire visual path within the brain is organized in a fashion that conforms to the peripheral optical system, so that the right hemisphere is presented with upside-down images of objects that lie to the left. This apparent distortion of position, however, is matched by the organization of other systems of the brain. Thus, the motor areas of the frontal lobes and the body image contained in the somesthetic zones of the parietal lobe also are inverted and reversed.

THE VISUAL PATHWAY

The human retina develops from the optic cup, which is an outgrowth of the diencephalon. Thus, the retina is an extension of the central nervous system. It contains two types of photoreceptors: **rods** and **cones**. Cones mediate color vision and provide high visual acuity. Rods mediate light perception; they provide low visual acuity with good perception of contrasts and are used chiefly in nocturnal vision. The **fovea centralis** within the **macula** is a specialized region in the retina adapted for high visual acuity; it contains the highest density of cones in the retina.

Both rods and cones respond to light because they contain visual pigments that are capable of trapping photons of light. In rods, the pigment is **rhodopsin**. Three different types of cones are characterized by three different forms of **iodopsin**, each of which absorbs light maximally in a different part of the visible light spectrum (i.e., light of a different color). The absorption of light by the visual pigments in both rods and cones isomerizes the pigment molecules. A cascade of chemical reactions initiated by this isomerization decreases the sodium conductance of the receptor cell membrane, which leads to a slow hyperpolarization, or a graded potential, across the cell. Although graded potentials are not as common as action potentials for transmitting information in the central nervous system, they are the characteristic mode of transmission in most retinal cells.

The five basic cell types in the retina and their interconnections are illustrated in simplified form in Figure 59. As this illustration shows, the activity of several **rods** converges onto single bipolar cells, which influence ganglion cells through the amacrine cell interneurons, whereas individual **cones** are connected singly and directly through bipolar cells to ganglion cells. The graded potentials through which these cells interact are generated at both electrical and chemical synapses, where

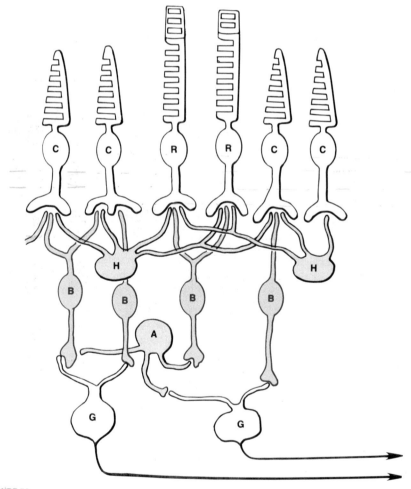

FIGURE 59

Five basic cell types form the circuitry of the retina. A = amacrine cell; B = bipolar cell; C = cone receptor cell; G = ganglion cell; H = horizontal cell; R = rod receptor cell.

numerous neurotransmitters have been identified. The **receptor cells** and **bipolar cells** are thought to use the excitatory amino acid glutamate at their chemical synapses as they transmit visual signals to the ganglion cells. The intervening interneurons, the **horizontal** and **amacrine** cells, transmit signals in all directions equally well, and apparently exert inhibitory actions by release of gamma-aminobutyric acid (GABA), although they also contain several other important neurotransmitter molecules, including dopamine, acetylcholine, and various neuropeptides.

The functional circuits that connect rods and cones to the **ganglion cells** process information about the color and contrast of images that fall on the retina. Thus, the

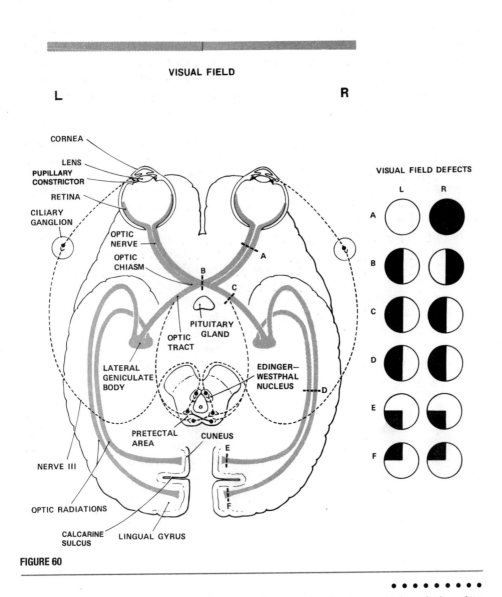

FIGURE 60

The visual pathways. Lesions along the pathway from the eye to the visual cortex (A through F) result in deficits in the visual fields shown as black areas on the corresponding visual field diagrams. The pathway through the pretectum and cranial nerve III, which mediates reflex constriction of the pupil in response to light, is also shown.

action potentials generated by ganglion cells provide highly processed information about visual images to the thalamus and brain stem. The axons of ganglion cells on the entire inner surface of the retina converge at the **optic disk**, where they exit from the eye, become myelinated, and form the **optic nerve** (Fig. 60). Axons from the macula, where visual acuity is sharpest, enter the temporal (lateral) side of the optic disk. Optic nerve fibers pass directly to the **optic chiasm**, which is located at the anterior part of the sella turcica of the sphenoid bone, immediately above the pituitary gland. A partial decussation (crossing) of fibers takes place in the chiasm. Fibers from the nasal halves of each retina cross; those from the temporal halves of each retina approach the chiasm and leave it without crossing. Optic fibers continue without any interruption behind the chiasm as two diverging **optic tracts** that go to the left and right lateral geniculate nuclei of the thalamus. The fibers in front of the chiasm are designated as optic nerves, while those behind it are the optic tracts. Optic fibers terminate in the **lateral geniculate bodies (LGBs)**, the **superior colliculus**, and the **pretectal area**, as well as other locations.

Large numbers of fibers in the optic nerve terminate in the LGBs. Each LGB receives inputs from the retina in an orderly, or topographic, pattern representing the contralateral visual half-field. In other words, ganglion cells in adjacent areas of the retina project systematically on adjacent neurons in the LGB. However, the visual field is not reconstructed equally in the LGB; the central visual field is represented more extensively than the peripheral field. Each LGB contains six layers of neurons, and each layer receives input from one eye only. The optic tract fibers originating in the ipsilateral eye distribute only to layers 2, 3, and 5 of the six layers; those from the contralateral eye distribute to the remaining three layers, 1, 4, and 6. Thus, there are no lateral geniculate cells with binocular receptive fields.

The **superior colliculus** receives direct visual input from the optic tracts and also projections from neurons in the visual cortex. The neurons in the superior colliculus receiving visual input project to motoneurons in the pons and spinal cord by way of the tectopontine and tectospinal tracts, respectively. The tectopontine projection relays visual information to the cerebellum. The tectospinal tract mediates the reflex control of head and neck movements in response to visual inputs. The superior colliculus also participates in the control of eye movements through projections to the paramedian pontine reticular formation (see Chap. 20).

The **pretectal area** is an important site for the mediation of pupillary reflexes. It is located just rostral to the superior colliculus, where the midbrain fuses with the thalamus. The pretectal area receives input from the optic tract (see Fig. 60). Pretectal neurons project into the mesencephalon, reaching the **Edinger-Westphal** nucleus, a component of the oculomotor complex bilaterally. Preganglionic parasympathetic neurons in the Edinger-Westphal nuclei project with the third nerve out of the brain stem to neurons in the **ciliary ganglion**. Ciliary postganglionic fibers project to the pupillary constrictor muscles and to the ciliary muscles, which control the shape of the lens. The reflexes mediated by the pretectal area are described in Chapter 20.

Neurons of the LGB give rise to fibers that form the **geniculocalcarine tract (optic radiations)** to the cortex of the occipital lobes. The radiating fibers from the lateral part of each LGB are directed downward and forward initially, they then bend backward in a sharp loop and form a flat band that passes through the temporal lobe in the lateral wall of the inferior horn of the lateral ventricle and sweep posteriorly to the occipital lobe. Fibers from the medial portion of the LGB travel adjacent to those from the lateral LGB but take a more direct, nonlooping course to the

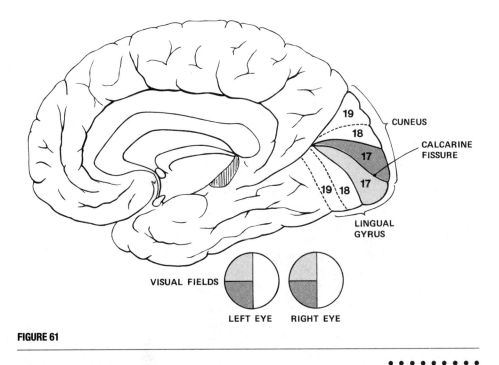

FIGURE 61

• • • • • • • • •

The visual cortex on the medial surface of the occipital lobe of the right hemisphere. Note that this brain area receives input from stimuli in the left half of the visual field of each eye.

occipital lobe. The area of cortex that receives the optic radiations surrounds the **calcarine fissure** (sulcus) on the medial side of the occipital lobe. The **cuneus**, which is the gyrus above the calcarine fissure, receives visual impulses from the dorsal, or upper, quadrant of the ipsilateral side of both retinas (this corresponds to the lower quadrant of the contralateral visual field); the **lingual gyrus**, below the calcarine fissure, receives impulses that arise from the ventral, or lower, quadrants of the retinas (Fig. 61). The **primary visual receptive area** (Brodmann's area 17) is also called the **striate area** because histologic sections of the cortex reveal a horizontal stripe of white matter (Gennari's line) within the gray matter. This stripe is created by the large number of myelinated fibers in layer IV of the cortex and is visible to the naked eye. Fibers from the LGB to the cortex maintain their topographic arrangement so that a retinal map is represented on the receptive areas of the cortex. The information from the upper quadrant of the left half of the visual field is projected onto the lower right quadrant of the retina, from there to the lateral portion of the right LGB, and from the LGB to the right visual cortex below the calcarine sulcus (see Figs. 60 and 61). The information within this quadrant is further organized so that the central retinal stimuli are projected to the posterior part of area 17, at the occipital pole. More peripheral visual stimuli reach the anterior part of area 17. Areas 18 and 19, which surround area 17, are important regions for visual perception (i.e., visual sensory processing). Areas 18 and 19 also play a role in visually guided saccades, ocular pursuit movements, accommodation, and convergence through connections with the frontal lobes and the midbrain. Areas 18 and 19 are the proximal **visual association areas**.

INFORMATION PROCESSING
IN THE VISUAL PATHWAYS

· · · · · · · · ·

Ganglion cells in the retina respond when light strikes the retina, and the most effective stimulus for each ganglion cell is a spot of light focused on a specific, small area of the retina. This area is termed the **receptive field** of a ganglion cell and is defined as the area in the retina that, on stimulation with light, induces maximal excitation or inhibition of the firing pattern of that ganglion cell. There are two types of **ganglion cells**: **on-center** and **off-center**. On-center cells have a central excitatory zone and an inhibitory surround (i.e., shining a focused beam of light in the center of the receptive field causes excitation of the cell, and shining a beam of light in a doughnut-shaped area around the center of the field causes inhibition of the cell). Off-center ganglion cells have reverse properties; they are inhibited when light falls on the center of their receptive fields and excited by illumination of the surrounding area. Diffuse light does not excite ganglion cells. Thus, ganglion cells are sensitive chiefly to contrasts.

Like ganglion cells, neurons in the lateral geniculate body respond to small spots of light and show on-center and off-center receptive fields. These neurons also do not respond to diffuse illumination.

The behavior of neurons in the striate cortex is more complex than that of neurons in the lateral geniculate body. Small spots of light are minimally effective in altering neuronal discharge; optimal light for cortical cell excitation must have linear properties (i.e., consist of a short line, a bar, or some other configuration with a clear edge). The stimuli also must have a specific axis of rotation. For an individual striate neuron, for example, a perfectly vertical bar of light falling on a specific part of the retina may be ineffective, but an oblique bar of light at a particular angle to the vertical falling on that same part of the retina is effective in altering neuronal discharge.

The functional organization of the visual cortex is based on narrow vertical columns of neurons running from the cortical surface to the white matter. Within each column, all of the neurons respond to bars or slits of light in essentially identical receptive field locations and with the same axis of rotation, but primarily from only one of the two eyes **(ocular dominance)**. The columns are arranged with respect to each other so that, in a series of adjacent columns, the neurons respond successively to a shifting axis of rotation of the visual stimulus. Neurons in an adjacent series of columns (forming a stripe) have all the same receptive field properties but are primarily activated by stimulation of the other eye. Neurons in the peristriate cortex (areas 18 and 19) also respond to edges of light, but the stimuli required to activate these neurons are more complex than those needed to activate most striate neurons.

Several separate streams of visual information flow from the retina to the LGB and then on to the striate cortex. The two major streams are named on the basis of the neurons in the LGB that process information. The **magnocellular stream** begins with large cells of the retinal ganglion cell layer (termed **Y-cells)** that project to the magnocellular layers (layers 1 and 2) of the LGB, which, in turn, project to the striate cortex. Most cortical neurons of the magnocellular stream respond to movement, orientation, and contrast, and do not respond to color. Thus, the magnocellular stream processes information required to locate quickly a moving object in visual space. The **parvocellular stream** begins with small cells of the retinal ganglion layer (termed **X-cells)** that project to the parvocellular layers of the LGB (layers 3 through 6). The parvocellular layers also project to the striate cortex. There are two functionally distinct types of cortical neurons of the parvocellular stream: those responsive to shape and orientation and those responsive to color.

EFFECTS OF LESIONS INTERRUPTING THE VISUAL PATHWAY

• • • • • • • • •

The **visual fields** can be measured in detail by tangent screen or perimetry. They can also be examined for defects at the bedside by using the **confrontation method**. While the patient fixes his or her gaze straight ahead, the examiner faces the patient and fixes on the patient's eyes. The patient covers one eye so that only a single eye is examined at one time. The examiner then introduces an object, usually a 4-mm white ball, from some point halfway between the examiner and the patient but beyond the normal periphery of vision and moves it slowly toward the line of vision. The examiner notes the points at which the object is first seen both in his or her own visual field and in the patient's visual field. After repeating the process in several directions, the examiner makes an estimate of the extent of the patient's field of vision. The examiner depicts the information obtained from this examination by drawing the patient's visual fields on paper. By convention, the visual fields are drawn from the patient's perspective. The confrontation method of testing the visual fields can also be used to screen the fields quickly for a gross defect. This is done by having the patient fix his or her gaze on the examiner's eye while the other eye is covered. The examiner then moves his or her index finger quickly in each visual quadrant, asking the patient to tell the examiner when a movement has occurred. The examiner can also ask the patient to count the number of fingers (usually 1 to 3) that the examiner holds up in each visual quadrant.

In Figure 60, the visual field defects are depicted as a patient with lesions in sites A to F would experience them. With partial damage of the optic nerves, both visual fields may be contracted, or a centrally located region with loss of vision may be found in each eye. Restricted visual fields, without any organic lesions, are encountered in some psychoneurotic patients, to whom everything appears as if viewed through twin gun barrels. These patients, however, do not stumble over objects, and if their visual fields are measured accurately on repeated occasions, gross inconsistencies may be demonstrated.

Complete destruction of one optic nerve produces blindness in the involved eye (see Fig. 60, lesion A). Some disease processes involving the optic nerves can affect some fibers but spare others, and instead of total blindness, there usually are areas of lost function in the central or peripheral parts of the fields of vision of each eye. An area of depressed function in the visual field is called a **scotoma**.

Lesions of the middle part of the optic chiasm frequently result from compression of these fibers by a tumor of the pituitary gland or from a craniopharyngioma lying near the midline immediately behind the chiasm. The decussating fibers of the optic nerves are injured, and visual impulses from the nasal halves of each retina are blocked. As a result, the left eye does not perceive images in the left half of its visual field, and the right eye does not perceive images in the right half of its visual field. The defect is in the temporal field of each eye and is therefore called **bitemporal hemianopia** (see Fig. 60, lesion B). The term hemianopia means that one half of the visual field is lost, and in the example shown in lesion B, the field defect respects the vertical meridian. The term bitemporal indicates that both temporal fields are affected. The term **heteronymous** might also be used in this case to indicate that both temporal fields are affected, as opposed to both right or both left fields, which would be a **homonymous defect**. Note that visual defects are always described with reference to the change in the **visual fields**.

A lesion of the optic tract disconnects fibers from one half of each retina. If the right optic tract is destroyed, visual function is lost in the right halves of both retinas. The result is blindness for objects in the left half of each field of vision, a condition known as left **homonymous hemianopia** (see Fig. 60, lesion C).

A lesion of the optic radiation usually results in a homonymous hemianopia (see Fig. 60, lesion D). Although the fiber bundles from the superior and inferior halves of the retina are separate in the optic radiation, the bundles are so close that they are rarely if ever damaged singly.

Lesions that destroy the entire visual area of the right occipital lobe also produce a left homonymous hemianopia. Visual acuity is not affected in the parts of the retina whose functions remain, and the patient may not be aware of the presence of a hemianopia. With small lesions in the occipital lobe, there may be **macular sparing**, which is preservation of central vision in the otherwise blind half of the visual field. The reason that macular sparing occurs is not known, but many experts believe that it results from the extensive representation of macular vision at the occipital pole and in the depths of the calcarine fissure.

As mentioned previously, the cuneus receives visual impulses from the upper halves of the retinas, and the lingual gyrus receives impulses from the lower halves (see Figs. 60 and 61). Thus, a lesion that is confined to the right lingual gyrus cuts off visual impulses from the lower part of the right half of each retina. This produces a loss of vision in one quadrant rather than a hemianopia. In this instance, an upper left quadrant visual field defect is found because the images that are focused on the lower part of the retina come from objects above the horizontal line (see Fig. 60F).

CHAPTER

20

Optic Reflexes and Eye Movements

LIGHT REFLEX

• • • • • • • • •

The normal pupil constricts promptly when light is flashed into the eye and dilates when the light is removed. This is the **direct light reflex**. The sensory receptors for this reflex are the rods and cones of the retina. The afferent pathway follows the course of the visual fibers through the retina, optic nerve, and optic tract almost to the lateral geniculate bodies, but instead of entering the geniculate body, the reflex fibers turn in the direction of the superior colliculus. They end in a region rostral to the superior colliculus known as the **pretectal area** (see Fig. 60 in Chap. 19). Interneurons located in this region send axons around the cerebral aqueduct to the **Edinger-Westphal nucleus**, a group of parasympathetic neurons in a rostral subdivision of the oculomotor nuclear complex. The efferent path begins with cells in the Edinger-Westphal nucleus whose **axons** leave the midbrain in the oculomotor nerve and end in the parasympathetic **ciliary ganglion**. Postganglionic fibers coming from the ganglion enter the eyeball and supply the sphincter muscle in the iris, which constricts the pupil when it contracts. When light is shined into one eye, the pupillary constriction of the ipsilateral eye (the **direct light reflex)** is accompanied by constriction of the pupil of the contralateral eye. This is the **consensual light reflex**. It is accomplished by crossing connections in the pathway at the level of the pretectum (see Fig. 60 in Chap. 19).

The direct light reflex is abolished by diseases that severely damage the retina or the optic nerve. Lesions of the visual pathway that are located in the optic tract, lateral geniculate bodies, optic radiations, or visual cortex of one side, however, do not interfere with this reflex. Even in cortical blindness produced by complete destruction of the primary visual areas of both occipital lobes, the direct and consensual light reflexes are preserved. The efferent path for the light reflex may be interrupted by damage to the oculomotor nuclear complex, the oculomotor nerve, or the ciliary ganglion. Neither a direct nor a consensual light reflex can be obtained on the affected side when the efferent path for the light reflex is interrupted.

The pupillary reflexes are important clinically. If light shined into one eye of a patient evokes a consensual response but no direct response, the afferent (receptive) limb of the reflex is intact but the efferent (effector) limb is defective, probably because of a third-nerve lesion of the eye being tested. If light shined into one eye evokes no direct or consensual response, but light shined into the opposite eye evokes both a direct and a consensual response, the afferent limb of the reflex is impaired in the first eye tested, most often because of a lesion in the retina or the optic nerve.

REFLEXES ASSOCIATED WITH THE NEAR-POINT REACTION

• • • • • • • • •

When the eyes are directed to an object close to the face, three different reflex responses are brought into cooperative action.

1. **Convergence**. The medial rectus muscles contract to move both eyes toward the midline so that the image in each eye remains focused on the fovea (the area of highest acuity within the macula). Without convergence, diplopia (i.e., double vision) occurs.
2. **Accommodation**. The lenses are thickened as a result of contraction of the **ciliary muscles**. This maintains a sharply focused image on the foveas. The ciliary muscles, like the pupillary sphincter, are innervated by postganglionic parasympathetic neurons in the ciliary ganglia.
3. **Pupillary constriction**. The pupils are narrowed as an optical aid to regulate the depth of focus. This constriction does not depend on any change in illumination and is regulated separately from the light reflex. The pathway mediating the pupillary response to accommodation and convergence reactions involves the optic nerve, optic tract, lateral geniculate body, optic radiations, occipital cortex, corticotectal projections, superior colliculus, Edinger-Westphal nucleus, oculomotor nerve, and ciliary ganglion. Pupillary responses to accommodation and convergence are separate phenomena in that pupillary constriction accompanies accommodation even when convergence is prevented by prisms, and it accompanies convergence when accommodation is eliminated by plus lenses.

All three reactions may be initiated by voluntarily directing the gaze to a near object, but an involuntary (reflex) mechanism will accomplish the same result if an object is moved slowly toward the eyes.

ADIE'S TONIC PUPIL AND ARGYLL ROBERTSON PUPIL

• • • • • • • •

Adie's tonic pupil is a benign condition often seen in young people, usually those younger than 30 years of age, consisting of a unilaterally dilated pupil, often in association with absent deep tendon reflexes. Over time, the pupil tends to become small and may appear to be an Argyll Robertson pupil (discussed later). Adie's tonic pupil shows minimal constriction to light, better constriction to a near target, and a pathologically slow ("tonic") redilatation. The pupil responds normally to drugs that cause **miosis** (constriction of the pupil) and **mydriasis** (dilation of the pupil). Adie's tonic pupil, however, constricts rapidly on instillation of 0.1 percent pilocarpine in the conjunctival sac, whereas the normal pupil does not respond to this drug.

Adie's tonic pupil results from a lesion of the parasympathetic postganglionic fibers of the ciliary ganglion or nerves. Most often, the cause is presumed to be viral. Orbital trauma or surgery also may be implicated.

In a clinical disorder of pupillary function known as the **Argyll Robertson pupil**, the pupil does not react to light but does react to accommodation. The pupil is small (usually 1 to 2 mm in diameter) and irregular, and usually does not dilate in response to the administration of atropine. The Argyll Robertson pupil results from syphilis of the central nervous system, but it can occur with other conditions, including diabetes mellitus. The site of the lesion causing the altered responses of the Argyll Robertson pupil is unclear. The region of the gray matter around the cerebral aqueduct was thought to be responsible, but more recently, damage to the ciliary ganglion or the iris has been implicated.

VISUAL FIXATION

• • • • • • • • •

Four visual subsystems are available to visualize an object in the optimal portion of the retina (the fovea) to permit scrutiny and keep the object in the optimal portion as the object or viewer moves. These subsystems include (1) **saccadic**, consisting of movement of the foveas to track a moving object by fast conjugate eye movements called "saccades"; (2) **pursuit**, which consists of slow conjugate eye movements to track a moving object; (3) **vergence**, involving converging or diverging the eyes to keep both foveas aligned to a target that moves closer or farther away; and (4) **vestibuloocular**, which uses vestibular signals to move the eyes in an equal and opposite direction if the viewer's head or body moves. These subsystems have distinct pathways and functional characteristics. They can be both stimulated and injured separately.

SACCADIC EYE MOVEMENTS

• • • • • • • • •

The **saccadic subsystem** locks the fovea on a target rapidly and accurately, establishing refixation. It can be assessed clinically by asking a patient to look in a particular direction at an object or directly at a stationary light. There are several types of saccades, which are divided into two classes: voluntary and involuntary. **Voluntary saccades** are willed eye movements searching for a target perceived on the peripheral retina ("visually guided") or an unseen or remembered target ("non–visually guided"). **Involuntary saccades** are spontaneous random eye movements, the saccades of rapid eye movement (REM) sleep, and the quick phases of nystagmus. **Visually guided voluntary saccades** are initiated principally by the cerebral cortex at the parietooccipital junction and visual cortex. **Non–visually guided volun-**

tary saccades are initiated mainly by the cerebral cortex of the frontal eye fields (Brodmann's area 8), with participation by the supplementary motor cortex and the prefrontal eye fields. The frontal eye fields and the parietooccipital junction are interconnected, and each can activate both kinds of voluntary saccades. **Involuntary saccades** are initiated in the brain stem, chiefly in the burst cells of the pons and mesencephalon.

For both visually guided and non–visually guided voluntary saccades, neuronal activity from the cerebral cortex travels downward to the contralateral pontine paramedian reticular formation (PPRF) (Fig. 62A). Impulse streams from the frontal eye field move directly to the PPRF, and impulses from the parietooccipital junction

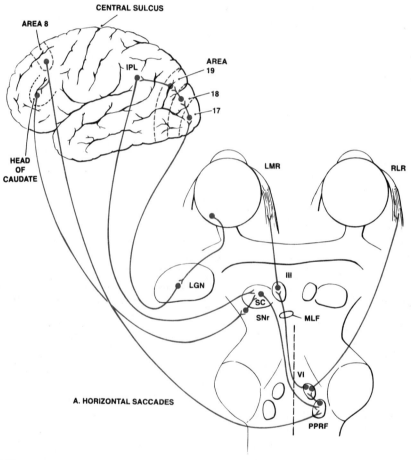

FIGURE 62

• • • • • • • • •

Pathways for visually guided and non–visually guided saccadic eye movements. Only eye movements to the right, which are initiated in the left cerebral hemisphere, are illustrated. (*A*) horizontal saccade pathways; (*B*) downward saccade pathways; (*C*) upward saccade pathways; INC = interstitial nucleus of Cajal; IPL = inferior parietal lobule; LGN = lateral geniculate nucleus; LIO = left inferior oblique muscle; LMR = left medial rectus muscle; LSO = left superior oblique muscle; MLF = medial longitudinal fasciculus; PC = posterior commissure; PPRF = paramedian pontine reticular formation; riMLF = rostral interstitial nucleus of the MLF; RIR = right inferior rectus muscle; RLR = right lateral rectus muscle; RSR = right superior rectus; SC = superior colliculus; SNr = substantia nigra reticulata; III = oculomotor nucleus; IV = trochlear nucleus; VI = abducens nucleus.

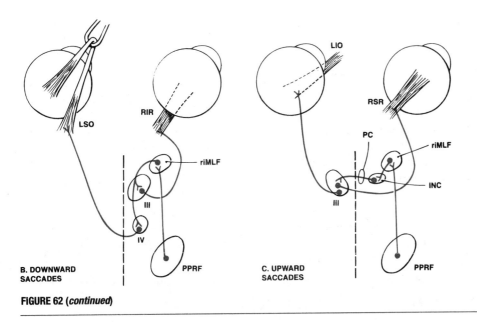

B. DOWNWARD SACCADES

C. UPWARD SACCADES

FIGURE 62 (*continued*)

synapse in the superior colliculus before moving on to the PPRF. An important downward pathway from the frontal eye field through the caudate nucleus to the substantia nigra pars reticulata and then to the superior colliculus provides inhibition that prevents this nucleus from responding to extraneous visual stimuli.

For horizontal gaze (see Fig. 62A), PPRF burst cells send signals to the nucleus of cranial nerve VI, where they synapse on both abducens motor neurons and on interneurons. Signals for horizontal ocular gaze proceed via abducens motor neurons to the lateral rectus muscle and through abducens interneurons through the medial longitudinal fasciculus (MLF) to the contralateral nucleus of cranial nerve III (the medial rectus subnucleus). For upward gaze (see Fig. 62C), PPRF impulses travel to the rostral interstitial nucleus of the medial longitudinal fasciculus (riMLF) in the mesencephalon. Burst cells in the riMLF send signals to the interstitial nucleus of Cajal and then through the posterior commissure to end on the superior rectus subnucleus of cranial nerve III and, through a separate but nearby pathway, signals reach the inferior oblique subnucleus of the third nerve. For downward gaze (see Fig. 62B), the pathway from the PPRF to the riMLF is the same as for upward gaze but the pathway out of the riMLF is through more ventral portions of the mesencephalon and then into the inferior rectus subnucleus of the third nerve and the trochlear nucleus (IV).

Lesions of the saccadic pathway in humans cause saccades that are too small **(hypometric)**, too slow, inaccurate **(dysmetric)**, delayed in onset, or completely absent **(gaze palsy)**. Large, acute lesions of the cerebral hemisphere result in absent, small, or slow saccades in the direction contralateral to the side of the lesion. The eyes are often deviated toward the side of the lesion. The disorder is temporary because other pathways can compensate. Lesions of the basal ganglia cause slow, small, long-latency saccades, or excessive saccades apparently unrelated to purposeful behavior **(saccadic intrusions)**. Pontine lesions cause disturbances similar to those caused by cerebral lesions but affect eye movements toward the side of the lesion. Cerebellar lesions cause small, dysmetric saccades and difficulty maintaining eccentric gaze.

PURSUIT EYE MOVEMENTS

• • • • • • • • •

The **pursuit subsystem** maintains fixation on slowly moving targets. If it fails, saccades are needed to catch up with the target. The pursuit subsystem can be assessed clinically by having the patient follow a slowly moving finger or light. Pursuit movements are initiated by visual inputs to the parietooccipital junction. Signals then go to nuclei in the ipsilateral dorsolateral pons. The pathway then leads to the cerebellar vermis, the nucleus prepositus hypoglossi, the medial vestibular nucleus, and then to cranial nerve VI and the medial rectus subnucleus of cranial nerve III for horizontal pursuit. The pathway for vertical pursuit is to the mesencephalon, but the precise route is unknown. Lesions of the pursuit pathway in humans result in "cogwheel" or "saccadic" pursuit eye movements. This is thought to occur because the saccadic system is more durable and substitutes for the ineffective pursuit system.

VESTIBULOOCULAR MOVEMENTS

• • • • • • • • •

The **vestibuloocular subsystem** prevents the image of interest from moving away from the fovea **(image slip)** during head movements. The vestibuloocular subsystem is assessed by stimulating vestibular receptors with head movement, body rotation, or introduction of warm or cold water into the external auditory canal (caloric testing; see Chap. 16). The **head rotation test** is performed in alert patients with a full range of eye movements. Patients are asked to identify the smallest line possible on a Snellen visual acuity card, shake the head quickly, and read the same line in reverse order. If **acuity falls**, the vestibuloocular subsystem is deficient. A similar test, the passive head movement maneuver, also known as the **doll's eye, doll's head**, or **oculocephalic maneuver**, can be applied to patients with reduced excursions of the eyes or to patients in a coma. The examiner grasps the patient's head and turns it in the horizontal and vertical planes, noting whether the oppositely directed ocular excursions are greater than the voluntary excursions. If so, the lesion causing the gaze disturbances must be rostral to the brain stem gaze regions **(supranuclear gaze palsy)**. The same maneuver is used in unconscious patients to determine whether the vestibuloocular reflex pathway from the medulla to the midbrain is intact.

The pathway for the vestibuloocular subsystem begins with signals generated by the semicircular canals, which travel to the vestibular nuclei. Projections from the vestibular nuclei reach the nucleus of cranial nerve VI and the medial rectus subnucleus of cranial nerve III for horizontal eye movements, and the subnuclei of cranial nerves III and IV for vertical eye movements.

Lesions of the vestibuloocular pathway in humans result in the symptom of oscillopsia, which is a sense that visual images are "jiggling." If the disease destroys both vestibuloocular pathways, the eyes cannot remain fixed in space as the head moves, and the patient complains of "bouncy" or blurred vision. If the lesion interrupts only one vestibuloocular pathway, the vestibular system becomes unbalanced, and the patient has a rhythmic oscillation of the eyes called nystagmus. The patient may report oscillopsia, vertigo, or dysequilibrium.

VERGENCE EYE MOVEMENTS

• • • • • • • • •

The **vergence subsystem** allows the continual presence of the image of interest on the fovea as the object moves closer or farther away. The vergence subsystem is assessed by having the patient focus on distant and near targets. Activation of the vergence subsystem results from a blurred image or from an image falling on non-corresponding retinal areas. Signals in the occipitoparietal areas bilaterally are conveyed to the mesencephalon and from there to cranial nerves III and VI. The pathway is not understood. Lesions of the vergence system in humans usually are located in the diencephalon or mesencephalon and cause excessive or insufficient convergence or divergence and excessive accommodation.

CHAPTER

21

The Thalamus

THE DIENCEPHALON

• • • • • • • • •

The **diencephalon** consists of an ovoid mass of gray matter situated deep in the brain rostral to the midbrain. It is separated from the **lentiform nucleus** by the fibers of the **internal capsule**. On its ventral surface, it extends from the **optic chiasm** to and including the **mammillary bodies**. The rostral limit may be demarcated on a hemisected brain by a line between the **interventricular foramen** and the optic chiasm. The caudal extent is demarcated by a line from the **pineal body** to the caudal edge of the mammillary bodies (see Fig. 3 in Chap. 1). The third ventricle separates the right half of the diencephalon from the left half, and the tela choroidea forming the roof of this ventricle bears a choroid plexus. In most but not all human brains, the two halves of the diencephalon are joined at a small area called the **massa intermedia** or **interthalamic adhesion**. Each half of the diencephalon is divided into the following regions: thalamus, hypothalamus, subthalamus, and epithalamus.

The thalamus comprises the dorsal portion of the diencephalon. It is bounded medially by the wall of the third ventricle and laterally by the posterior limb of the internal capsule. It is separated from the hypothalamus below by the shallow **hypothalamic sulcus** on the wall of the third ventricle. A groove, the **terminal sulcus**, which contains the **stria terminalis** and terminal vein, separates the thalamus from the caudate nucleus along the dorsolateral margin of the thalamus.

The thalamus is subdivided into three unequal parts by the **internal medullary lamina**. This band of myelinated fibers demarcates the medial and lateral nuclear masses and bifurcates at its rostral extent to encompass the anterior nucleus (Fig. 63A). The **centromedian nucleus** and other **intralaminar nuclei** are enclosed within the internal medullary lamina in the center of the thalamus (Fig. 63B).

The thalamus serves as the station from which, after synaptic processing, neuronal activity from all types of peripheral sensory receptors, from the basal ganglia, and from the cerebellum is relayed to the cerebral cortex. It is an important general principle that thalamic nuclei projecting to a specific region of the cerebral cortex also receive afferents (corticothalamic fibers) from that same cortical region.

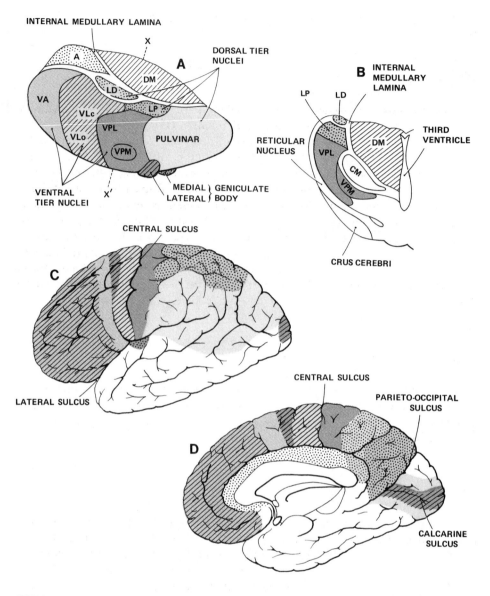

FIGURE 63

• • • • • • • • •

The thalamocortical connections in the human brain. (*A*) A dorsolateral view of the thalamus, which has been dissected from the left side of the brain, showing the boundaries of the major nuclei. The reticular nucleus has been omitted to expose the ventral nuclei. (*B*) A coronal section through the thalamus and subthalamus, showing the plane of a section through X to X' in A. Also shown is the centromedian nucleus (CM), which is one of the intralaminar nuclei. (*C*) The lateral surface of the cerebral cortex. Shaded and colored areas on the cortex designate the correspondingly shaded thalamic nuclei with which these cortical areas are interconnected. Note that the projection area of the ventral anterior nucleus (VA) covers the territory of the dorsomedial nucleus (DM) anteriorly and also overlaps with the territory of the ventral lateral pars caudalis (VLc) and the ventral lateral pars oralis (VLo) posteriorly. (*D*) The medial surface of the cerebral cortex. A = anterior nuclear group; LD = lateral dorsal nucleus; LP = lateral posterior nucleus; VPL = ventral posterolateral nucleus; VPM = ventral posteromedial nucleus.

THALAMIC NUCLEI AND THEIR CONNECTIONS

• • • • • • • • •

Medial Nuclear Mass

The **medial nuclear mass**, located medial to the internal medullary lamina, contains one major nucleus, the **dorsomedial nucleus (DM)** (see Fig. 63A and B), which is subdivided into **small-cell (parvicellular)** and **large-cell (magnocellular)** components. The small-cell portion has a reciprocal relation with the prefrontal cortex on the dorsal and lateral surfaces of the frontal lobe (Fig. 63C and D). This cortex is involved in sensory integration necessary for abstract thinking and long-term, goal-directed behavior. The large-cell component is interrelated with limbic structures, including the amygdala and the orbital portion of the frontal lobe. It also relays processed olfactory signals from the primary olfactory cortex (paleocortex) to the orbitofrontal cortex (neocortex). The dorsomedial nucleus has many interconnections with other thalamic nuclei, including the intralaminar and midline nuclei and the lateral thalamic nuclear mass. It is also one of the three thalamic nuclei through which the basal ganglia are connected with the cerebral cortex.

Midline Nuclei

The midline nuclei are diffuse, small nuclei located in the periventricular region surrounding the third ventricle and in the interthalamic adhesion. They are interconnected with structures in the basal ganglia and limbic system. These nuclei are not illustrated in Figure 63.

Anterior Thalamic Nucleus

The **anterior thalamic nucleus (A)** is actually a complex of three nuclei located in the conspicuous anterior tubercle of the thalamus (see Fig. 63A). This nucleus, in which the mammillothalamic tract and fibers from the hippocampal formation terminate (see Figs. 64 and 65 in Chap. 22), has reciprocal connections with the anterior part of the cingulate gyrus (see Fig. 63A and D and Fig. 65 in Chap. 22) and the hypothalamus. Like the magnocellular part of the dorsomedial nucleus, the anterior nucleus is an important relay nucleus in the limbic system, and because of its prominent connections with the hippocampal formation, its function is presumed to be related to attention, memory, and learning.

Intralaminar Nuclei

Intralaminar nuclei are numerous, small, diffuse collections of nerve cells within the internal medullary lamina. In the caudal aspect of the lamina, there are two circumscribed intralaminar nuclei that can be delineated: the **centromedian nucleus (CM,** see Fig. 63B), which lies adjacent to the ventral posterior complex, and the **parafascicular nucleus (PF)**, which is located immediately medial to the centromedian nucleus.

The intralaminar nuclei are considered to represent the rostral extent of the ascending reticular system. They are interconnected with other thalamic nuclei and receive bilateral input from the anterolateral system of the spinal cord (see Chap. 6).

The intralaminar nuclei are also integrated into the circuitry of the basal ganglia (see Figs. 57 and 58 in Chap. 18). The centromedian nucleus receives fibers from the globus pallidus and area 4 of the cerebrum and, in conjunction with the parafascicular nucleus, projects to the putamen and caudate nucleus. The parafascicular nucleus receives fibers from area 6 of the cerebrum. Axon collaterals of the parafascicular fibers to the putamen and caudate project onto the cerebral cortex.

Lateral Nuclear Mass

The **lateral nuclear mass**, located lateral to the internal medullary lamina, is subdivided into a dorsal and a ventral tier of nuclei (see Fig. 63A).

The **dorsal tier of nuclei** is closely related to the association areas of the cerebral cortex (see Chap. 24) and is involved in the integration of sensory information. The dorsal tier includes, in a rostrocaudal direction, the following nuclei:

1. The **lateral dorsal nucleus (LD)** can be considered the caudal extension of the **anterior thalamic nuclei (A)** and interconnects with the posterior part of the **cingulate gyrus** and the anterior part of the **precuneus** (see Fig. 63B and D).
2. The **lateral posterior nucleus (LP)** is reciprocally connected with the posterior aspect of the **precuneus** and the **superior parietal lobule** (areas 5 and 7) on the lateral surface of the hemisphere (see Fig. 63A, C, and D). It receives input from the superior colliculus and from other thalamic nuclei.
3. The **pulvinar nucleus** is the largest nucleus in the human thalamus. It is located in the posterolateral portion of the thalamus and connects reciprocally with large **association areas** of the parietal, temporal, and occipital lobes of the cerebral cortex. Similar to the lateral posterior nucleus, it receives input from the superior colliculus, retina, cerebellum, and the thalamic nuclei that relay sensory information.

In the **ventral tier of nuclei**, the more posterior nuclei are concerned with essentially all sensory modalities, including somatic sensation, vision, hearing, and taste. These nuclei integrate and transmit sensory information to the cerebral cortex. The more anterior nuclei of the ventral tier nuclei receive information from the basal ganglia, reticular formation, and cerebellum, processing the information and projecting it to the cerebral cortex, especially the motor areas of the cortex. The ventral tier of nuclei includes, in a rostrocaudal direction, the following nuclei:

1. The **ventral anterior nucleus (VA)** is subdivided into **small-** and **large-cell** populations. The large-cell component receives its input from the substantia nigra, and the small-cell portion receives fibers from the internal segment of the globus pallidus. The ventral anterior nucleus also receives fibers from other thalamic nuclei (intralaminar and midline) and the brain stem reticular formation. It projects diffusely to the frontal lobe, particularly to area 6, including the **premotor cortex** on the lateral surface of the hemisphere and the **supplementary motor cortex** located on the medial aspect of the superior frontal gyrus immediately rostral to area 4 (see Figs. 67 and 68 in Chap. 24).
2. The **ventral lateral nucleus (VL)** is similar to the ventral anterior nucleus in that it contains both **small-** and **large-cell components** that receive fibers from the

globus pallidus and substantia nigra, respectively. The projections from the basal ganglia terminate in the oralis (anterior) portion of the VL (VLo; see Fig. 63A). The caudal (posterior) part of the VL (VLc) receives a major input from the cerebellum. Thus, within the VL, the pallidal, nigral, and cerebellar afferents are segregated. The VL also receives fibers from other thalamic nuclei and the brain stem reticular formation. It is reciprocally connected to area 4 of the precentral gyrus, the **primary motor region**, and to the **premotor** and **supplementary motor regions** in area 6 of the cerebral cortex.

3. The **ventral posterior nuclear complex (VP)** is referred to as the ventrobasal complex by physiologists and consists of two major subdivisions: the **ventral posteromedial nucleus (VPM)**, which is also called the semilunar or arcuate nucleus, and the **ventral posterolateral nucleus (VPL)**. Some authorities include a third, smaller component, the **ventral posteroinferior nucleus (VPI)**, which is sandwiched between the VPL and VPM. The VP is the main somatosensory and taste region of the thalamus. Many of the cells in this complex are both place- and modality-specific and have small receptive fields. The VP is a synaptic station for the medial lemniscus, the gustatory pathways, the secondary trigeminal tracts, and part of the spinothalamic system. The sensory tracts from the head, including the gustatory pathways, terminate in the ventral posteromedial nucleus, whereas those from the remainder of the body synapse in the VPL. Consequently, the VP is **somatotopically organized**, such that the input from the lower portion of the body is most laterally represented and the input from the upper part is most medially represented. Taste fibers from the nucleus of the solitary tract terminate in the most medial part of the VPM. The VP projects primarily to the **postcentral gyrus** areas 3, 2, and 1, or the **primary somesthetic cortex**. The postcentral gyrus is also somatotopically organized such that the face is represented ventrolaterally (thus receiving the projection from the VPM), and the leg dorsomedially (receiving its input from the VPL). The VP, especially the neurons receiving gustatory information, also project to a region in the most ventral aspect of the precentral gyrus (the superior lip of the lateral or Sylvian fissure), which continues onto the anterior insular cortex. This gustatory region is continuous with the **secondary somesthetic** cortical areas caudally (see Fig. 70 in Chap. 24).

4. The **metathalamic nuclei** include the medial and lateral geniculate bodies.

   a. The **medial geniculate body (MGB)** lies adjacent to the superior colliculus and receives bilateral auditory impulses from the nucleus of the inferior colliculus (IC) and some fibers from more caudal auditory nuclei through the brachium of the inferior colliculus. It projects, through the auditory radiations, to the auditory cortex of the superior temporal gyrus, specifically to the **transverse gyrus of Heschl**, or area 41 (see Fig. 67 in Chap. 24).

   b. The **lateral geniculate body (LGB)** is the main portion of this nuclear complex in primates. It is reciprocally connected by way of the optic radiations (the geniculocalcarine tract) to the **visual cortex** of the occipital lobe (area 17), which is on the medial surface of the hemisphere (see Fig. 63; see also Figs. 60 and 61 in Chap. 19 and 67 and 68 in Chap. 24). The LGB also is interconnected with the pulvinar and other thalamic nuclei.

Thalamic Reticular Nucleus

The **thalamic reticular nucleus** is a thin layer of cells sandwiched between the posterior limb of the internal capsule and the external medullary lamina (see Fig. 63B).

It is actually a derivative of the ventral thalamus. There is disagreement regarding whether this nucleus should be considered part of the reticular system. It does not project fibers to the cerebral cortex; instead, it sends fibers to the thalamic nuclei, the brain stem reticular formation, and other parts of the thalamic reticular nucleus. Nearly all thalamic efferent fibers to the cortex must pass through this nuclear complex. In doing so, they send collaterals to its neurons. Similarly, corticothalamic projections to the thalamic nuclei send collaterals to the reticular nucleus. Thus, although it is not directly connected to the cortex, this nucleus monitors both thalamocortical and corticothalamic activity. Consequently, the reticular nucleus may be important in the regulation of thalamic activity, although its precise function has not been defined. The thalamic reticular nucleus has a large proportion of neurons containing gamma-aminobutyric acid (GABA), indicating that this nucleus probably has largely inhibitory effects.

FUNCTIONAL CATEGORIZATION OF THALAMIC NUCLEI

Functionally, the thalamic nuclei have been categorized as either specific or nonspecific. This nomenclature was based on electrophysiologic responses evoked in the cerebral cortex after stimulation of individual thalamic nuclei. "Nonspecific" nuclei were those that produced evoked potentials over large areas of the cortex, in contrast to localized responses following stimulation of "specific" nuclei.

A somewhat different way of categorizing thalamic nuclei, the anatomic nomenclature, is based on similarities in patterns of connections. In this system, three groups of nuclei are frequently identified.

1. **Specific nuclei** have reciprocal relations with areas of the cerebrum known to have specific sensory or motor functions. They receive an input from the ascending sensory pathways, basal ganglia, or cerebellum and include most of the ventral tier nuclei of the lateral nuclear mass: the lateral geniculate body, medial geniculate body, and ventral anterior, ventral lateral, and ventral posterior nuclei.
2. **Association nuclei** do not receive their major direct inputs from sensory or motor systems. They receive projections from other thalamic nuclei, including the specific nuclei, and have reciprocal connections with the association areas of the cerebral cortex. The main structures in this group are the dorsal tier nuclei in the lateral nuclear mass: the lateral dorsal, lateral posterior, and pulvinar nuclei. The parvicellular component of the dorsomedial nucleus and the anterior nuclei also are included.
3. **Subcortical nuclei** do not have reciprocal connections with the cerebral cortex. The best example is the thalamic reticular nucleus, although parts of other thalamic nuclei also lack direct cortical projections.

EPITHALAMUS

The epithalamus is the most dorsal division of the diencephalon. The major structures of this region are the pineal body (epiphysis), the habenular nuclei and habenular commissure, the posterior commissure, the striae medullaris, and the roof of the third ventricle.

The **pineal body** is the dorsal diverticulum of the diencephalon. It is a cone-shaped structure that overlies the tectum of the midbrain. Microscopically, the pineal body consists of glial cells (i.e., astrocytes) and parenchymal cells (i.e., pinealocytes). No neurons are present, but there is an abundance of nerve fibers that are the terminals of postganglionic sympathetic neurons in the superior cervical ganglion. Calcareous accumulations (i.e., corpora arenacea) are conspicuous features of the pineal body after middle age. Because the pineal body is normally a midline structure and its calcifications are often radiopaque, its position can be a useful diagnostic aid on routine skull radiographs. The function of the pineal body is better understood in other vertebrates than it is in the human. In many vertebrates, the secretions of the pinealocytes, including melatonin, are involved in the cyclical maintenance and regression of the gonads associated with seasonal breeding. The function of the pineal body in humans is not known.

The **habenular nuclei** are located in the dorsal margin of the base of the pineal body. Afferent fibers to the habenula originate in the septal area, the ventral pallidum (see Chap. 18), the lateral hypothalamus, and the brain stem, including the interpeduncular nucleus, the raphe nuclei, and the ventral tegmental area. The brain stem afferents reach the habenula in the **habenulopeduncular tract**, whereas the more rostral afferents are carried in the **stria medullaris**. The stria medullaris forms a small ridge on the dorsomedial margin of the thalamus. The efferent fibers of the habenula in the **habenulopeduncular tract**, or **fasciculus retroflexus**, are contained in a conspicuous, dense bundle that terminates in the interpeduncular nucleus in the ventral midline area of the midbrain. Fibers from the interpeduncular nucleus include ascending projections to the thalamus, hypothalamus, and septal area and descending fibers that terminate in the central gray matter and serotonergic raphe nuclei of the brain stem.

The **habenular commissure** consists of stria medullaris fibers crossing over to the contralateral habenular nuclei. The **posterior commissure**, located ventral to the base of the pineal body, carries decussating fibers of the superior colliculi and pretectum (visual reflex fibers), and possibly fibers from other sources.

CENTRAL PAIN ("THALAMIC SYNDROME")

• • • • • • • • •

Injury of the central nervous system, usually affecting the spinothalamic or trigeminothalamic tracts, can result in severe, spontaneous pain in portions of the body represented in the damaged tracts **(central pain)**. Often, central pain is triggered or worsened by cutaneous stimulation of the region of the body affected, although the pain can also occur without provocation. Commonly, the affected portions of the body have an elevated threshold to the perception of pain and temperature. Lesions of many portions of the central nervous system can lead to central pain, including the cerebral cortex, thalamus, brain stem, and spinal cord.

A frequently encountered form of central pain occurs after injury to the thalamus, which often results from vascular disease (stroke) and causes clearly recognizable symptoms. The VPL and the VPM are usually involved, and correspondingly, the patient develops a marked decrease of all modalities of sensation on the contralateral side of the body. Usually, the affected limbs are paralyzed because of damage to the corticospinal tract, which is located in the internal capsule adjacent to the thalamus. After a brief interval, generally several weeks, the patient develops a burning, agonizing pain in the affected parts of the body, worsened by any sort of sensory stimulation of the painful areas. The combination of hemianesthesia with spontaneous pain and hemiparesis is called the **thalamic syndrome**. Fortunately, medical therapy can sometimes relieve the pain that occurs with this syndrome. The thalamic syndrome results in one of the more severe forms of pain that follows damage to the central nervous system.

CHAPTER

22

The Hypothalamus and Limbic System

One of the major functions of the nervous system is to maintain the constancy of the internal environment of the body, a process termed **homeostasis**. Although essentially the entire brain participates in this process, neurons vitally important to homeostasis are concentrated in the **hypothalamus** and the **limbic system**. These neurons maintain homeostasis through three closely related processes: (1) the secretion of hormones, (2) central control of the autonomic nervous system, and (3) the development of emotional and motivational states. Hypothalamic and limbic structures also interact with neurons in the **reticular formation** and the neocortex for the maintenance of **arousal**, which is a general state of awareness.

THE HYPOTHALAMUS

• • • • • • • • •

The **hypothalamus**, in the ventral diencephalon, forms the floor and the ventral part of the walls of the third ventricle. The shallow **hypothalamic sulcus** on the wall of the third ventricle demarcates the hypothalamus from the thalamus.

The hypothalamus includes a number of well-defined structures. The **optic chiasm** is located in the rostral portion of the hypothalamic floor. The **tuber cinereum** is the portion of the hypothalamic floor between the optic chiasm and the mammillary bodies. The **infundibulum**, or stalk of the pituitary, extends ventrally from the tuber cinereum to the pars nervosa of the hypophysis. The lumen of the third ventricle may evaginate into the infundibulum for a variable distance, forming the infundibular recess (see Figs. 3 and 4 in Chap. 1). The **median eminence** is a part of the tuber cinereum and is located in the portion of the hypothalamic floor between the optic chiasm and the infundibulum. The **mammillary bodies** are paired, spherical nuclei located caudal to the tuber cinereum and rostral to the **posterior perforated substance**.

HYPOTHALAMIC NUCLEI

The hypothalamus is divided rostrocaudally into four regions: the **preoptic region**, which is most rostral; the **anterior hypothalamus**; the **tuberal region**; and the **mammillary region**, which is most caudal. The hypothalamus is also divided sagittally into three zones: periventricular, medial, and lateral. The **periventricular zone** is a narrow lamina of evenly distributed cells adjacent to the third ventricle. The suprachiasmatic, paraventricular, and arcuate nuclei are the most conspicuous cell groups within this narrow zone. The **medial zone**, in contrast, contains numerous, well-differentiated cell groups, which are described in the following sections of this chapter. The **lateral zone** is characterized by sparsely distributed neurons and, like the periventricular zone, contains only a few discrete nuclei, including the lateral tuberal nuclei. The boundary between the medial and lateral zones is a parasagittal plane through the fornix. The fornix is a bundle of fibers that connects the hypothalamus with the hippocampus. It enters the hypothalamus at the anterior commissure and passes ventrolaterally to the mammillary bodies.

Although discrete nuclei can be identified in the human hypothalamus, particularly in the medial zone, little definitive information is available about their connections and functions. At present, neurophysiologists can do little more than make assumptions based on the study of brains of other mammals. These functional associations are described later in this chapter in the section entitled Hypothalamic and Limbic System Function.

The preoptic area is developmentally a part of the telencephalon, but it is histologically indistinguishable from the hypothalamus and is so closely associated with it functionally that many authorities describe it as part of the hypothalamus. The **preoptic area** consists of a periventricular zone, a **medial preoptic area** in the medial zone, and a **lateral preoptic area** in the lateral zone. This region forms the wall of the third ventricle from the lamina terminalis to an imaginary line running from the interventricular foramen to the midportion of the optic chiasm (see Fig. 3 in Chap. 1). Caudal to the preoptic area, and combined with it in some accounts of the hypothalamus, is the **anterior region**, which contains several distinctive nuclear groups, including the suprachiasmatic, supraoptic, and paraventricular nuclei, as well as the more diffuse anterior and lateral hypothalamic areas. The **suprachiasmatic nucleus** lies immediately dorsal to the center of the optic chiasm and receives input directly from the retina. The **supraoptic and paraventricular nuclei** of this area develop from the same anlage. Both of these nuclei include magnocellular neurosecretory cells with axons that terminate in the posterior pituitary, where they secrete oxytocin and vasopressin into the systemic circulation.

In the **tuberal region** of the human hypothalamus, the best-differentiated cell group is the **ventromedial nucleus**, which is surrounded by a cell-sparse capsule. Like its counterpart in other mammals, the ventromedial nucleus consists of two somewhat separate subnuclei. In the floor and ventral walls of the third ventricle, adjacent to the ventromedial nucleus, is the **arcuate nucleus**, which, like the other parts of the periventricular zone, plays a particularly important role in regulating the anterior pituitary. The **dorsomedial nucleus**, located above the ventromedial nucleus, and the adjacent lateral hypothalamic area are not easily delineated from one another, although within the lateral area lie the easily defined **lateral tuberal nuclei**.

In the **mammillary region**, the medial mammillary nucleus is the most prominent structure. The **mammillary bodies** are surrounded by the **tuberomammillary nuclei** and the **posterior hypothalamus**. A distinctive group of large cells in the lateral zone of the mammillary region blends rostrally with the lateral tuberal nuclei and caudally with the fields of Forel in the subthalamus. These cells constitute a caudal extension of the basal nucleus of Meynert and provide extensive cholinergic projections to the neocortex (see Chap. 25) and noncholinergic projections to the remaining allocortex. Other cells in this lateral hypothalamic group give rise to descending projections to the brain stem and spinal cord.

FIBER CONNECTIONS OF THE PREOPTIC AREA AND HYPOTHALAMUS

The hypothalamus is interconnected with the limbic system in the telencephalon, with cranial nerve nuclei and the reticular formation in the brain stem, and with the spinal cord.

Pathways connecting the hypothalamus with telencephalic limbic system structures include the stria terminalis, ventral amygdalofugal pathway, and fornix (see the Telencephalic Limbic System).

Connections with the brain stem and spinal cord follow a number of different fiber systems. The **medial forebrain bundle (MFB)** is probably the largest of these systems. It is a somewhat diffuse tract that extends from the septal area through the lateral hypothalamic zone to the brain stem, particularly to the reticular formation. Of particular importance are fibers arising from cells in the paraventricular nucleus and lateral hypothalamus that descend through the MFB to visceral sensory neurons (nucleus solitarius) and preganglionic parasympathetic nuclei in the brain stem (dorsal motor nucleus of the vagus and nucleus ambiguus) and to both sympathetic and parasympathetic cell groups in the spinal cord. Many fibers join the MFB and others leave it in all areas through which the tract travels. In other words, this system provides both afferent and efferent connections for the hypothalamus.

The brain stem is also connected with the hypothalamus by several smaller fiber bundles. The **mammillary peduncle** is a pathway carrying input from the tegmentum of the midbrain to the mammillary bodies; the **dorsal longitudinal fasciculus** parallels the MFB but passes through the medial zone of the hypothalamus.

The **fasciculus mammillary princeps** is a fiber bundle that arises from neurons of the mammillary body. These axons pass dorsally for a very short distance and then bifurcate into two collateral systems: **mammillothalamic tract**, which in humans is the much larger of the two, projects to the anterior nuclear group of the thalamus, and the **mammillotegmental tract** turns caudally and terminates in the tegmentum of the midbrain.

THE HYPOTHALAMUS AND RETICULAR FORMATION

● ● ● ● ● ● ● ● ●

The reticular formation consists of clusters of interconnected neurons throughout the brain stem, with projections to the spinal cord, hypothalamus, cerebellum, and cerebral cortex. In the medial reticular formation, many neurons have extensive axonal projections. Single large neurons with bifurcating ascending and descending axons reach both the hypothalamus and the spinal cord. Other neurons with only ascending or descending axonal projections are nonetheless integrated with each other within the reticular formation so that they also contribute to the distribution of its influence along the entire neuraxis.

The lateral part of the reticular formation contains many short-axon interneurons that integrate reflexes through the cranial nerve nuclei. In this capacity, the reticular formation can be viewed as the rostral extension of the interneuronal pool of the spinal cord.

The reticular formation is involved in the control of posture, visceral motor function, and sleep and wakefulness. An essential ingredient in motivational states controlled by the hypothalamus is the phenomenon of wakefulness. In experimental animals, lesions of the rostral (mesencephalic) reticular formation lead to constant behavioral stupor, whereas lesions of the caudal (pontine) reticular formation result in constant wakefulness. The reticular formation is also necessary for sleep to occur; although the complex circuitry responsible for sleep has been identified only partially, the nuclei of the pontine reticular formation are clearly important.

THE TELENCEPHALIC LIMBIC SYSTEM

• • • • • • • • •

The hypothalamus is central to the organization of the limbic system, which is a collection of interconnected but not contiguous structures in the telencephalon, diencephalon, and brain stem. In the telencephalon, these structures include the three cortical areas of the limbic lobe: the cingulate gyrus, the septal area, and the parahippocampal gyrus (see Chap. 1), as well as several gray matter areas beneath the limbic lobe cortex, including the amygdala and hippocampal formation, which lie deep to the cortex of the parahippocampal gyrus.

The Amygdala

The amygdala forms the **uncus** on the parahippocampal gyrus (see Fig. 5 in Chap. 1 and Fig. 56B in Chap. 18). It is a spherical mass of neurons that are subdivided into two functional units: the corticomedial and basolateral divisions.

The **corticomedial amygdala**, including the cortical, medial, and central nuclei, is interconnected with the olfactory bulb, olfactory cortex, hypothalamus, and brain stem. It also receives cortical information indirectly through the basolateral amygdala. Its connections with the hypothalamus and brain stem are established through the **stria terminalis** and the **ventral amygdalofugal pathway** (Fig. 64). Through these routes, the corticomedial amygdala modulates activity in both the autonomic nervous system and hypothalamic neurons that control pituitary function.

The **basolateral amygdala**, including the basal and lateral nuclei, receives highly processed sensory information from sensory association areas of the frontal, temporal, occipital, and insular lobes, and is reciprocally connected to limbic lobe cortex, orbitofrontal cortex, and temporal neocortex (see Chap. 24). The neuronal morphology, connections, and neurotransmitters in this part of the amygdala show striking similarities to those of the cerebral cortex, suggesting that it is a displaced cortical area. Like the cortex, the basolateral amygdala has connections with the thalamus (especially the dorsomedial and midline nuclei) and the striatum (the ventral

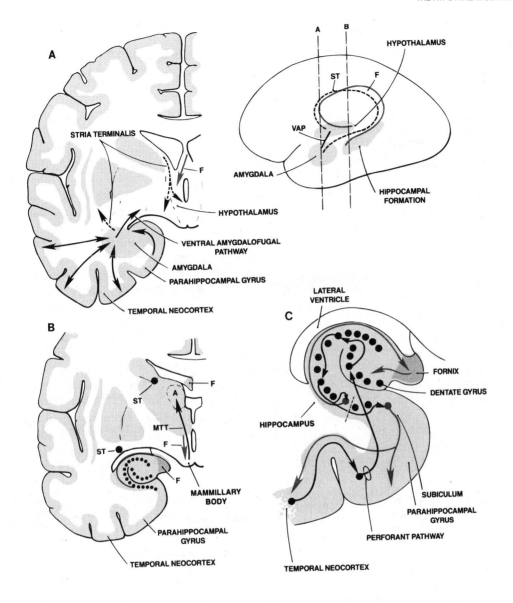

FIGURE 64

• • • • • • • • •

The amygdala and hippocampal formation. The lateral view of the hemisphere in the upper right shows the position of these limbic structures and their major efferent pathways. (*A*) and (*B*) on this small diagram indicate the levels of the corresponding coronal sections illustrated in *A* and *B* on the left. The drawing on the lower right (*C*) is an enlarged view of the hippocampal formation. A = anterior nucleus of the thalamus; F = fornix; MTT = mammillothalamic tract; ST = stria terminalis; VAP = ventral amygdalofugal pathway. (Adapted from Heimer, L: The Human Brain and Spinal Cord. Springer-Verlag, New York, 1983.)

striatum, including nucleus accumbens). The chemical neuroanatomy of this amygdaloid area also shows cortical characteristics. It receives glutamatergic inputs from other cortical regions and acetylcholine inputs from the cholinergic basal forebrain system (see Chap. 25). It also contains numerous GABAergic interneurons.

The functions of the amygdala in the primate remain controversial, although both experimental and clinical evidence suggests that it is important in linking emotional and motivational responses to external stimuli. In this context, the amygdala is believed to contribute to the establishment of memories associated with specific constellations of sensory stimuli. Through its connections with the autonomic nervous system, the neuroendocrine system, and the ventral striatum, the amygdala is in an ideal position to influence both visceral and somatic components of behavior.

The Hippocampal Formation

Just caudal to the amygdala is the beginning of the inferior horn of the lateral ventricle, in the floor of which is the **hippocampal formation**. This structure, consisting of the **dentate gyrus, hippocampus** proper **(Ammon's horn)**, and the **subiculum**, is a large gray matter area that extends from the rostral end of the inferior horn of the lateral ventricle to the back (splenium) of the corpus callosum (Fig. 64B and C).

The hippocampal formation is recognized as a simple cortical structure that is folded into the most medial edge of the cortical mantle. Because of this infolding, it appears to lie deep to the parahippocampal gyrus (see Fig. 64B). The hippocampal formation is connected to other brain areas through two main pathways: the **fornix** and the **perforant pathway**. Both of these fiber connections are two-way systems; that is, they provide both afferent and efferent projections of the hippocampal formation.

The organization of this brain area into three subunits is related not only to its cytoarchitecture but also to its circuitry. Inputs from other brain areas are processed serially through the hippocampal formation. Afferent fibers from the fornix and the perforant pathway are directed first to the dentate gyrus, which in turn projects to the hippocampus. The hippocampus then projects to the subiculum, which is the major source of efferent fibers from this region, although some output also arises from the hippocampus proper.

Through the fornix, the hippocampal formation is reciprocally connected to the septal area, the thalamus (particularly the anterior nuclear group), and the hypothalamus, where many of its fibers terminate in the mammillary bodies. Through the perforant pathway, the hippocampal formation is interconnected with cortical association areas in the temporal lobe, specifically with the temporal neocortex and the entorhinal cortex (see Fig. 64). The entorhinal cortex (Brodmann's area 28) is a specific area within the parahippocampal gyrus (see Fig. 68 in Chap. 24). Through both the fornix and the perforant pathway, the hippocampal formation, like the amygdala, receives highly processed sensory information about the external and internal environment.

The hippocampal formation is also like the amygdala in that a great deal more is known about the connections, the neurotransmitters, and the electrophysiologic properties of the region than about its function. Experimental and clinical observations indicate clearly that it is important in learning and memory. In this capacity, and as recipient of the most highly processed sensory information from the cerebral cortex, this region appears to provide a cognitive map through which humans recognize their position in space and time in relation to external stimuli and events.

THE HYPOTHALAMUS AND LIMBIC SYSTEM

HYPOTHALAMIC AND LIMBIC SYSTEM FUNCTION

The hypothalamus integrates descending influences from the cerebral cortex by way of the amygdala and hippocampal formation, with ascending influences from the spinal cord and brain stem (from somatic and visceral sensory systems and the reticular formation). With this integrated information, the hypothalamus coordinates visceral function with a constellation of behaviors that are essential for the survival of the individual and the species.

For example, coordination of sexual behavior with neuroendocrine regulation of the gonads and reproductive organs ensures survival of the species. Coordination of feeding and drinking behavior with gastrointestinal function ensures the survival of the individual. Similarly, thermoregulatory behavior must be coordinated with body metabolism, peripheral vascular tone and sweating for control of body temperature within the narrow range compatible with human life. The hypothalamus and limbic system also influence many aspects of emotional expression, such as anger, rage, placidity, fear, and social attraction, some of which are associated with survival behaviors, but all of which can occur independently.

To control all of these complex behaviors requires integration of the endocrine system and the autonomic nervous system with the somatic motor system. The hypothalamus regulates endocrine activity through two mechanisms: (1) directly, by secretion of neuroendocrine products into the general circulation through the vasculature of the posterior pituitary (neurohypophysis); and (2) indirectly, by secretion of releasing hormones into the local portal plexus, which drains into the blood vessels of the anterior pituitary (adenohypophysis). Conversely, the autonomic nervous system is controlled by neural pathways that project to the reticular formation and by direct projections through the medial forebrain bundle from the hypothalamus to the parasympathetic and sympathetic neurons in the cranial nerve nuclei and the spinal cord.

Similarly, the inputs to the hypothalamus are both blood borne and neural. Information conveyed in the bloodstream, such as body core temperature, water and salt content of the blood, and circulating hormone and glucose levels, is as important for the functioning of the hypothalamus as neural activity relayed from the limbic system and brain stem.

Endocrine Activity: Hypothalamic–Pituitary Relationships

Cells in the **supraoptic and paraventricular nuclei** produce the peptide hormones **oxytocin** and **vasopressin** (antidiuretic hormone), which are transported down the **hypothalamohypophyseal tract** and secreted from axon terminals directly into the systemic circulation in the posterior pituitary (neurohypophysis). Both hormones are produced initially as prohormones in neurons of the hypothalamic nuclei. During transport along the axons of the neurons, cleavage of the hormones occurs, yielding a **neurophysin** with oxytocin and another neurophysin with vasopressin. The hormones and neurophysins are released at axonal terminals in the posterior pituitary. Vasopressin stimulates water reabsorption by the kidney, and oxytocin stimulates uterine contraction and milk ejection.

Cells in the hypothalamus also control the anterior pituitary, but by a fundamentally different mechanism. Cells primarily localized in the **arcuate nucleus** and other parts of the **periventricular zone of the hypothalamus** produce peptide-releasing hormones, which are transported to their terminals and secreted into capillaries in the median eminence and pituitary stalk. These capillaries collect into very short portal veins that deliver the releasing hormones to cells of the anterior pituitary (adenohypophysis). Some of the substances produced by the hypothalamus are actually release-inhibiting molecules. In response to appropriate releasing hormones, subpopulations of cells of the anterior pituitary synthesize and secrete thyroid-stimulating hormone, follicle-stimulating hormone, luteinizing hormone, growth hormone, adrenocorticotropic hormone, and prolactin. These substances are collectively termed **trophic hormones** because they have a stimulating effect on the target tissues. In response, many of the target tissues (e.g., thyroid, adrenal glands) produce hormones that serve as negative feedback regulators of the hypothalamus and pituitary. This is not true, however, of the regulation of growth hormone and prolactin, which are controlled by a balance of stimulating and inhibiting substances from the hypothalamus. Prolactin, for example, is produced and released in response to prolactin-releasing hormone, and its secretion is inhibited by the release of dopamine from hypothalamic neurons into the hypophyseal portal system. Similarly, the release of growth hormone is regulated in part by the inhibitory action of somatostatin cells.

Reproductive Physiology and Behavior

Neurons in the **preoptic region, anterior hypothalamus, ventromedial nucleus**, and **arcuate nucleus** are involved in gonadal regulation and sexual behavior in the male and female. Both anatomic and physiologic differentiation of these brain areas occur in response to gonadal hormones circulating before birth, leading to a postpubertal pattern of cyclical (female) or noncyclical (male) secretion of gonadotropin-releasing hormone (Gn-RH). In the human, neurons in the arcuate nucleus and throughout the extent of the periventricular zone synthesize Gn-RH, transport it down their axons, and secrete it into the portal capillaries in the infundibulum. Through this pathway, the hypothalamus regulates the pituitary–gonadal axis.

Neurons in the **medial preoptic area, anterior hypothalamus**, and **ventromedial nucleus** profoundly influence sexual behavior in all experimental animals studied, but the pathways out of the hypothalamus by which sexual behavior is coordinated are not fully known. Obviously, some of this behavioral integration involves hypothalamic output to the parasympathetic and sympathetic preganglionic neurons that control genital reflexes (see Chap. 5).

The neuronal inputs to the preoptic area and hypothalamus that regulate sexual behavior come from the amygdala and the brain stem. In addition, the blood-borne gonadal hormones, estrogen and progesterone or testosterone, provide feedback to the brain. Androgen and estrogen receptors are abundant in neurons of all limbic areas that control reproduction, including the amygdala, periventricular and medial zones of the hypothalamus, and the brain stem. Through the action of sex steroids in these areas during neonatal development, the male and female brains become sexually differentiated both structurally and functionally.

Body Temperature

The **preoptic region** and the **anterior hypothalamic area** are important for temperature regulation. Damage to these areas of the brain can lead to complete loss of the integration of autonomic reflexes (e.g., peripheral vasoconstriction, vasodilation and sweating) and somatic motor or behavioral responses (e.g., shivering, seeking a warmer or cooler environment) that regulate body temperature. In addition, local cooling or warming of the blood supply in these brain areas produces an appropriate set of compensatory responses to maintain the body temperature at 37°C. Neurons in the preoptic and anterior hypothalamic regions appear to be directly responsible for this regulatory function. These neurons probably control the production of fever as well, but the mechanisms involved are not fully understood.

Food Intake

Damage to the ventromedial nucleus of the hypothalamus causes an experimental animal to eat voraciously. If allowed continuous access to food, such an animal quickly becomes obese. Conversely, a lesion placed in the lateral hypothalamic zone of the tuberal region abolishes eating and drinking behavior, at least temporarily, and may lead to death from lack of water and nourishment. These experimental findings led investigators to designate the neurons of the ventromedial nucleus as "the satiety center" and those of the lateral hypothalamic area as "the feeding center."

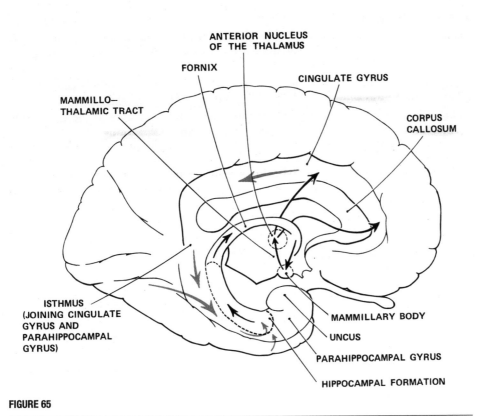

FIGURE 65

The Papez circuit (*arrows*) diagrammed on a schematic view of the limbic system on the medial surface of the cerebral hemisphere. *Black arrows* indicate the circuit described by Papez in 1937. The connections from the cingulate cortex through the parahippocampal gyrus to the hippocampal formation, which complete the circuit (*colored arrows*), were discovered later.

Further experiments, however, have suggested that pathways passing through these areas, particularly noradrenergic pathways destined for more rostral regions of the hypothalamus, may be as important as the ventromedial and lateral hypothalamic neurons in controlling appetite.

Emotion

The hypothalamus clearly regulates the autonomic discharge of nerve impulses that evoke the physical expressions of emotion: acceleration of the heart rate, elevation of blood pressure, flushing or pallor of the skin, sweating, "goose-pimpling" of the skin, dryness of the mouth, and disturbances of the gastrointestinal tract. Emotional experience, however, includes subjective aspects, or "feelings," that involve the cerebral cortex. Furthermore, mental processes in the cerebral cortex possessing strong emotional content can bring forth hypothalamic reactions. Pathways that connect the cerebral cortex and hypothalamus are intimately involved in the mechanisms of emotion. These conduction pathways are diverse and circuitous, and many of them involve the amygdala or the hippocampal formation. One of the most direct is a pathway known as the Papez circuit. Papez's description of this pathway and his proposal that it is concerned with emotion led the way in the development of the concept of the limbic system. The pathway begins with projections from the hippocampal formation to the mammillary body by way of the fornix. From the mammillary body, the prominent mammillothalamic tract projects to the anterior nuclear group of the thalamus, and from these nuclei, axons distribute to the cingulate gyrus (see Fig. 64B; Fig. 65).

Although the limbic system as a whole has been shown to be concerned with emotion, the hippocampus itself, as discussed previously, appears to be an area of the brain responsible for integrating sensory and other messages in the processing of memories—an area, therefore, of prime importance in learning.

23

The Rhinencephalon and Olfactory Reflexes

The **rhinencephalon** consists of the **olfactory nerves, bulbs**, and **tracts**, a portion of the **anterior perforated substance**, the **pyriform region of the cortex**, the **entorhinal cortex of the parahippocampal gyrus**, and the **corticomedial division of the amygdala**. The rhinencephalon is relatively prominent in the brain of macrosmatic vertebrates such as carnivores and rodents. In microsmatic vertebrates such as primates, the visual sense is used more extensively than the olfactory sense for locating food and communicating with other members of the species.

PERIPHERAL OLFACTORY APPARATUS

The peripheral olfactory receptors are found in a specialized area of the nasal mucosa designated as the **olfactory epithelium**. In humans, this tissue consists of pseudostratified columnar olfactory epithelium located on the superior concha, the roof of the nasal chamber, and the upper portion of the nasal septum. The receptor cells are bipolar neurons. Although olfactory transduction is not well understood, it appears that the chemical moieties that serve as olfactory stimuli alter the membrane potential of the receptor neurons, in some cases through direct action on voltage-sensitive channels in the membrane, and in others through ligand-receptor–mediated second-messenger mechanisms. Coding of discrete stimuli for discrimination of different odorants is also poorly understood, but experimental observations suggest that temporal and spatial patterns of activation over the surface of the olfactory mucosa play an important role. The axons of the receptor neurons, grouped into fascicles, pass through the fenestrae of the **cribriform plate** as the **olfactory nerve**. The olfactory nerve terminates in the **olfactory bulb**, which is an extension of the telencephalon.

OLFACTORY BULBS AND PATHWAYS

• • • • • • • • •

The paired olfactory bulbs rest on the cribriform plate. Layers of different neuronal cell types make the laminar architecture of the bulb prominent in histologic preparations of most vertebrate brains, but this organization is less distinct in humans. The bulb contains several types of neurons, including interneurons and **mitral cells**. The mitral cells receive direct synaptic input from **olfactory nerve fibers** and project their axons into the **lateral olfactory tract**.

The **anterior olfactory nucleus**, in the **olfactory stalk**, consists of a number of groups of neurons (Fig. 66). It contains the cells of origin of the **olfactory portion of the anterior commissure**. These cells receive input from the ipsilateral olfactory bulb and send their axons across the anterior commissure to the contralateral olfactory bulb.

The olfactory stalk lies in the **olfactory sulcus** of the frontal lobe. The olfactory tract in the stalk bifurcates into medial and lateral striae. Some of the fibers of the medial olfactory stria are the axons of anterior olfactory nucleus neurons, which enter the rostral portion of the anterior commissure to be returned to the opposite olfactory bulb. The remainder of the fibers, which terminate in the ipsilateral **olfactory trigone** (olfactory tubercle) within the anterior perforated substance, are believed to be mitral cell axons from the olfactory bulb. All of the projections of the mitral cells are ipsilateral.

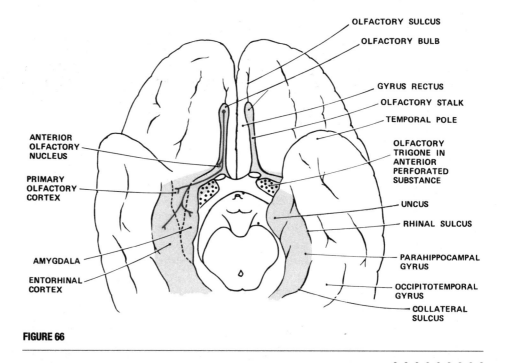

FIGURE 66

• • • • • • • • •

The structures of the olfactory system. On the left, the temporal lobe has been pulled to the left to expose more of the ventral surface of the brain. The projections of the mitral cells of the olfactory bulb are indicated in color.

The lateral stria, or lateral olfactory tract, composed primarily of mitral cell processes, skirts the lateral margin of the anterior perforated substance to reach the **pyriform cortex (primary olfactory cortex)**, the **entorhinal cortex**, and the **amygdala** (see Fig. 66). The olfactory system is unusual in that it is the only sensory system in which second-order neurons (the mitral cells) project directly to the cortex. The **primary olfactory cortex** is three-layered paleocortex, which is phylogenetically older than the six-layered neocortex in which visual, auditory, and somatosensory systems terminate. Like these other sensory systems, however, the olfactory system does use a thalamocortical connection to the **neocortex** for discriminative functions. This connection includes projections from the primary olfactory cortex to the orbitofrontal cortex directly, and indirectly through projections to the magnocellular portion of the **dorsomedial nucleus of the thalamus**, which relays information to the **orbitofrontal cortex**. Experimental animals in which this system has been damaged can still be trained to distinguish between the presence and the absence of an odorant, but they cannot discriminate one odorant from another. Corticocortical connections between the temporal lobe and the orbitofrontal cortex may also be important in olfactory discrimination performance.

Olfactory impulses that reach the amygdala are involved in the regulation of chemosensory control of social behaviors in macrosmatic vertebrates. These behaviors include sexual, aggressive, and maternal responses to other members of the same species. The functional significance of olfactory projections to the amygdala in primates is not clear, nor is the function of the olfactory input to the entorhinal cortex. It is likely that in both of these regions, olfactory information is integrated with visual, auditory, and somatosensory impulses arriving from the respective association cortices. The entorhinal area projects heavily to the hippocampal formation. Thus, both the amygdala and the hippocampal formation may be involved in the integration of multisensory inputs into meaningful and appropriate emotional and physiologic responses to external stimuli. This may serve as the groundwork for the development of learned emotional responses to specific stimuli, which is an aspect of motivation.

DAMAGE TO THE OLFACTORY APPARATUS

• • • • • • • • •

Anosmia, a loss of the sense of smell, can result from a number of conditions, including trauma (e.g., fracture of the cribriform plate with injury to the olfactory bulbs or tracts); infections (the common cold, other systemic viral infections such as viral hepatitis, syphilis, bacterial meningitis, abscesses of the frontal lobe, and osteomyelitis of the frontal or ethmoid regions); neoplasms (e.g., olfactory groove meningiomas, frontal lobe gliomas); metabolic diseases (e.g., pernicious anemia, disorders of zinc metabolism); and drug ingestion (especially amphetamines or cocaine). People with complete anosmia lose the ability to recognize flavors, because the olfactory and taste systems function together in the perception of flavors. Hyperosmia, an increase in olfactory sensitivity, occurs commonly in early pregnancy and also occurs frequently in hysteria and some psychoses.

The subarachnoid space on the cranial side of the cribriform plate is located in close approximation to the olfactory mucosa. A fracture through the cribriform plate that tears the mucosa can result in a leak of cerebrospinal fluid (CSF) through the nose **(CSF rhinorrhea)**. This condition can result in meningitis caused by the spread of microorganisms from the nose to the CSF.

CHAPTER

24

The Cerebral Cortex

The advanced intellectual functions of the human depend on the activity of the cerebral cortex and interactions of this structure with other portions of the nervous system. The cerebral cortex is involved in many aspects of memory storage and recall. It is necessary for the comprehension and execution of language and for certain special talents such as musical and mathematic abilities. The cerebral cortex is involved in most higher cognitive functions. It is responsible for the perception and conscious understanding of all sensations, and it is a site in which one modality of sensation can be integrated with others. The cerebral cortex is involved in the planning and execution of many complex motor activities, particularly fine digit and hand movements.

NEURONS OF THE CEREBRAL CORTEX

• • • • • • • • •

The convoluted surface of the cerebral hemispheres contains a mantle of gray matter densely populated with cells that are arranged in layers. The cerebral cortex can be divided into five types based on the complexity of structure: (1) **idiotypic isocortex**, (2) **homotypical isocortex**, (3) **mesocortex**, (4) **allocortex**, and (5) **corticoid areas**. The idiotypic isocortex consists of the primary motor region in the precentral gyrus and the primary sensory areas, including the primary somatosensory cortex in the postcentral gyrus, the primary auditory cortex in Heschl's gyrus of the superior part of the temporal lobe, and the primary visual cortex in the occipital pole. The homotypical isocortex constitutes the association areas of the cerebral cortex and includes areas that are (1) modality specific or unimodal (i.e., the areas that respond physiologically to only one type of sensory input) and (2) modality nonspecific or heteromodal (i.e., the areas that respond to multiple types of sensory input). The unimodal area for somatosensory input is located in the superior parietal lobule (Brodmann's area 5); the area for auditory input is located in the superior temporal gyrus (Brodmann's area 22); and the area for visual input is located in the peristriate regions of the occipital lobe (Brodmann's areas 18 and 19). The heteromodal areas are located in (1) the prefrontal region, including the rostral orbitofrontal and dorsolateral regions of the frontal lobe; (2) the superior (Brodmann's area 7) and inferior parietal lobules; and (3) parts of the lateral and medial temporal lobe cortices.

The idiotypic isocortex and homotypical isocortex constitute the **neocortex**. These areas have six well-differentiated layers of neurons. From the pial surface, the layers of the neocortex have been named: **I, molecular; II, external granular; III, external pyramidal; IV, internal granular; V, internal pyramidal;** and **VI, multiform**. In general, afferents to the cortex synapse in layers I through IV, whereas efferents from the cortex arise from layers V and VI. The afferents from the specific thalamic nuclei terminate primarily in layer IV of the primary sensory areas, and the efferents projecting to the brain stem and spinal cord arise chiefly in layer V. In addition to this horizontal lamination, the cells of the cortex are functionally organized into vertical columns. Afferent fibers to the cortex run radially toward the surface (i.e., along the length of the vertical columns) and provide branches that form sheets between the horizontal layers of cells. The vertical columns are considered to be the functional units of the cortex. Short axons make connections between neurons within each column to form a great variety of closed chains, or loops. Some of the fibers that terminate on the cells of the cortex come from the thalamus **(projection fibers)**; others arrive from widely dispersed areas of the cortex by way of long or short **association fibers**. A third group of fibers projects to the cortex from several specific subcortical structures outside the thalamus. These include the **locus ceruleus** (origin of noradrenergic fibers), the **raphe nuclei** of the brain stem (origin of serotonergic projections), and the **basal nucleus of Meynert** in the basal telencephalon (origin of cholinergic projections). The corpus callosum and anterior commissure contain **commissural fibers** that link corresponding and, to some degree, noncorresponding regions of the two hemispheres.

The cerebral cortex contains three types of neurons: **pyramidal cells, stellate cells,** and **fusiform cells.** Pyramidal cells are found in layers II, III, and V, and they serve as the major efferent pathway of the cerebral cortex. Small pyramidal cells in layers II and III project to other cortical regions, and large pyramidal cells in layer V project to the brain stem and spinal cord. Stellate cells can be found in all layers but are most common in layer IV. They are the interneurons of the cerebral cortex. Fusiform cells are found in layer VI and project primarily to the thalamus.

The relative thickness of each of the six cortical layers and the density of neuron cell bodies within each layer vary in different regions of the cortex. On the basis of such morphologic characteristics—some obvious, others subtle—several cytoarchitectural maps have been developed that divide the surface of the cerebrum into distinct areas. Some areas have recognized functions, but for many others, no clear correspondence with a specific function has been proved. Based on the differences in cytoarchitecture, Brodmann designated a total of 52 anatomic areas. Many of these numbered areas are referred to frequently for descriptive purposes (Figs. 67 and 68).

The **mesocortex** consists of the **paralimbic areas**, which surround the medial and basal parts of the cerebral hemispheres. There are five paralimbic areas, including the (1) **cingulate complex** (cingulate gyrus, retrosplenial area, and subcallosal area, which includes the paraterminal gyrus); (2) **parahippocampal gyrus;** (3) **temporal pole;** (4) **insula;** and (5) **caudal orbitofrontal cortex.** The mesocortex has three to six layers of neurons; six in zones that lie adjacent to isocortex and three in zones next to the allocortex.

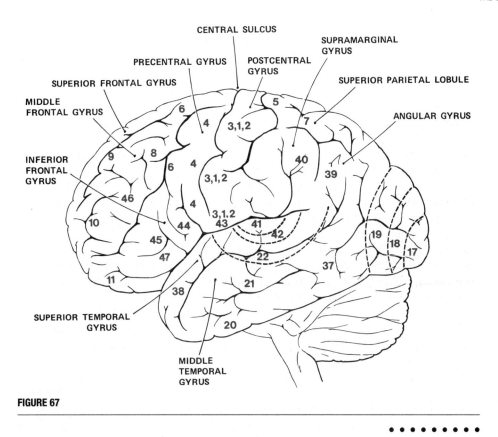

FIGURE 67

A lateral view of the surface of the brain, showing the numbered Brodmann's areas.

The **allocortex** consists of the **hippocampal formation**, which is also known as **archicortex** because phylogenetically the structure is very old, and the **pyriform** or **primary olfactory cortex**, which is also known as **paleocortex** because it is older than neocortex but not as old as the archicortex of the hippocampal formation. The allocortex is a three-layered structure.

The **corticoid areas** include the **septal region** (deep to the paraterminal gyrus), **substantia innominata**, and parts of the **amygdaloid complex**. These regions are at the base of the forebrain and contain simple, poorly differentiated cortex, which nonetheless shares the neurotransmitter and connectional characteristics of other cortical areas.

MOTOR FUNCTIONS OF THE CEREBRAL CORTEX

The **primary motor region** (MI) is located in the precentral gyrus on the convexity of the cerebral hemisphere, extending from the Sylvian fissure laterally into the interhemispheric fissure medially. This region is Brodmann's area 4. The largest neuronal cell bodies of the cerebral cortex, the Betz cells, are located in layer V of this region. These cells give rise to only a small percentage (about 3 percent) of the fibers in the corticospinal tract. The smaller neurons in MI give rise to approximately

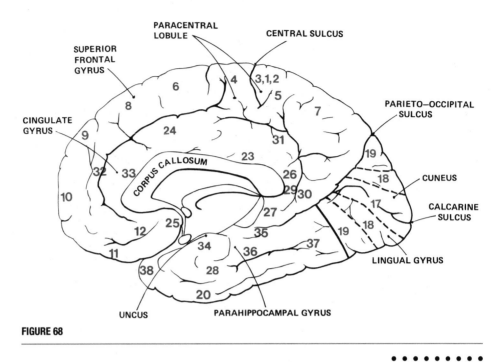

FIGURE 68

A medial view of the surface of the cerebral hemisphere showing the numbered Brodmann's areas.

30 percent of the corticospinal tract. Neurons of MI influence the motor system through projections that pass through the extrapyramidal as well as the pyramidal pathways. As described in previous chapters, neurons in this area project to the putamen and the red nucleus as well as to the spinal cord. As shown by the effects of electrical stimulation in humans and animals, this area of the cerebral cortex contains a representation of the muscles of the body in an orderly arrangement (Fig. 69). The toes, ankle, leg, and genitalia are represented on the medial wall of the brain; the knee, hip, and trunk follow in sequence on the convexity; the shoulder, elbow, wrist, and fingers occur next; and the neck, brow, face, lips, jaw, and tongue are represented most laterally. The amounts of cortex devoted to various parts of the body are unequal. The parts of the body capable of fine or delicate movement have a large cortical representation, whereas those performing relatively gross movements have a small representation.

The primary motor cortex is organized into radially arranged columns of neurons extending vertically from the surface into the depths of the cortex. A single column is a functional entity responsible for directing a group of muscles acting on a single joint. With this organization, movements, not individual muscles, are represented in the motor cortex. Individual neurons within these clusters innervate individual muscles; thus, individual muscles are represented repeatedly, in clusters of neurons in different combinations, among the columns. Neurons of the motor cortex having axons in the pyramidal tract function chiefly in the control of the distal muscles of the limbs.

Lesions in the primary motor region result immediately in paresis of the contralateral musculature with hypotonia (i.e., decreased resistance to passive manipulation) and diminished muscle stretch reflexes. This is followed in a few weeks by

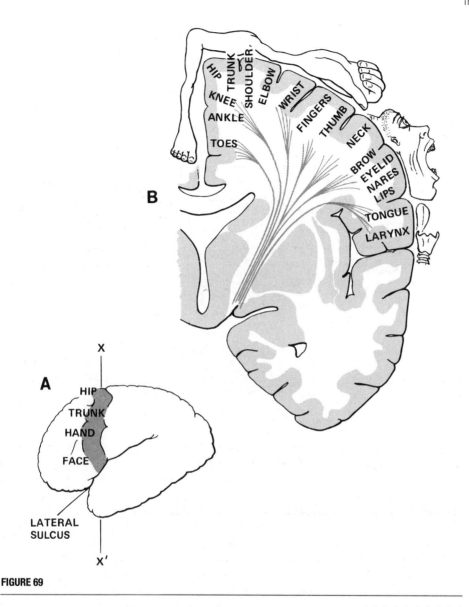

FIGURE 69

• • • • • • • • •

(*A*) Lateral surface of the left cerebral hemisphere. The precentral gyrus is colored, and the functional organization of upper motor neurons is indicated. (*B*) A coronal section taken through X to X′ provides a more detailed representation of the opposite side of the body in the motor area. (Adapted from Penfield, W and Rasmussen, H: The Cerebral Cortex in Man. Macmillan, New York, 1950.)

partial recovery of muscle strength, the development of spasticity of the affected musculature (i.e., increased resistance to passive manipulation), enhanced muscle stretch reflexes, and an extensor plantar response **(Babinski's sign)**.

A secondary motor area (MII), termed the **supplementary motor area**, is located on the medial surface of the frontal lobe in area 6, just anterior to MI (Fig. 70). This area contains a complete somatotopic representation of the body, as shown by the results of electrical stimulation in animals and humans. The supplementary motor area is thought to participate in the advance planning of movements, particularly for movements involving both sides of the body.

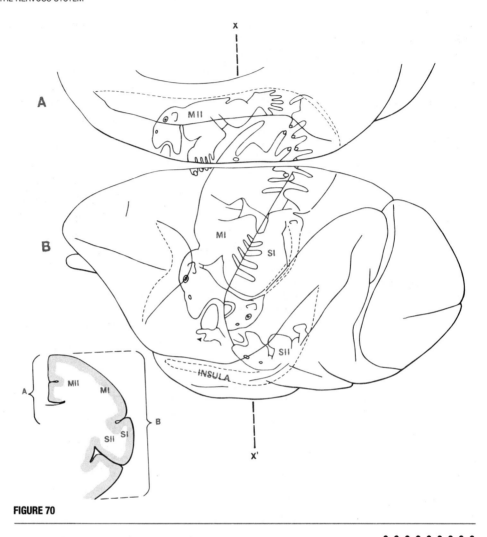

FIGURE 70

• • • • • • • • •

Diagram of the cerebral cortex of the monkey, showing the location of four principal motor areas: precentral motor (MI); supplementary motor (MII); somatic sensory I (SI); and secondary sensory (SII). (*A*) The medial surface of the cortex. (*B*) The lateral surface of the cortex. X to X′ indicates the plane of section through the brain that reveals the cortical relationship shown in the inset (lower left). The animal outlines in the diagram indicate the segments of the body induced to move by electrical stimulation. The motor regions SI and SII coincide with the primary and secondary somatosensory areas. (Adapted from Harlow, HF and Woolsey, CN (eds.): Biological and Biochemical Bases of Behavior. University of Wisconsin Press, Madison, 1958.)

Neurons projecting through the corticospinal pathway also arise in the postcentral gyrus of the cerebral cortex, where a third motor representation exists. The body components of this representation coincide with the primary somatic sensory pattern in the same area (SI in Fig. 70). A fourth motor representation has been found in the parietotemporal region, coinciding with the secondary sensory area (SII). All four of the areas of cerebral cortex containing motor representation contribute fibers to the pyramidal tract and probably provide inputs to extrapyramidal motor pathways as well.

The **premotor area** (area 6) lies immediately in front of area 4 on the lateral surface of the hemisphere. This area contains neurons projecting into the primary motor cortex and provides inputs both to the pyramidal tract and to extrapyramidal pathways. Area 8 lies rostral to area 6 and, on the lateral surface of the hemisphere, contains the **frontal eye field**. Stimulation of this area results in conjugate deviation of the eyes to the opposite side. This region is responsible for voluntary conjugate movement of the eyes independent of visual stimuli. Another motor eye field is located in a large region of the occipital lobe, including the visual receiving areas and adjacent zones of the cerebral cortex. The site of lowest threshold for a response to electrical stimulation is area 17. This area subserves movements of the eyes induced by visual stimuli.

Lesions of the premotor cortex result in complex defects of movement in the absence of weakness. Experimental animals with lesions in area 6 lose the ability to alter the type of limb and body movement in response to different types of sensory inputs. Visual guidance of motor performance is also impaired. Unilateral lesions that include area 8 result in defective scanning and exploration of the opposite side of the visual environment.

PREFRONTAL CORTEX

• • • • • • • • •

The large remaining part of the frontal lobe lying rostral to the motor and premotor areas is known as the **prefrontal region** and includes Brodmann's areas 8 through 12 and 45 through 47. The prefrontal cortex is best defined by the extent of its reciprocal connections with the dorsomedial nucleus of the thalamus, but it is also reciprocally connected with the ventral anterior and intralaminar nuclei. The other reciprocal connections of the prefrontal area are differentially distributed to its two main subregions: the ventral (or orbital) region and the dorsolateral region. The orbital area is widely connected to structures of the limbic system, including limbic cortex, amygdala, hypothalamus, and midbrain. Conversely, the dorsolateral region projects to and receives from the sensory association areas of the parietal, occipital, and temporal lobes. Both ventral and dorsolateral regions send projections to the basal ganglia, primarily to the caudate nucleus.

The neurons of the prefrontal cortex respond to many different types of sensory inputs and thus are known as heteromodal neurons, but they are also highly responsive to the behavioral importance of the inputs. A neuron that responds strongly to a sensory input that is associated with a pleasant reward may respond differently when the same input is associated with a noxious stimulus. Thus, the neurons of the prefrontal region are thought to integrate motivational events with complex sensory stimuli. These neurons also are involved in inhibitory responses to stimuli that require a delay in the motor responses.

Injury to the prefrontal cortex in experimental animals impairs the ability to perform tasks requiring the animal to alternate responses to stimuli with a delay. Unilateral ablation of the frontal eye fields results in neglect of stimuli in the opposite side of extrapersonal space. In humans, lesions of the prefrontal cortex result in disruption of some of the most complex aspects of behavior. Unilateral lesions lead to neglect of the contralateral side of extrapersonal space. Bilateral lesions cause the patient to show markedly disturbed behavior. These patients are frequently unconcerned with their illness, inappropriately jocular, slovenly, and unclean. Their social graces and concern for others are lost. They may eat from the floor, drop food on their clothing without concern, and ignore the ordinary standards of cleanliness. Often, they are apathetic, although they may be irascible. They cannot exercise foresight or good judgment and have essentially no insight. They are easily distracted and cannot perform complex tasks requiring several steps.

PRIMARY SENSORY RECEPTIVE AREAS

• • • • • • • • •

Three primary receptive areas of the cerebral cortex contain the terminations of projections relaying somatosensory, auditory, and visual information. The postcentral gyrus (areas 3, 1, and 2) contains the primary (unimodal) somatosensory area, SI. This gyrus receives projections from the ventral posterior lateral nucleus of the thalamus, which is the thalamic relay for the somatosensory projections. The SI region contains a map of the surface of the contralateral half of the body, with the leg and foot represented medially; the thigh, trunk, arm, and hand dorsolaterally; and the mouth and face ventrolaterally. Studies in animals show that neurons of area 3a (the most rostral strip of area 3, in the depths of the central sulcus) are activated by muscle spindle afferents, area 3b (caudal to 3a) and area 1 by cutaneous afferents, and area 2 by joint receptors. Neurons of these areas are especially stimulated by active tactile exploration. In humans, lesions of SI result in impairment of "cortical sensation," that is, two-point discrimination, localization of touch, position sense, and stereognosis. The primary modalities of sensation (i.e., touch, pain, and temperature) are preserved but poorly localized in humans with lesions of SI.

Heschl's gyrus (areas 41 and 42), which is in the superior part of the superior temporal gyrus, contains the primary auditory area, A1. This gyrus receives projections from the medial geniculate body, which is one of the relays for the auditory projections. A1 is organized tonotopically, with low frequencies represented more rostrally and laterally than high frequencies. Neurons of A1 respond not only to the frequency but also to the localization of sound. The ascending auditory pathway has many decussations in the brain stem; the A1 of each hemisphere receives information from both ears, although the input from the contralateral ear is more strongly received than input from the ipsilateral ear. Unilateral lesions of A1 in the human are undetectable clinically and can be discovered only with specialized tests such as auditory evoked potentials or dichotic listening tasks. Complete cortical deafness results only from bilateral damage to the A1 area and the adjacent auditory association areas of both cerebral hemispheres.

The striate cortex (area 17), which lies along the banks of the calcarine fissure medially and along the occipital pole laterally, is the primary visual cortex (VI). This area receives projections from the lateral geniculate nucleus, which mediates visual input from the retina. The striate area of each hemisphere receives information from the contralateral visual field, with the dorsal parts of the striate cortex responding to stimuli in the contralateral lower field and the ventral parts responding to inputs from the contralateral upper field. Neurons of the striate cortex respond to the shape of objects as well as to their color, size, location, and direction of movement. In humans, focal lesions of the striate cortex result in visual field defects (see Chapter 19). Complete bilateral destruction of the striate cortex results in **cortical blindness**. The pupillary light reflexes remain intact, but the patient has no useful vision. Some patients with cortical blindness claim that they can see when it is obvious that they cannot. This is termed **Anton's syndrome** and results from lesions that destroy area 17 as well as the peristriate cortex in areas 18 and 19.

Primary sensory areas for the chemical senses, olfaction and taste, are less well studied and less well understood. As described in Chapters 12 and 23, there is a taste or gustatory cortical area in the parietal operculum and adjacent insular cortex (Brodmann's area 43; see Fig. 67). Olfactory sensation is processed in the primary olfactory cortex (see Fig. 66 in Chap. 23), but the ability to discriminate among odorants appears to depend on an intact orbitofrontal cortex.

SECONDARY SENSORY AREAS

• • • • • • • • •

Near each primary receptive area are cortical zones that receive sensory inputs directly or indirectly from the thalamus as well as connections from the adjacent primary sensory areas. These secondary sensory areas contain somatotopic representations of parts of the body, but the areas are smaller than the primary areas, and the order of representation is different. A secondary somatic sensory area (SII; see Fig. 70) is located in the cerebral cortex on the inner part of the parietal operculum, adjacent to the dorsal insula. Parts of the body are represented there bilaterally, although the contralateral representation predominates. This area is involved in the perception of several sensory modalities, including touch, pressure, position sense, and pain. A secondary auditory area (AII) is located in the cortex immediately surrounding AI, and a secondary visual area (VII) is contained within area 18, which is located in the occipital lobe adjacent to area 17 (see Figs. 67 and 68).

SENSORY ASSOCIATION AREAS

• • • • • • • • •

Sensory information channeled into the primary and secondary sensory cerebral cortical areas is subjected to elaboration and analysis in extensive cortical zones, the **sensory association areas**, which are adjacent to the primary and secondary sensory areas. The sensory association areas consist of modality-specific (i.e., unimodal) and modality-nonspecific (i.e., heteromodal) areas. Lesions of the unimodal association areas lead to complex defects in sensory perception with the elemental sensations remaining intact. Lesions of the heteromodal areas result in complex defects involving both cognitive and affective (emotional) components.

The somatosensory unimodal association area lies in the superior parietal lobule (area 5 and the anterior part of area 7). Most of the neurons in this region respond only to somatosensory stimuli. This area is thought to be important in touch localization, exploration of the environment with the body surface, synthesis of personal and extrapersonal space, and memory of the somesthetic environment. Neurons of this region project to the heteromodal association area in the posterior part of area 7 and the inferior parietal lobule.

The auditory unimodal association area lies in area 22 of the superior temporal gyrus. Most of the neurons in this area respond only to auditory stimuli. This area is thought to be important in the discrimination of auditory frequency and sequence of sound. The area is also important in the retention of auditory information. Neurons in this region project to the heteromodal association areas in the prefrontal and temporoparietal areas of cerebral cortex and also to the paralimbic and limbic structures of the temporal lobe. In the human, bilateral lesions of the auditory association areas or a unilateral left-sided lesion that disconnects area 22 from Wernicke's area results in **pure word deafness**. Patients with this disorder cannot understand or repeat spoken language, but they respond appropriately to environmental sounds (indicating that they are not deaf) and they can understand written language (indicating they are not aphasic).

The visual unimodal association area is located in the peristriate cortex (areas 18 and 19) and the middle and inferior temporal gyri (areas 20, 21, and 37). Neurons in the visual unimodal association area respond only to visual stimuli and are capable of responding to complex aspects of visual stimuli such as form, motion, and color. In experimental animals, lesions of this area result in defects of depth perception, distance judgment, spatial orientation, and hue discrimination thresholds. In humans, lesions in areas 20, 21, and 37 can result in discrete deficits in naming visual stimuli, affecting some categories of objects and not others. For example, a patient may easily recognize and name man-made tools but be unable to identify correctly items of food or types of animals.

The information processed within the primary and secondary sensory areas and within the unimodal association areas is confined to single sensory modalities such as touch, hearing, and vision. A separate type of processing occurs at the next stage and is termed heteromodal because several different sensory modalities can activate a single neuron. Many neurons in heteromodal regions also change their discharge rate during specific motor acts, indicating that these neurons function in the integration of complex sensory input with motor output. Heteromodal association areas are required for many cognitive processes, including language, but they also have extensive connections with paralimbic and limbic structures and therefore are involved in emotional states, including mood and motivation. Injury to heteromodal areas leads to complex neurologic disorders with combinations of cognitive defects and emotional disturbances. There are two major heteromodal association areas: (1) temporoparietal areas and (2) prefrontal areas.

The **temporoparietal heteromodal association areas** are located in areas 39 (the angular gyrus) and 40 (the supramarginal gyrus) of the inferior parietal lobule, the cortex along the superior temporal sulcus, and the posterior parts of area 7. Many neurons in these regions respond to a single sensory modality, whereas neighboring neurons respond to a single sensory modality of another type, and other neurons respond to multiple types of sensory modalities. Many neurons in this region alter their discharge during performance of tasks with a strong motivational component such as a reward. In experimental animals, unilateral lesions in these areas result in neglect of objects and stimuli in personal and extrapersonal space on the contralateral side of the body. Bilateral lesions in animals lead to impairment in exploring extrapersonal space, with defects in determining spatial relationships between objects and negotiating relatively simple mazes. Visual, auditory, and somatosensory perceptions remain intact, but these sensory modalities cannot be integrated.

Lesions of the temporoparietal heteromodal association areas in the human result in complex disturbances that depend on the side of the lesion. Damage in the right cerebral hemisphere causes disturbances in the integration of personal and extrapersonal space, whereas damage in the left cerebral hemisphere leads to disorders of language and disturbed spatial integration. An important part of the temporoparietal heteromodal association area in the left hemisphere is **Wernicke's area**, which is located in the posterior part of the superior temporal gyrus. This area integrates the sensory modalities needed to understand written and spoken language. Injury to this area results in **Wernicke's aphasia**, which is described later in this chapter. If Wernicke's area is spared but a left cerebral hemisphere lesion damages the inferior parietal lobule, complex disorders occur consisting of varying combinations of alexia (inability to read), anomia (inability to name objects), constructional apraxia (inability to construct simple figures such as a clock or a house with pencil and paper), agraphia (inability to write), finger agnosia (inability to name individual fingers), and confusion between the left and right sides of personal and extrapersonal space. These disorders are termed the **angular gyrus syndrome**, and the combination of acalculia, agraphia, finger agnosia, and right-left disorientation is known as the **Gerstmann syndrome**.

Unilateral lesions in the temporoparietal heteromodal association areas of the right cerebral hemisphere result in dressing apraxia (difficulty in dressing, particularly the left side of the body), constructional apraxia (difficulty constructing simple figures with pencil and paper, usually with inattention to the left side of the figure), neglect of the left side of personal and extrapersonal space, and lack of insight about these difficulties.

Bilateral lesions of the temporoparietal heteromodal association areas lead to complex disorders including visual, spatial, and language defects. One such disorder, usually resulting from bilateral lesions of the dorsal parts of these areas, is the **Balint syndrome**, which consists of (1) inability to gaze toward the peripheral field (even though eye movements are intact), (2) difficulty in reaching out and touching objects accurately with visual guidance, and (3) inattention to objects in the peripheral parts of the visual field.

In addition to the cognitive, perceptive, and motor disturbances produced by lesions of the temporoparietal heteromodal association areas, there are also affective disorders. Mood alterations ranging from anger to apathy are seen in patients with these disturbances. These emotional disturbances result from interruption of the connections between heteromodal association areas and parts of the limbic system.

The **prefrontal region** contains a second large expanse of heteromodal association cortex. This region receives inputs from all the unimodal association areas and from all the heteromodal association areas. Integration with limbic inputs occurs here because the cingulate, caudal orbitofrontal, and insular areas project here. The behavior of neurons and the effects of lesions in this region have been described earlier in this chapter.

PARALIMBIC AREAS

• • • • • • • • •

The **paralimbic areas**, which are considered to be mesocortex based on their structure, are located on the basal and medial aspects of the cerebral hemispheres. These areas include the (1) temporal pole (area 38); (2) insula; (3) caudal orbitofrontal cortex (caudal parts of areas 11 and 12); (4) parahippocampal regions (areas 27, 28, 34, and 35); and (5) retrosplenial area (areas 26, 29, and 30), cingulate gyrus (areas 23, 24, 31, and 33), and the precallosal and subcallosal regions (areas 32 and 25). The paralimbic areas receive information from heteromodal association areas of the cerebral cortex and from limbic areas. The paralimbic areas are thought to be involved in memory and learning, drive and affect, and processing of information relevant to the autonomic nervous system. Damage to the parahippocampal cortex as well as to the hippocampus, amygdala, and subcortical limbic structures in humans leads to severe disorders of memory. Damage to the paralimbic areas of the orbitofrontal region as well as to the amygdala results in a reduced level of aggressiveness, which in some patients can lead to severe apathy. The paralimbic cortex is thought to influence autonomic regulation in the hypothalamus, reticular formation, dorsal motor nucleus of the vagus, and the nucleus of the solitary tract. The paralimbic areas of the orbitofrontal and insular regions are also involved in processing olfactory and gustatory information, as noted previously in this chapter.

LIMBIC AREAS

• • • • • • • • •

The limbic areas, composed of allocortex and corticoid areas, include the (1) septal area, (2) substantia innominata, (3) piriform cortex, (4) amygdala, and (5) hippocampal formation. Some of these areas (the medial septal nucleus, the vertical and horizontal nuclei of the diagonal band of Broca, and the nucleus basalis of Meynert) provide cholinergic innervation for the whole surface of the cerebral cortex. Limbic structures are thought to be important in memory and motivation. The pyriform cortex receives incoming olfactory information and is probably involved in feeding. The amygdala is connected with the hypothalamus, hippocampus, and substantia innominata. It also receives inputs from extensive areas of the cerebral cortex, including paralimbic areas, heteromodal association cortex, and unimodal association cortex. The amygdala, a key structure in motivation and affect, is also involved in regulating autonomic, endocrine, and immune functions. In experimental animals, lesions of the amygdala result in the Kluver-Bucy syndrome, which consists of (1) excessive sexual activity, often with inappropriate objects, (2) loss of aggressiveness, and (3) compulsive oral exploration of objects in the environment. An equivalent syndrome has been observed in humans. The hippocampus receives input from the paralimbic areas, hypothalamus, amygdala, and septal region. The hippocampus is involved in memory formation, control of the endocrine system, and regulation of the immune system. Patients with bilateral lesions of the hippocampal formation, who usually have involvement of the parahippocampal regions as well, develop severe disturbances of memory.

CORTICAL NETWORKS

• • • • • • • • •

In recent years, the understanding of the processing of information in the cerebral cortex has altered dramatically. The earlier concept of serial, unidirectional processing from primary sensory areas through association areas to motor areas suggested that the cortex functioned as an elaborate reflex arc. With increasing knowledge of anatomic connections in the primate cortex and activity patterns of various cortical areas from human imaging studies, the concept of large-scale functional networks for a variety of specific cognitive functions has emerged. This concept of cortical function takes into account that heteromodal association areas are reciprocally connected not only with the unimodal sensory association areas and with each other but also with the paralimbic and limbic areas necessary for learning, memory, and motivation. The resulting concept is one of essentially simultaneous activation of the nodes in a functional cortical network and its related subcortical structures associated with particular sensory stimuli or cognitive tasks. Separate but overlapping networks for attention, learning and memory, and language have been proposed and, with the advent of functional imaging studies, will be amenable to confirmation and clarification.

DISORDERS OF HIGHER CEREBRAL FUNCTION

• • • • • • • • •

Agnosia

The process of comprehension ("knowing" or "gnosis") must entail a comparison of present sensory phenomena with past experience. For example, the visual association areas must be called on when an old friend is recognized in a crowd. **Agnosia** is a failure to recognize stimuli when the appropriate sensory systems are functioning adequately. Agnosia commonly occurs in visual, tactile, and auditory forms.

Visual agnosia is the failure to recognize objects visually in the absence of a defect of visual acuity or intellectual impairment. The patient often can see the object clearly but cannot recognize or identify it visually. In a pure visual agnosia, the same object can be identified by other sensibilities such as touch. Bilateral lesions of visual unimodal association areas usually are associated with visual agnosia.

Tactile agnosia is the inability to recognize objects by touch when tactile and proprioceptive sensibilities are intact in the part of the body being tested. Lesions of the supramarginal gyrus (area 40) usually are responsible for tactile agnosia. Patients with tactile agnosia often have disturbances of body image.

Auditory agnosia is the failure of a patient with intact hearing to recognize what he or she hears, including speech, musical sounds, or familiar noises. Bilateral lesions of the posterior part of the superior temporal convolution (area 22) are frequently responsible for this condition.

Apraxia

Apraxia is the loss of the ability to carry out correctly certain movements in response to stimuli that normally elicit these movements. This deficit is present even though the patient has no weakness, sensory loss, or disturbance of language comprehension. Accomplishing a complex act requires the integrity of a large part of the cerebral cortex. There must first be an idea—a mental formulation of the plan. This formulation must then be transferred by association fibers to the motor system, where it can be executed. Apraxias often result from lesions interrupting connections between the site of formulation of a motor act and the motor areas responsible for its execution. A lesion of the supramarginal gyrus of the dominant parietal lobe leads to an **ideomotor apraxia**, in which a patient knows what he or she wants to do but is unable to do it. The patient can perform many complex acts automatically but cannot carry out the same acts on command. **Ideational apraxia** refers to failures in carrying out sequences of acts, although individual movements are correct. This form of apraxia may also result from lesions in the dominant parietal lobe or the corpus callosum. **Kinetic apraxia** (i.e., the inability to execute fine acquired movements) and **gait apraxia** often result from disease of the frontal lobe.

Aphasia

Facile use of language and speech is a remarkable attribute of the human brain—one that is shared by no other animal. **Language** refers to the vocabulary and syntactic rules needed for communication. **Speech** refers to the production of spoken language. **Dysarthria** is a disturbance in the execution of speech and often occurs without a disorder of language. **Aphonia** is the inability to produce sounds. **Aphasia** is a disorder of language caused by a defect in either the production or comprehension of vocabulary or syntax. Beginning early in life, nearly every individual selectively develops one hemisphere of the brain more intensively than the other in the processes of language function. Usually, the left side of the brain assumes the leading role, and the person becomes right-handed. Right-handedness indicates the preferential use of the right hand in most or all unimanual activities. Approximately 90 percent of people in the United States are right-handed, and essentially all of them have left-hemisphere dominance for language. About 10 percent of people are left-handed, but about half of them also have left-hemisphere dominance. The remaining left-handed people have right-hemisphere dominance or mixed left and right dominance. Aphasia appears only if a lesion is located in the dominant hemisphere. It is unclear when cerebral dominance for language occurs; children display a preference for the use of the right or left hand from an early age. Cerebral dominance for language is a plastic phenomenon up to the age of 7 years. Thus, a right-handed child 5 years of age who suffers an injury in the language areas of the left hemisphere will learn to speak again in 1 or 2 years. An adult can rarely recover to this extent.

Three regions of the dominant cerebral hemisphere are of particular importance in aphasia: **Broca's area, Wernicke's area,** and the intervening area of parietal lobe (the parietal operculum). Broca's area, the anterior speech region, is located in the inferior frontal gyrus just rostral to the site of the motor representation of the face (Fig. 71). This is in the region of Brodmann's areas 44, 45, and 47. As mentioned previously, Wernicke's area lies in the posterior part of the superior temporal gyrus on the convexity of the brain and extends onto the upper surface of the temporal lobe. The posterior part of Brodmann's area 22 is central to Wernicke's area. It is connected with Broca's area through the **arcuate fasciculus**, a fiber bundle coursing from the temporal lobe around the posterior end of the Sylvian fissure into the lower parietal lobe and running forward into the frontal lobe. The function of Wernicke's area is to make the individual capable of recognizing speech patterns relayed from the left primary auditory cortex. Information about incoming speech patterns is forwarded to Broca's area, which generates the proper pattern of signals to the speech musculature for the production of meaningful speech. Three general forms of aphasia are recognized that relate to Broca's area, Wernicke's area, and the parietal operculum containing the arcuate fasciculus.

Lesions of Broca's area lead to an **executive** (also termed **motor, nonfluent, anterior**, or **Broca's) aphasia** (see Fig. 71). The patient produces spoken language slowly and effortfully, with poorly produced sounds and ungrammatical, telegraphic speech. Many prepositions, nouns, and verbs are deleted. The patient has extreme difficulty in expressing certain grammatical words and phrases. "No ifs, ands, or buts" is a particularly difficult phrase for affected persons to speak. Repetition of phrases or sentences is poor. The patient has good comprehension of spoken and written language but is frustrated and discouraged by his or her difficulty with speech. Vascular lesions of Broca's area often involve the internal capsule. Consequently, a right hemiplegia usually accompanies an executive aphasia.

Lesions of Wernicke's area lead to a **receptive** (also termed **sensory, fluent, posterior**, or **Wernicke's) aphasia** (see Fig. 71). The patient produces spoken language more rapidly than normal, with preserved grammatic construction. The patient cannot find the correct words to express thoughts, however, and may omit words or use circumlocutions, words without precise meanings, or substitute words. Substitutions of one word for another are called **verbal paraphasias. Literal para-**

phasia is the substitution of a well-articulated but inappropriate phoneme in a word (e.g., saying pork for cork). Words may be produced that are random collections of sounds; these are termed **neologisms**. The patient has poor comprehension of speech and poor repetition of phrases or sentences. The patient often is unaware of this speech difficulty and may show no concern about it. Because lesions of Wernicke's area are far removed from the primary motor area and the internal capsule, patients with receptive aphasia usually are not hemiplegic.

Lesions of the white matter underlying the parietal operculum lead to a **conduction aphasia** by disconnecting Wernicke's area from Broca's area. The patient has a fluent aphasia with poor repetition of spoken language. Despite phonetic errors, the patient tends to have good comprehension of spoken language.

Patients with posteriorly placed vascular lesions affecting speech may have damage to the angular gyrus (area 39) associated with injury to Wernicke's area. Infarction of the angular gyrus of the dominant hemisphere results in loss of the ability to read (alexia) and write (agraphia) in the absence of primary visual or motor impairment.

The preceding paragraphs describe the regions in which control of various aspects of language are localized. Individual patients vary greatly, however, in the precise location of small subregions of cortex that are responsible for various language skills within these large areas. Individual brains also appear to vary in the number of cortical loci within these regions through which language can be controlled. The result of this individual variability is that partial lesions of these general cortical regions in the dominant hemisphere do not produce predictable language deficits. The

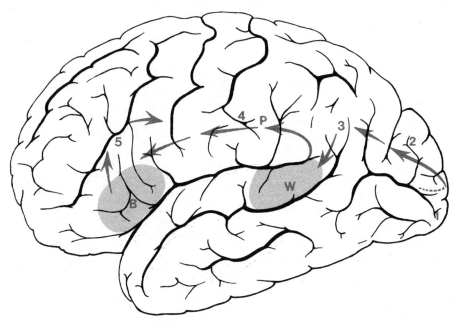

FIGURE 71

Cerebral cortical areas that are important for language. A visual image of a word is projected from the calcarine cortex (*1*) into the visual association areas 18 and 19 (*2*) to the region of the angular gyrus (*3*). Information is then transferred to Wernicke's area (*W*) to arouse the learned auditory form of the word. This information is then transferred via the arcuate fasciculus (*4*) under the parietal operculum (*P*) to Broca's area (*B*), which contains programs that control (*5*) the cortical motor region in the precentral gyrus involved in speech.

effects of any given lesion depend on the number and distribution of language processing sites within Broca's and Wernicke's areas in the afflicted individual.

THE INTERNAL CAPSULE

• • • • • • • • •

Afferent and efferent fibers of all parts of the cerebral cortex converge toward the brain stem, forming the **corona radiata** deep in the medullary substance of the hemisphere. As these fibers course ventrally from the cortex, the rostral fibers pass down between the head of the caudate nucleus and the rostral end of the lentiform nucleus. These rostral fibers form the **anterior limb of the internal capsule**. Caudally, the fibers pass between the thalamus and the lentiform nucleus as the **posterior limb of the internal capsule**. At the level of the interventricular foramen, the transition between the anterior and posterior limbs is called the **genu (knee)** of the internal capsule (Fig. 72). Descending fibers of the pyramidal system pass through the posterior limb of the internal capsule. The corticobulbar fibers for movements of the muscles of the head are located rostral to the corticospinal fibers. Motor fibers to the upper extremity are rostral to those to the lower extremity. Fibers passing to

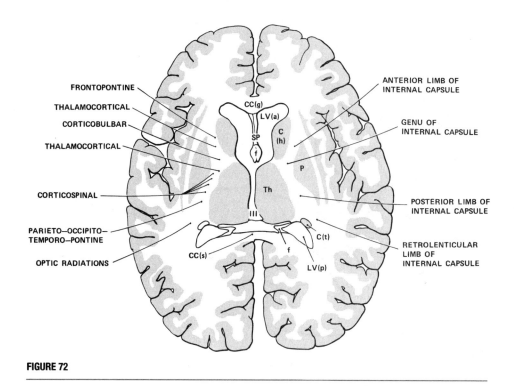

FIGURE 72

• • • • • • • • •

A horizontal section through the cerebrum showing the location of the internal capsule fibers (*right*) and the various bundles that make up the capsule (*left*). CC(g) = corpus callosum, genu; CC(s) = corpus callosum, splenium; C(h) = caudate head; C(t) = caudate tail; f = fornix; LV(a) = lateral ventriseptum pellucidum; Th = thalamus; III = third ventricle.

and from the frontal lobe, other than pyramidal fibers (e.g., connections between the dorsomedial thalamic nucleus and the prefrontal cortex), make up the anterior limb of the internal capsule, whereas those of the parietal lobe occupy the posterior part of the posterior limb. Optic radiation fibers are located in the retrolenticular portion of the internal capsule (i.e., "behind" the lentiform nucleus). Auditory radiation fibers are found in the sublenticular part of the internal capsule (i.e., "underneath" the lentiform nucleus), which is below the plane of section in the brain slice pictured in Figure 72.

CHAPTER

25

Chemical Neuroanatomy

Communication between neurons in the human nervous system is accomplished primarily by the release of neurotransmitters at chemical synapses. The chemicals that have been tentatively or definitively identified as neurotransmitters include several different classes of molecules and dozens of individual substances. Some of these, such as acetylcholine and the monoamines, have been studied extensively. Conversely, many of the neuropeptides have only recently been localized in neural tissue; in these cases, little is known about their physiologic significance.

Most of the neurotransmitters that have been identified fall into one of four different groups of compounds: acetylcholine, a derivative of the lipid cholesterol; biogenic amines or monoamines, derived from aromatic amino acids; neuropeptides, which are short chains of amino acids; and amino acids themselves. To function effectively as a neurotransmitter, a compound must be: synthesized in the presynaptic neuron; stored in presynaptic vesicles; released by calcium-dependent mechanisms from the presynaptic neuron; active at selective receptors on the postsynaptic element, where it alters the membrane potential; and finally, removed from the synaptic site or destroyed biochemically. The neurotransmitters that are discussed in this chapter are examples of molecules for which sufficient data currently exist to satisfy these criteria.

Although the action of a neurotransmitter at the chemical synapse is influenced by factors that control its synthesis and release, the nature of that action (excitation or inhibition) is determined by the types of receptors on the postsynaptic cell. In addition, the intensity of that action is influenced by the number of receptors present. Chemical synapses, and chemical systems in the brain, are therefore characterized not only by the transmitter released but also by the subtype or subtypes of receptors available for that transmitter. These subtypes are defined experimentally by the selective binding of specific pharmacologic agents acting as agonists or antagonists of the transmitter.

In general, two very different mechanisms have been found to account for the actions of neurotransmitters at their receptors, and individual receptor subtypes are characterized accordingly. At **ionotropic receptors**, neurotransmitters produce rapid, phasic responses by altering the state of ion channels in the postsynaptic membrane. In contrast, longer-lasting effects are mediated by the action of neurotransmitters at **G protein–coupled (metabotropic) receptors**, where a cascade of enzymatic reactions alters the metabolism of the postsynaptic cell through activation of second messengers. Both of these receptor mechanisms are used by receptor subtypes identified for acetylcholine and the amino acid transmitters glutamate and gamma-aminobutyric acid (GABA). However, the receptors identified to date for monoamines and neuropeptides are all G protein–coupled receptors, with the exception of the ionotropic 5-HT$_3$ serotonin receptor.

Although it is obvious that detailed maps of the distribution of various receptor subtypes are essential for fully understanding the chemical systems of the central nervous system (CNS), this chapter attempts to describe only the known receptor subtypes and to outline the neuronal origins and projections of several of the major chemical systems.

ACETYLCHOLINE

• • • • • • • • •

Acetylcholine (ACh) is synthesized from acetylcoenzyme A and choline in a reaction catalyzed by the enzyme **choline acetyltransferase (ChAT)**. Upon release from a presynaptic terminal, ACh is destroyed in the synaptic cleft by the enzyme **acetylcholinesterase (AChE)**. Both of these enzymes are synthesized in the cell body of an ACh neuron and moved by axoplasmic transport to the terminals, where ACh is synthesized.

The CNS distribution of both enzymes has been studied to define the acetylcholine system, but these studies indicate that AChE is produced in neurons that do not make ChAT. Thus, the description in this chapter is based, as much as possible, on the more limited information available from ChAT localization.

Acetylcholine is the primary neurotransmitter of the peripheral nervous system. It is released at the neuromuscular junction by **all alpha, beta, and gamma motoneurons** of the brain stem and spinal cord. Within the cord, axon collaterals of the alpha motoneurons activate the Renshaw cells at cholinergic synapses. Acetylcholine is also released in the autonomic ganglia by **all preganglionic sympathetic and parasympathetic neurons**. In these locations, the primary cholinergic receptor is the nicotinic subtype. Additionally, **all postganglionic parasympathetic neurons** and one population of postganglionic sympathetic fibers, those to the sweat glands of the skin, are cholinergic. At these postsynaptic autonomic sites, the muscarinic receptors predominate.

Acetylcholine neurons within the brain, with the exception of the motoneurons in the cranial nerve nuclei, are limited to a cluster of nuclear groups in the ventral forebrain and hypothalamus, a smaller group of nuclei in the tegmentum of the brain stem, and interneurons of the striatum (Fig. 73). In the brain areas that receive input from these cells, muscarinic receptors predominate. The projection neurons of the ventral forebrain include those in the **septum**, the **nucleus of the diagonal band of Broca**, and the **basal nucleus of Meynert**. From these neurons arise an extensive system of axons to the hippocampal formation (from the more rostral neurons in the septal area and diagonal band) and to the neocortex (from the diagonal band and the basal nucleus). The basal nucleus also provides cholinergic fibers to the basolateral amygdala.

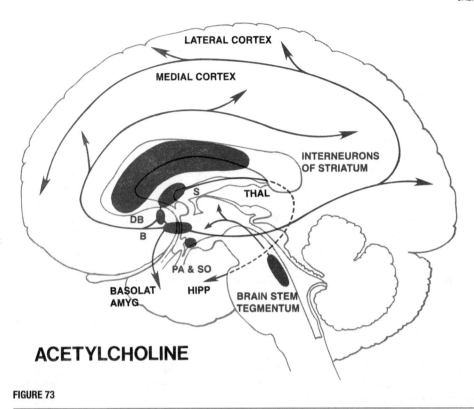

ACETYLCHOLINE

FIGURE 73

● ● ● ● ● ● ● ● ●

The location of the acetylcholine neurons in the central nervous system and their projections. In Figures 73 through 77, areas containing cell bodies are shown and labeled in color. The projection pathways of these neurons are indicated with colored arrows. The regions that receive the cholinergic input are labeled in black. B = basal nucleus of Meynert; BASOLAT AMYG = basolateral amygdala; HIPP = hippocampal formation; PA & SO = paraventricular and supraoptic nuclei of the hypothalamus; S = septum; THAL = thalamus.

A projection found in the rat from cholinergic neurons in the medial habenula to the interpeduncular nucleus has not been demonstrated in the primate brain. Data from the rat are also the only source of information to date on the projections of ACh neurons in the **pedunculopontine and laterodorsal tegmental brain stem nuclei**. In the rat, these neurons project rostrally to the thalamus and hypothalamus and caudally to the paramedian medullary reticular formation. These caudal projections have been implicated in control of rapid eye movement sleep.

ChAT immunoreactive neurons have been localized in the **magnocellular neuronal populations of the paraventricular and supraoptic nuclei of the hypothalamus** and in the posterior lateral hypothalamus.

The best-established functional significance of ACh neurons in the CNS is the role of the cholinergic interneurons of the striatum in motor control (see Chap. 16). In addition, changes in ACh terminals in the cerebral cortex are a major factor in the dementia of Alzheimer's disease, although this is only part of the complex pathology of this disease.

MONOAMINES

• • • • • • • • •

The monoamines, or biogenic amines, that have been identified as neurotransmitters include the catecholamines **dopamine, norepinephrine**, and **epinephrine**; the indoleamine **serotonin**; and histamine.

Catecholamines are produced in the brain and in the sympathetic ganglia from their amino acid precursor **tyrosine** by a sequence of enzymatic steps in which dopamine appears first. In the presence of the appropriate enzymes, dopamine can be converted to norepinephrine, and it, in turn, can be converted to epinephrine. Serotonin is produced in brain and other tissues of the body from the amino acid **tryptophan**; histamine is synthesized from histidine. The activity of the monoamine neurotransmitters in the synaptic cleft is limited by their reuptake into the presynaptic ending, where they are recycled into vesicles for future release.

In the human brain, the dopaminergic and adrenergic neurons contain melanin pigment and can often be visualized microscopically without special stains.

Dopamine

Dopamine is localized in the CNS in a number of sites where it is confined to interneurons. These sites include the **retina** and the **olfactory bulb**, where the dopamine neurons selectively inhibit transmission of sensory information to enhance the signal-to-noise ratio. This physiologic process is known as **lateral inhibition**, and it is an important part of information processing in all sensory systems.

Projection neurons that produce dopamine are found in the diencephalon and the brain stem. In the diencephalon, dopamine cell bodies give rise to the **tuberoinfundibular and tuberohypophysial dopamine projections**, which inhibit the release of prolactin and melanocyte-stimulating hormone from the anterior and intermediate lobes of the pituitary, respectively, and the **incertohypothalamic projections**, which connect the zona incerta in the posterior diencephalon with the anterior hypothalamus, medial preoptic area, and septal area. A third dopamine projection system arises from neurons in the caudal diencephalon that send descending projections to the dorsal motor nucleus of the vagus, the nucleus solitarius, and the spinal cord.

Longer dopamine projection systems arise from the **substantia nigra** and the **ventral tegmental area (VTA)** of the midbrain (Fig. 74). The former, the nigrostriatal dopamine system, is particularly important in the control of motor function. Parkinsonism is caused by damage to these neurons and the loss of their inhibitory input to the neurons of the caudate and putamen (see Chap. 18). The function of the VTA's dopamine projections to the forebrain, called the mesolimbic and mesocortical systems, is related to the limbic system and ventral striatum, in which these projections have dense terminations. This system has been linked to the complex group of diseases referred to as schizophrenia. Antipsychotic drugs, which have long been known to alleviate symptoms effectively in schizophrenic patients, are now known to bind to and block one of the two major dopaminergic receptor subgroups.

At least six dopamine receptor subtypes have been identified. All are G protein–coupled (metabotropic) receptors that affect the activity of adenyl cyclase. However, on the basis of their specific actions on this enzyme and their individual agonists and

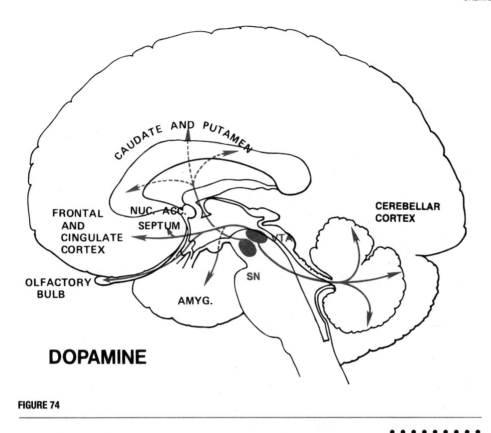

DOPAMINE

FIGURE 74

• • • • • • • • • •

The locations and projections of two of the major dopaminergic systems in the brain are illustrated in color. Other dopaminergic systems are described in the text. AMYG. = amygdala; NUC. ACC. = nucleus accumbens; SN = substantia nigra; VTA = ventral tegmental area.

antagonists, they have been divided into two major subgroups, for which the D1 and D2 receptors are prototypes. The D2 receptor subgroup (D2a, D2b, D3 and D4) has a higher affinity for antipsychotic drugs than does the D1 subgroup (D1 and D5).

Norepinephrine

Norepinephrine, or noradrenalin (NA), cell bodies are found in the sympathetic ganglia, where they give rise to all of the postganglionic fibers except those to sweat glands. In the CNS, norepinephrine cell bodies are confined to the brain stem, but their axons, which are highly branched, extend to all parts of the CNS (Fig. 75). These cell bodies are found in the medulla and pons. In the medulla, they are located in the **medullary reticular formation**, closely associated with the dorsal motor nucleus of X and the nucleus solitarius. In the pons, NA neurons are located in the central gray area surrounding the fourth ventricle and in the locus ceruleus.

Although the **locus ceruleus** contains only several hundred neurons, it sends axons to all parts of the CNS: rostrally to the forebrain, dorsally to the cerebellum, and caudally to the medulla and spinal cord. The rostral projections of the locus ceruleus follow three different routes, including the central tegmental tract, the dor-

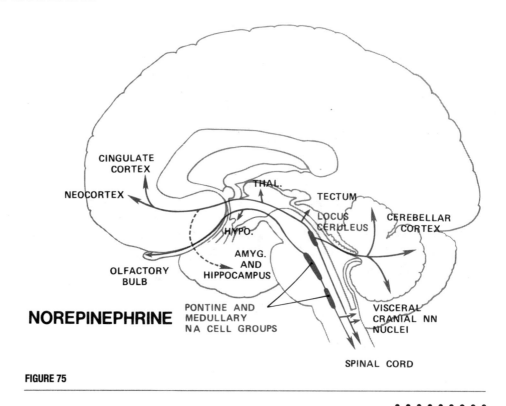

FIGURE 75

• • • • • • • • •

Norepinephrine (noradrenalin) neurons in the brain stem and their projections are illustrated in color. AMYG. = amygdala; HYPO. = hypothalamus; NA = norepinephrine; NN = nerves; THAL. = thalamus.

sal longitudinal fasciculus, and the medial forebrain bundle (these three tracts are not shown separately in Fig. 75), to terminate extensively in the tectum, thalamus, and outermost (molecular) layer of the cerebral cortex, including the hippocampus. A projection through the superior cerebellar peduncle leads to a similar terminal field in the molecular layer of the cerebellar cortex. The projections of the lateral tegmental norepinephrine groups of cells are distributed to more limited areas in the basal telencephalon and the spinal cord.

Like dopamine, NA has been found to have inhibitory influences on postsynaptic neurons. In some locations, its primary action appears to be to inhibit spontaneous activity. Thus, like dopamine's action in the retina and olfactory bulb, NA may enhance the signal-to-noise ratio in its terminal field. This influence is spread widely, not only because of the extensive branching of the NA neurons but also because it can be secreted into the neuropil from varicosities along the axons, as well as at conventional synaptic sites.

Epinephrine

Although the role of this catecholamine hormone in the physiologic response to stress has been established for many years, its identification as a transmitter in the CNS is much more recent. In the periphery, norepinephrine and epinephrine are released by both the adrenal medulla and postganglionic sympathetic nerve endings. In the CNS, epinephrine neurons are restricted to the lower brain stem, where they are found in the **dorsal tegmentum**, near the floor of the fourth ventricle, and in the **lateral reticular nucleus**, in the ventrolateral tegmentum (see Fig. 77A). The ascending projections from these cells comprise part of the central tegmental tract and, in the human, appear to project primarily to the locus ceruleus and the midbrain periaqueductal gray area. Caudal projections into the spinal cord terminate in the intermediolateral cell column of sympathetic neurons. Little is known of the action of epinephrine as a central neurotransmitter except in the locus ceruleus, where it inhibits firing of the neurons.

Both epinephrine and norepinephrine act on a common set of receptors ($\alpha1$, $\alpha2$, $\beta1$, and $\beta2$). Of these, the beta receptors predominate in the brain, where $\beta1$ receptors are found in highest density in the cerebral cortex and $\beta2$ receptors in the cerebellum. However, both in the brain and other tissues, especially the heart, $\beta1$ and $\beta2$ receptors coexist in the same location and cannot be differentiated with regard to their physiologic functions.

Serotonin

Serotonin (5-hydroxytryptamine, or 5-HT) is an indolamine found in many cells of the body (e.g., mast cells, platelets, and enterochromaffin cells of the gut) as well as in neurons of the CNS. It is synthesized from tryptophan and released from synaptic vesicles in the neuronal endings, and like the catecholamines, its action in the synaptic cleft is limited by active reuptake into the same terminal.

Cell bodies of origin for the serotonin pathways are found only in the brain stem. The vast majority of these neurons are within the eight raphe nuclei, which extend along the midline throughout the length of the brain stem and are bounded laterally by nuclei of the reticular formation (Fig. 76). Although there is some overlapping, the efferent projections of the raphe nuclei can be divided into two distinct groups. The rostral nuclear groups project rostrally to the forebrain and to the cerebellum. The caudal raphe nuclei send their axons into the spinal cord. Serotonin endings are also found in the ependyma lining the ventricles. Axons of the rostral raphe nuclei ascend in the medial forebrain bundle and distribute to the diencephalon and to both the striatum and the cortex of the telencephalon. In the cerebral cortex, the 5-HT terminals are less extensive than the norepinephrine terminals, but both 5-HT and norepinephrine terminal systems are rather diffuse, in contrast to the discrete and topographically organized endings of the dopamine system. Serotonin terminals are particularly dense in limbic cortical areas and in the sensory cortical areas such as the primary visual cortex.

Multiple factors influence the firing of the raphe nuclei, including pain stimuli and changes in blood pressure and body temperature. Through its diffuse projections, the serotonin system, in turn, influences multiple systems. In the spinal cord, for example, descending raphe–spinal axons inhibit afferent input from pain fibers and, at the same time, facilitate motoneurons. Although important physiologic roles have been proposed for serotonin in sleep, pain transmission, mood (and affective disorders), and aggression, much remains to be learned about the specific physiologic functions of 5-HT.

Serotonin receptors now include at least seven described subtypes (5-HT$_{1A-D}$, 5-HT$_2$, 5-HT$_3$, and 5HT$_4$). Of these, all but the 5-HT$_3$ receptors are G protein–coupled receptors.

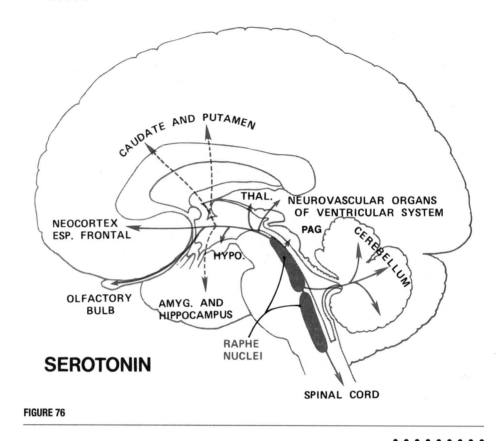

SEROTONIN

FIGURE 76

• • • • • • • • •

Serotonin fibers arising from the raphe nuclei of the brain stem are illustrated in color. AMYG. = amygdala; HYPO. = hypothalamus; PAG = periaqueductal gray area; THAL. = thalamus.

NEUROPEPTIDES

• • • • • • • • •

Neurons that produce neuropeptides for release at their terminals employ a fundamentally different system for neurotransmitter synthesis than do neurons that produce ACh and monoamines. The latter substances are synthesized by enzymatic alterations of molecules that are delivered to the cell. In contrast, peptides are produced de novo in the cell body, through RNA-directed preparation of a protein, from which the active peptide is later cleaved by peptidases.

Neuropeptides also appear to differ significantly from other groups of transmitters in the variability of their distribution in different species. Given this variability, it is particularly important to present information derived from human brains. However, definitive localization of the cell bodies containing neuropeptides is rarely obtained from human postmortem material. Even under experimental conditions, neuropeptide-producing cell bodies are often visualized only when the peptide has been artificially accumulated by blocking axonal transport. Thus, the descriptions of neuropeptide systems in this chapter summarize the current state of knowledge with the caveat that definitive information from the human brain is limited.

Opioid Peptides

Many peptides have been studied as putative neurotransmitters. Among the most intensively studied are the opioid peptides, which are now recognized as three genetically distinct peptide families. The opioid peptide neurotransmitters come from three precursors: proopiomelanocortin (POMC) [the beta-endorphin/adrenocorticotropic hormone (ACTH) precursor], proenkephalin, and prodynorphin. Each of these precursors contains several active peptides that are differentially produced and regulated in different brain areas. In addition, there are several biologically active sites within a single peptide, and multiple opioid receptors have been identified. Thus, the opioid peptides constitute an entire class of transmitters.

The opioid transmitters appear to be important in neural systems that respond to stress. This is especially noteworthy in the involvement of opioids in pain pathways and cardiovascular control circuits. Many of the opioid cells have been localized in neural systems that process somatic and visceral pain information and in the limbic system. The opiatergic system is also of great importance in regulating hypothalamo-pituitary neuroendocrine function.

Enkephalin can be produced from all three of the opioid peptide precursors. Met-enkephalin is derived from both POMC and proenkephalin, whereas leu-enkephalin originates from proenkephalin and prodynorphin. Taken together, met-enkephalin and leu-enkephalin neurons are widely distributed in the CNS. Figure 77B shows the location of some of the major groups of **enkephalin cell** bodies in the striatum, the limbic system, and the raphe nuclei of the brain stem. One of these groups, the striatal neurons, provides projections to the external segment of the globus pallidus and substantia nigra. In these cells, the enkephalin is coexistent with GABA. In many other areas, the enkephalin-containing neurons are interneurons. This includes the cerebral cortex (not illustrated in Fig. 77B).

Dynorphin-containing cells, like enkephalin neurons, are heavily concentrated in limbic system structures and the hypothalamus. In general, dynorphin cells are less widely distributed in the brain than cells containing enkephalin but are much more numerous than the beta-endorphin neurons.

Beta-endorphin cell bodies are restricted in distribution (Fig. 77C) and are found almost exclusively in the hypothalamus. One group of beta-endorphin cells not discussed in this chapter has been localized in some species in the nucleus solitarius of the medulla.

The best studied of the multiple opioid receptor subtypes are the mu, delta, and kappa receptors, which preferentially bind beta-endorphin, enkephalins, and dynorphins, respectively. This preferential binding is, however, by no means exclusive. Each of the three receptor subtypes has been found in areas to which few, if any, projections from cells produce the preferred ligand. The mu receptors appear to be the most abundant and widely distributed opioid receptors in the human brain. All three opioid receptor subtypes are found in the neocortex, limbic cortex, basal ganglia, and cerebellum, but they are differentially distributed within these areas.

Gut-Brain Peptides

A number of peptides that were first identified in the gastrointestinal tract have now been localized in specific cell groups within the brain. These include substance P, cholecystokinin, vasoactive intestinal peptide, and neurotensin.

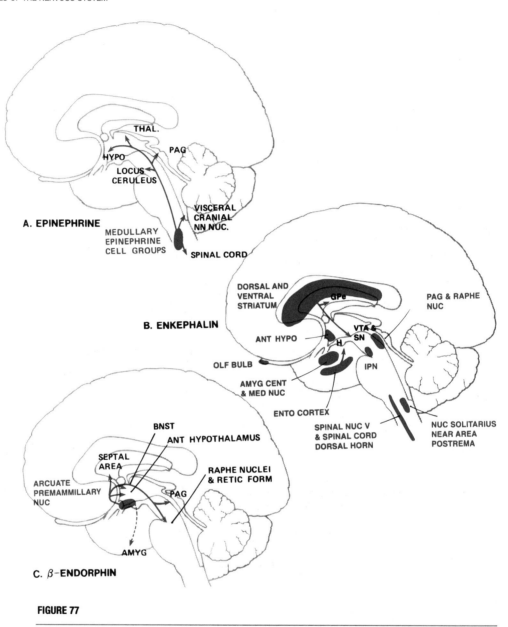

A. EPINEPHRINE

B. ENKEPHALIN

C. β-ENDORPHIN

FIGURE 77

• • • • • • • • •

Composite of a variety of central nervous systems producing epinephrine, peptides, and amino acids as neurotransmitters. Colored areas indicate the locations of cell bodies; colored arrows show projections away from the area of origin. Areas of termination of these projections are labeled in black. AMYG = amygdala; AMYG CENT & MED NUC = central and medial nuclei of the amygdala; BNST = bed nucleus of the stria terminalis; ENTO CORTEX = entorhinal cortex; GPe = globus pallidus external; GPi = globus pallidus internal; H or HIPP = hippocampal formation; HYPO = hypothalamus; IPN = interpeduncular nucleus; PAG = periaqueductal gray area; RN = red nucleus; RETIC FORM = reticular formation; SN = substantia nigra; SpV = spinal nucleus of V; THAL = thalamus; VTA = ventral tegmental area.

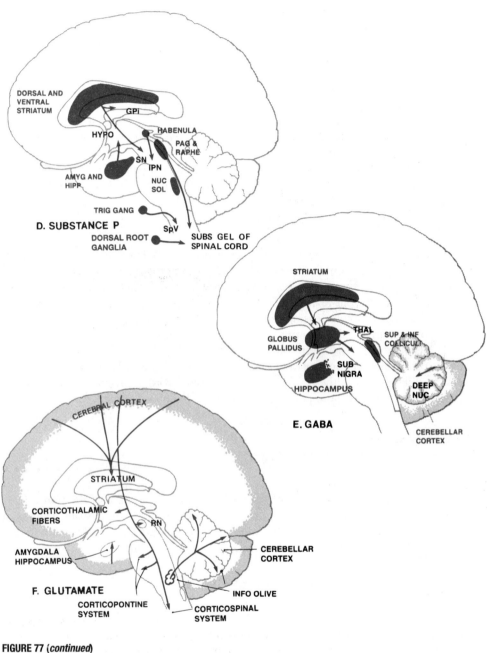

FIGURE 77 (*continued*)

• • • • • • • • •

SUBSTANCE P

Substance P is a member of the family of neuropeptides called neurokinins, which are the tachykinins of the mammalian nervous system. Substance P is an undecapeptide for which the exact chemical structure has been known for some time. It has an excitatory effect of long duration in CNS areas where it is active. One of these areas is the substantia gelatinosa of the spinal cord, where dorsal root ganglion cells conveying information from Aδ and C fibers secrete substance

P. Another important system containing substance P is a specific population of neurons in the striatum that projects to the internal segment of the globus pallidus and the substantia nigra. These cells, like the enkephalinergic striatal cells, contain GABA as well as the neuropeptide. Figure 77D shows other areas where radioimmunoassay and immunohistochemical studies have demonstrated high concentrations of this peptide. Not shown in Figure 77D are areas where substance P fibers and terminals of as yet unknown origin are observed. These areas include the anterior nucleus, centromedian nucleus, and ventral posteromedial nucleus of the thalamus, as well as the deep layers of the superior colliculus and the parabrachial nucleus of the brain stem.

There are three major subtypes of receptors at which substance P and the other neurokinins are believed to act. These are the NK-P, NK-A, and NK-B receptors.

Hypophysiotrophic Peptides

A third group of neuropeptides that act as neuromodulators in the brain consists of the peptides first identified as neuroendocrine secretory products. These peptides are produced by neurons that control pituitary function. They include vasopressin, oxytocin, corticotropin-releasing factor, gonadotropin-releasing hormone, somatostatin, and thyrotropin-releasing hormone.

Although many of the neurons containing these peptides are found in the hypothalamus, they have also been found in numerous other areas of the brain, and their axons provide projections not only to the median eminence and neurohypophysis but also to distant areas of the CNS, including the spinal cord. Only some of the specific projection systems of these peptidergic cells have been determined.

AMINO ACIDS

• • • • • • • • •

Amino acid neurotransmitters are probably the most plentiful of the transmitters identified to date, in terms of the number of synapses at which they act. The major molecules in this group include the inhibitory transmitters GABA, glycine, and taurine, and the excitatory amino acids glutamate and aspartate.

Gamma-Aminobutyric Acid and Glycine

In mammals, GABA is found almost exclusively in the CNS. It is produced in neurons in reactions that are related to carbohydrate metabolism; its immediate precursor is L-glutamic acid, which is decarboxylated by an enzyme that is unique to the mammalian CNS. The inactivation of GABA's transmitter action is not known in detail but appears primarily to involve enzymatic breakdown in the synaptic cleft or postsynaptic cell.

GABA is widely distributed in inhibitory interneurons and projection neurons over much of the CNS. Two of the best known sites of GABAergic neurons are the cerebellar cortex, where Purkinje cells produce GABA for inhibition of the deep nuclei, and in the striatum, where GABAergic cells project to the substantia nigra and globus pallidus (Fig. 77E). In Huntington's disease, the loss of GABAergic neurons in the caudate nucleus and putamen reduces the GABA-mediated inhibition of the substantia nigra, which in turn causes an increase in dopamine produced by the nigrostriatal neurons. This unbalances the dopamine–acetylcholine relationship in the striatum and is associated with uncontrolled involuntary (choreic) movements. In a sense, this is the reverse of the loss of nigrostriatal dopamine innervation, which decreases the dopamine–acetylcholine ratio in the striatum and is associated with the difficulty in initiating movement seen in parkinsonism. GABA is also the major transmitter of the globus pallidus and its projections to the thalamus and subthalamic nucleus and substantia nigra.

GABAergic inhibitory interneurons are also important in the circuitry of the cerebral cortex, cerebellar cortex, olfactory bulb, hippocampus, and hypothalamus, most of which are not shown in Figure 77E. In many of these cell populations, GABA coexists with a variety of neuropeptides. Although cells containing GABA and a neuropeptide compose less than 20 percent of the total population of GABA neurons, it has been estimated that more than 90 percent of the substance P, cholecystokinin, neuropeptide Y, and somatostatin cells in the monkey brain also produce GABA as a transmitter. In the primate brain, GABA has also been found in neurons of most of the thalamic nuclei and in the substantia nigra.

Two major types of GABA receptors, the ionotropic $GABA_A$ and the G protein–coupled $GABA_B$ receptors, have been described. The $GABA_A$ receptors are distributed throughout the brain and are thought to mediate the sedative effects of the benzodiazepines and the actions of the barbiturates.

Glycine, like GABA, functions as an inhibitory neurotransmitter in the CNS, but unlike GABA, which is widely distributed in the brain, glycine appears to be used primarily by inhibitory neurons in the spinal cord and brain stem. It is plentiful in the brain stem auditory pathways.

Glutamate and Aspartate

Glutamic acid (glutamate) is the most plentiful amino acid transmitter in the adult CNS. It does not cross the blood–brain barrier and is synthesized from glucose in a metabolic pathway that includes glutaminase. Glutamate functions as an excitatory neurotransmitter in many areas of the CNS. Initially, its status as a neurotransmitter was difficult to establish because of its widespread distribution and its role in other metabolic pathways (e.g., synthesis of GABA). Because the available evidence does not allow aspartate to be ruled out as the active amino acid in many cases, the use of "glutamate" in the following paragraphs should be understood to mean "glutamate/aspartate."

The highest concentrations of glutamate synapses in the mammalian brain appear to be in the dentate gyrus of the hippocampus, the cerebral cortex, and the striatum. The hippocampal formation not only receives glutamatergic input from the entorhinal cortex but also contains pyramidal cells in the hippocampus proper that use glutamate as a transmitter. In the cerebral cortex, glutaminase-immunoreactive neurons have been localized in layers V and VI, the layers of origin of projections to the striatum, brain stem, spinal cord, and thalamus. The striatum receives excitatory glutamatergic inputs from all areas of the cortex (Fig. 77F). Changes in this corticostriatal system may, in fact, be the first step in the development of Huntington's disease and may be a clue to the involvement of glutamatergic pathways in other neurodegenerative disorders.

Virtually all major efferent systems of the cerebral cortex use glutamate. This includes not only the corticostriate pathway but also the corticobulbar, corticopontine, and corticothalamic pathways. The climbing fiber afferents to the cerebellar cortex from the inferior olivary complex are thought to use glutamate as a transmitter. In this case, experimental evidence from nonprimate species suggests specifically that aspartate may be the transmitter.

Although the excitation provided by these fibers is essential for normal brain function, hyperactivation of the excitatory amino acid systems, or failure of the normal rapid uptake mechanisms for glutamate, can be more deleterious than inactivation of the pathways. Both experimental and clinical data demonstrate that, in excess, these amino acids can function as excitotoxins, causing neuronal cell death.

Like other neurotransmitter systems, glutamate has been found to act at a variety of different receptors that are defined by their specific agonists. These include the kainate, quisqualate, and N-methyl-D-aspartate (NMDA) receptors. The NMDA receptors are the only receptors of the three that open channels in the membrane highly permeable to calcium, and it is thought to be through this mechanism that NMDA receptors are primarily responsible for the long-term damage in excitotoxicity.

6

Circulation of Blood and Cerebrospinal Fluid

CHAPTER

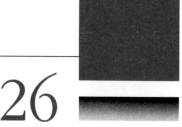

26

Cerebral Arteries

BLOOD SUPPLY TO THE FOREBRAIN

The arterial supply to the brain is provided by the paired common carotid arteries, which supply the "anterior circulation" and the paired vertebral arteries, which supply the "posterior circulation." The posterior circulation has been described in Chapter 10. This chapter deals with the anterior circulation.

The common carotid arteries of each side divide into an **external carotid artery**, which supplies the face, scalp, and meninges, and an **internal carotid artery**. The internal carotid artery ascends into the cranial cavity and divides into the **middle cerebral artery** and the **anterior cerebral artery**. Before reaching this branch point, the internal carotid artery gives off the **ophthalmic artery**, which supplies blood to the eye. Occlusion of the ophthalmic artery can lead to complete unilateral blindness. **Amaurosis fugax** consists of temporary unilateral blindness, often because of emboli (small particles of cholesterol and platelets from a diseased heart or carotid artery) that pass through the ophthalmic artery to the eye.

The **middle cerebral artery** (Fig. 78), a terminal branch of the internal carotid, enters the depth of the lateral fissure and divides into cortical branches that spread in a radiating fashion to supply the insula and the lateral surface of the frontal, parietal, occipital, and temporal lobes. The **lateral and medial striate arteries**, sometimes termed the **lenticulostriate arteries**, are small branches, variable in position and arrangement, that come from the basal part of the middle cerebral artery and the anterior cerebral artery to supply the internal capsule and portions of the basal ganglia (Figs. 79 and 80).

Blockage of a lateral striate artery by atherosclerosis causes infarction of the internal capsule that manifests clinically as a "stroke" (i.e., a neurologic deficit of sudden onset that has a vascular cause). Because all corticospinal fibers are contained

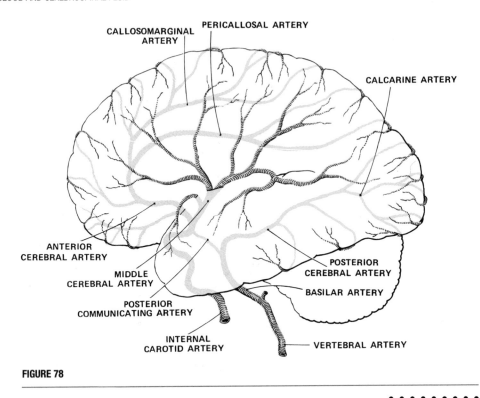

FIGURE 78

● ● ● ● ● ● ● ● ●

A left lateral view of the cerebral hemisphere, showing the principal arteries. The anterior cerebral and posterior cerebral arteries are on the medial surface and are shown as though projected through the substance of the brain.

in one small area of the internal capsule, a relatively small infarct (less than 1.5 cm in diameter) in this structure may result in complete paralysis of the opposite side of the body. Initially, the patient has a hypotonic hemiplegia with decreased muscle stretch reflexes; with time, the patient develops a spastic hemiplegia with increased muscle stretch reflexes and an extensor plantar response. Occasionally, a lateral striate artery may rupture in a patient with hypertension, resulting in hemorrhage into the internal capsule. If the hemorrhage is small, the neurologic deficit usually consists of hemiplegia from which the patient may recover, but a large hemorrhage may be fatal (see Fig. 27 in Chap. 9).

An occlusion of the main trunk of the middle cerebral artery by the formation of a clot **(thrombosis)** produces paralysis of the opposite side of the body with a preponderant effect in the face and upper extremity, hypesthesia (decreased sensation) in the same regions, and aphasia if the occlusion is located in the dominant hemisphere. When individual branches of the middle cerebral artery are occluded, the symptoms are limited to the loss of function in that particular region. For example, if the branch of the middle cerebral artery supplying the inferior frontal gyrus on the left is occluded, weakness is noted in the lower part of the right face and tongue, and the patient has Broca's aphasia.

The **anterior cerebral artery**, one of the two terminal branches of the internal carotid artery, turns medially to enter the medial longitudinal cerebral fissure. On reaching the genu of the corpus callosum, it curves dorsally and turns

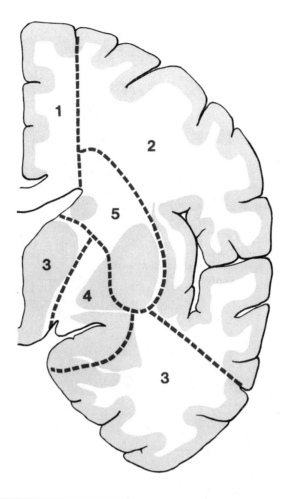

FIGURE 79

• • • • • • • • •

A cross section through the brain at about the level of the central sulcus, showing the areas of distribution of (*1*) the anterior cerebral artery, including the callosomarginal and pericallosal arteries; (*2*) the middle cerebral artery; (*3*) the posterior cerebral artery to the diencephalon and inferior temporal lobe; (*4*) the medial striate arteries to the internal capsule, globus pallidus, and amygdala; and (*5*) the lateral striate arteries to the caudate nucleus, putamen, and internal capsule.

backward close to the body of the corpus callosum, supplying a callosomarginal branch and continuing as the pericallosal artery. These arteries supply the medial surface of the frontal and parietal lobes and also an adjoining strip of cortex along the medial edge of the lateral surface of these lobes (see Figs. 78 and 79). A small recurrent branch (medial striate artery, or recurrent artery of Huebner), given off near the base of the artery, supplies the anterior limb of the internal capsule (see Figs. 79 and 80). Thrombosis along the course of the anterior cerebral artery produces paresis and hypesthesia of the opposite lower extremity because of damage to the paracentral lobule.

The paired posterior cerebral arteries are the terminal branches of the basilar artery (see Fig. 80; see Fig. 40 in Chap. 10). The posterior cerebral arteries curve dorsally around the cerebral peduncles and send branches to the medial and in-

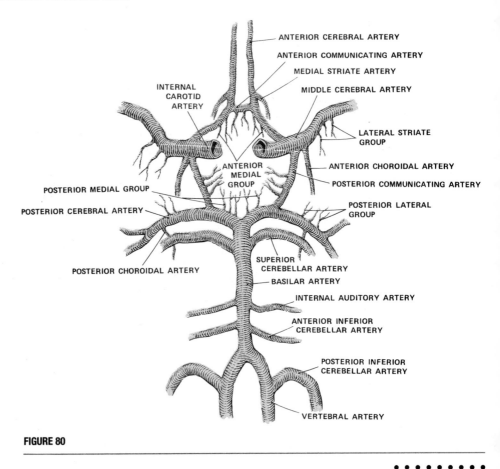

FIGURE 80

• • • • • • • • •

The origin of the branches from the circulus arteriosus, or circle of Willis.

ferior aspects of the temporal lobe and to the occipital lobe (see Fig. 78). A separate branch of the posterior cerebral artery, the **calcarine artery**, supplies the visual cortex. A number of perforating branches (posterior medial and posterior lateral groups in Fig. 80) supply the posterior and lateral parts of the thalamus and the subthalamus (see Fig. 79). Occlusion of the posterolateral thalamic branches produces partial to complete loss of sensation in the opposite half of the body. Often, there is an accompanying paresis of the affected side of the body. In time, the **thalamic syndrome** may appear, consisting of severe, constant pain in the regions with limited sensation. The pain is agonizing and often has a burning quality. Sensations of touch, pain, and temperature are decreased in the affected limbs. In addition to the sensory changes, symptoms of cerebellar ataxia and tremor may be produced in the extremities of the opposite side from damage to fibers of the superior cerebellar peduncle ascending to the ventral lateral nucleus of the thalamus. The calcarine branch of the posterior cerebral artery may be occluded independently of the thalamic branches. In this case, the only sign produced will be contralateral homonymous hemianopia.

FORMATION OF THE CIRCULUS ARTERIOSUS AND ITS CENTRAL BRANCHES

• • • • • • • • •

The **circulus arteriosus (circle of Willis)** is formed by the junction of the terminal branches of the basilar artery and the two internal carotid arteries. This is achieved through a pair of **posterior communicating arteries** and an **anterior communicating artery** (see Fig. 80). All of the major cerebral vessels have their origin in the arterial circle.

The **central arteries** supply the structures within the interior of the brain: the diencephalon, corpus striatum, and internal capsule. These vessels are direct branches of the circle of Willis. They are illustrated in Figure 80 and may be conveniently considered in four groups:

1. The **anterior medial group** of central arteries originates from the anterior cerebral and anterior communicating arteries. Distribution through the anterior perforated substance supplies the anterior hypothalamic region (i.e., the preoptic and supraoptic regions).
2. The **posterior medial group** originates from the posterior cerebral and posterior communicating arteries. Distribution is through the posterior perforated substance. The rostral group supplies the tuber cinereum, infundibular stalk, and hypophysis. Deeper branches penetrate the thalamus. The caudal group supplies the mammillary bodies, subthalamus, and medial portion of the thalamus and midbrain.
3. The **anterior lateral group** consists of the **lateral striate arteries**, which originate primarily from the middle cerebral arteries, and the **medial striate artery** or **recurrent artery of Huebner**, which originates from the anterior cerebral arteries. The medial striate artery supplies the anterior limb of the internal capsule. The lateral striate vessels supply the basal ganglia and part of the posterior limb of the internal capsule. These vessels are also known as lenticulostriate arteries.
4. The **posterior lateral group** originates from the posterior cerebral artery. Distribution is to the caudal portion of the thalamus (i.e., the geniculate bodies, pulvinar, and lateral nuclei).

The **anterior and posterior choroidal arteries** are also considered to be central branches. The anterior choroidal artery arises from the internal carotid or the middle cerebral artery and supplies the choroid plexus of the lateral ventricles, the hippocampus, some of the globus pallidus, and part of the posterior limb of the internal capsule. The posterior choroidal artery arises from the posterior cerebral artery and supplies the choroid plexus of the third ventricle and the dorsal surface of the thalamus.

CHAPTER

27

The Cerebrospinal Fluid

The brain and spinal cord are suspended in cerebrospinal fluid, a clear, watery liquid that fills the subarachnoid space surrounding them. The four ventricles of the brain also are filled with this fluid. The average total quantity of fluid in adults is estimated to be 100 to 150 ml. The cerebrospinal fluid is constantly being renewed by production and reabsorption so that the total volume is replaced several times daily. Small amounts of protein, sugar, electrolytes, and a very few lymphocytes (no more than 5 per mm³) are present in the fluid. It differs from plasma in that it contains very little protein, and it differs from an ultrafiltrate of plasma in that the concentrations of various ions are maintained at levels different from those in plasma.

FORMATION AND CIRCULATION OF CEREBROSPINAL FLUID

The cerebrospinal fluid is formed mainly by the **choroid plexuses**, which are capillary networks surrounded by cuboidal or columnar epithelium and projecting into the ventricles. There are two large plexuses, one in the floor of each lateral ventricle, supplemented by smaller ones in the roofs of the third and fourth ventricles (Fig. 81). On the average, the rate of formation of cerebrospinal fluid is 0.37 ml per minute. Cerebrospinal fluid is not simply an ultrafiltrate of serum; its formation is controlled by enzymatic processes.

Cerebrospinal fluid moves slowly from the ventricles into the subarachnoid spaces, from which it passes into the dural venous sinuses and is removed by the blood stream. The fluid leaves the lateral ventricles through the **interventricular foramina (foramina of Monro)**, traverses the third ventricle, and reaches the fourth ventricle by way of the **cerebral aqueduct**, which is the narrowest passageway of its entire route (see Fig. 81). Three openings in the fourth ventricle allow the cerebrospinal fluid to pass from the ventricle into the subarachnoid space outside the brain. The two **lateral ventricular foramina (foramina of Luschka)** are located in the roof of the lateral recesses of the fourth ventricle; the **median ventricular foramen (foramen of Magendie)** is in the midline of the roof of the fourth ventricle. The subarachnoid space, which lies between the arachnoid membrane externally and the pia mater internally, provides a route by which the fluid can flow from its site of production in the ventricles to the points of absorption. Cerebrospinal fluid flows from the outlet foramina of the fourth ventricle over the whole surface of the brain and spinal cord. In places where the brain surface is not close to the bone of the skull, collections of cerebrospinal fluid are found within the subarachnoid space, particularly around the base of the brain. The largest of these is the **cisterna magna**, which is located between the inferior surface of the cerebellum and the medulla. Other cisterns—the pontine, interpeduncular, and chiasmatic—lie between the base of the brain and the floor of the cranial cavity. The cisterna ambiens lies dorsal and lateral to the midbrain.

Cerebrospinal fluid also fills the tubular extension of the subarachnoid space that forms a sleeve around the spinal cord. The lower limit of this space is variable, but on the average, it lies at the body of the second sacral vertebra, considerably below the end of the spinal cord. Only a small amount of cerebrospinal fluid reabsorption occurs in **spinal arachnoid villi**. Thus, the spinal subarachnoid space is in effect a blind pocket, and exchange of spinal fluid takes place over the cerebral hemispheres through a slow mixing process induced by changes in posture.

Cerebrospinal fluid flows slowly upward from the spinal cord and basal areas of the brain over the convexities of the hemispheres until it reaches the **arachnoid villi (pacchionian granulations)** in the walls of the superior sagittal sinus. It passes through

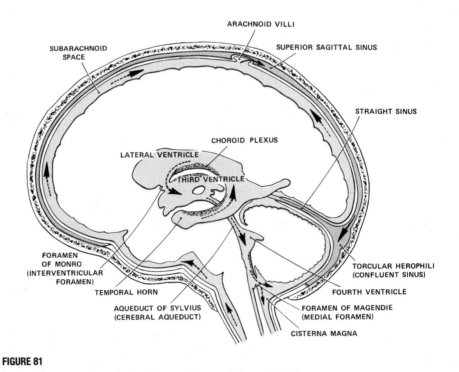

FIGURE 81

The circulation of the cerebrospinal fluid. The foramina of Luschka, in the lateral recesses of the fourth ventricle, are not shown.

these villi into the venous blood stream in the sinus. The arachnoid villi function as valves, allowing one-way flow of cerebrospinal fluid from the subarachnoid spaces into the venous blood. All constituents of the fluid leave with the fluid, a process termed **bulk flow**. Cerebrospinal fluid also is absorbed from the subarachnoid space surrounding the brain stem and spinal cord by the vessels in the sheaths of emerging cranial and spinal nerves. The veins and capillaries of the pia mater also may be capable of removing some cerebrospinal fluid by diffusion across their walls.

The subarachnoid space extends into the substance of the nervous system through extensions around blood vessels known as perivascular spaces, or **Virchow-Robin** spaces. Every blood vessel entering the nervous system passes across the subarachnoid space and carries with it a sleeve of arachnoid immediately surrounding the vessel. As the blood vessel enters the brain, it carries both this arachnoid covering and more externally, a sleeve of pia mater, for a short distance into the tissue. The cerebrospinal fluid of the subarachnoid space probably receives a contribution from the perivascular spaces. Small solutes diffuse freely between the extracellular fluid and the cerebrospinal fluid in these perivascular spaces, and also across the ependymal surface of the ventricles, so that metabolites can move from brain tissue to the subarachnoid space. Within the depths of the central nervous system, the layers of pia and arachnoid fuse, so that the perivascular space does not continue to the level of the capillary beds.

COMPOSITION AND FUNCTION OF CEREBROSPINAL FLUID

• • • • • • • • •

Cerebrospinal fluid is formed by a combination of capillary filtration and active epithelial secretion. The fluid is similar to an ultrafiltrate of blood plasma but contains lower concentrations of potassium, bicarbonate, calcium, and glucose, and higher concentrations of magnesium and chloride. The pH of cerebrospinal fluid is lower than that of blood.

Cerebrospinal fluid has several functions. (1) Cerebrospinal fluid preserves homeostasis in the nervous system. The constituents of cerebrospinal fluid are in equilibrium with brain extracellular fluid and thus maintain a constant external environment for the cells of the nervous system. (2) Cerebrospinal fluid provides buoyancy for the brain, decreasing the weight of the brain on the skull, and serves as a mechanical cushion, protecting the brain from impact with the bones of the skull. (3) Cerebrospinal fluid drains unwanted substances away from the brain. This is important because the brain has few if any lymphatic vessels.

THE BLOOD–BRAIN BARRIER

• • • • • • • • •

The brain is able readily to absorb some substances from the blood, such as glucose and oxygen, but other substances cannot be absorbed. The barrier to passage of molecules from the blood into the brain is known as the **blood–brain barrier**. This is a physical barrier resulting from a combination of membrane properties and cellular transport systems. A similar barrier exists between blood and cerebrospinal fluid and is called the **blood–cerebrospinal fluid barrier**. The blood–brain barrier provides selective mechanisms for exclusion or transport of any given solute depending on the functional characteristics of brain capillaries and the biochemical characteristics of the solute. The primary locus of the blood–brain barrier is the capillary endothelium. Brain capillaries are unique in having (1) **tight junctions** between capillary endothelial cells, (2) few pinocytotic vesicles, (3) glial foot processes of astrocytes encasing capillaries, and (4) an exceptionally high number of mitochondria (and thus the capability for high levels of oxidative metabolism) in the endothelial cells. These features make brain capillary endothelium more like a secretory membrane than the capillary endothelium in other organs.

Several characteristics of solutes can affect their ability to penetrate the blood–brain barrier. These characteristics are important in determining how well drugs enter the central nervous system: (1) Small molecules enter the central nervous system more rapidly than large molecules. Most larger proteins do not enter at all, and ordinarily, substances bound to serum protein cannot penetrate. (2) Substances that are highly soluble in lipid enter the central nervous system more readily than those that are poorly soluble in lipid. (3) Some substances, such as glucose and some amino acids, are transported by carrier-mediated mechanisms into the brain. These transport systems can affect both entry and exit of substances.

The permeability barriers provide mechanisms to preserve the homeostasis of the nervous system by promoting entry of needed substances and by excluding or removing unwanted substances. The blood–brain barrier breaks down under certain conditions, including infections, stroke, brain tumors, and trauma.

PRESSURE OF CEREBROSPINAL FLUID

Any obstruction to the normal passage of cerebrospinal fluid causes the fluid to back up in the ventricles and leads to a general increase in intracranial pressure. After the pressure has been elevated for some time, usually a matter of days or weeks, the effect can be seen by inspecting the fundus of the eye with an ophthalmoscope. Because of the high cerebrospinal fluid pressure in the subarachnoid space inside the sleeve of dura mater that surrounds the optic nerve, the retinal veins are dilated and the optic nerve head (optic disk) is pushed forward above the level of the retina. This is known as **papilledema**. If papilledema persists for a long time, the fibers of the optic nerve will be damaged and the disk will assume a chalk-white color instead of the normal pale-pink hue.

The most common cause of papilledema is a brain tumor. Tumors far removed from the ventricles in the supratentorial cranial cavity often do not cause papilledema or increased intracranial pressure until they become large. Tumors of the brain stem and cerebellum, however, often cause increased intracranial pressure while they are still relatively small. Because the posterior fossa is roofed by the semirigid tentorium cerebelli, there is little room for expansion in this fossa. Thus, tumors in this region often cause early obstruction to the flow of cerebrospinal fluid through the aqueduct or fourth ventricle, resulting in increased intracranial pressure. Other cardinal signs of brain tumor, in addition to papilledema, are persistent headache and vomiting, which are often worse in the early morning. The headache probably results from the stretching of nerve endings in the dura mater and intracranial blood vessels. The cause of the nausea and vomiting is not clear, but stimulation of the area postrema and vagal nuclei in the floor of the fourth ventricle may be involved.

Idiopathic intracranial hypertension (benign intracranial hypertension or pseudotumor cerebri) is a condition of undetermined cause usually affecting obese young women. The disease causes headaches and papilledema resulting from a marked increase of intracranial pressure. The condition can be treated effectively and usually resolves after a few weeks or months. If untreated, the disease can cause blindness.

Hydrocephalus is an increase in the volume of cerebrospinal fluid within the ventricular system and can be divided into **obstructive hydrocephalus** and **communicating hydrocephalus**. **Obstructive hydrocephalus** results from an obstruction to the normal flow of cerebrospinal fluid out of the ventricles. Obstruction most commonly occurs at the foramina of Monro, the aqueduct, or at the outlet of the fourth ventricle. Many types of pathology may cause obstructive hydrocephalus, including developmental abnormalities, brain tumors, and inflammatory processes. In **communicating hydrocephalus**, there is free communication between the ventricles and subarachnoid space. Communicating hydrocephalus results from a disturbance in the circulation of cerebrospinal fluid through the subarachnoid space or in the reabsorption of cerebrospinal fluid at the arachnoid villi. In young children in whom the cranial sutures are unfused, hydrocephalus usually causes cranial enlargement. Children with hydrocephalus often fail to achieve normal mental and motor milestones. In older children and adults, the fused sutures do not readily permit cranial enlargement. As a result, the head may be normal in size, but the intracranial pressure is often elevated. In these instances, hydrocephalus may cause lethargy, headaches, vomiting, and unsteadiness of gait.

Normal-pressure hydrocephalus is a syndrome of adults characterized by the triad of dementia, unsteady gait, and urinary incontinence. It is a type of communicating hydrocephalus. In some cases, it is a sequel of inflammatory disorders, but in most cases its cause is unknown. The cerebrospinal fluid is usually normal in composition, and cerebrospinal fluid pressure is normal. Computed tomography and magnetic resonance imaging show abnormalities in the periventricular regions, which are thought to result from increased water content (edema) adjacent to the ventricles. The edema is thought to result from passage of cerebrospinal fluid from the ventricles into adjacent brain, where it is reabsorbed. A test called **isotope cisternography** may be useful in diagnosing this condition. With this test, an inert radiopharmaceutical injected into the lumbar subarachnoid space can be demonstrated with a gamma camera to enter the lateral ventricles. Normally, the radiopharmaceutical is expected to pass over the cerebral convexities and be reabsorbed into the arachnoid villi but not to enter the ventricular system. Detection of the radiopharmaceutical in the ventricles assists in the diagnosis of normal-pressure hydrocephalus. A shunt to divert cerebrospinal fluid from the ventricles to the peritoneal cavity in the abdomen can relieve the symptoms of this condition.

Approaches to Patients with Neurologic Symptoms

CHAPTER

28

Clinical Evaluation of Patients with Neurologic Disorders

Physicians evaluating patients with symptoms referable to the nervous system use the same approach as physicians evaluating patients with any other medical problem. The basis of the neurologic evaluation includes the history of the illness and the physical and neurologic examination.

The **history** consists of a chronologic account of the patient's complaints and should provide clues to the **type of pathology** underlying the complaint. For example, the symptoms in vascular disease such as stroke generally have a sudden onset and improve with time. Patients with progressive symptoms that do not show improvement often have neoplastic diseases such as brain tumors or degenerative diseases such as Alzheimer's disease. Patients with relapsing and remitting symptoms often have demyelinative diseases such as multiple sclerosis.

The **neurologic examination** provides information that assists in localizing the **site of the pathology**. For example, a right-handed patient with an executive aphasia and a right hemiplegia probably has disease involving the left frontal lobe, including Broca's area and the white matter underlying the precentral region. Other types of aphasia, apraxia, and agnosia also commonly result from disease of the cerebral cortex. Patients with a unilateral cranial nerve disorder and a contralateral hemiplegia often have disease involving one side of the brain stem. Patients with spastic paraparesis and loss of sensation below a specific level on the trunk usually have disease of the spinal cord.

After completing the history, general physical examination, and neurologic examination, the physician makes a formulation of the patient's illness by first predicting the localization of the lesion. Then the physician evaluates the possible cause of the lesion; that is, whether it is the result of vascular disease, trauma, neoplasm, degenerative changes, or demyelination. The next step is to determine the differential diagnosis; that is, the most likely disease processes that could account for both the history and the localization. Usually, if the formulation is correct, the list of possible diseases is small. The physician then uses selective laboratory investigations to further the diagnostic process. In most cases, completion of these steps results in a clear diagnosis so that appropriate treatment can be administered.

Since the advent of anatomic imaging techniques such as computed tomography and magnetic resonance, some physicians request imaging procedures for their patients before fully exploring the history and examination. This often results in misleading or inconclusive findings. It is essential to obtain a full history and examination initially, and then formulate the problem before ordering any laboratory test. Considerable time, effort, and expense can be saved in this way. Moreover, disease processes that move rapidly, such as meningitis or encephalitis, can be treated much more quickly if the physician does not waste time obtaining tests that are not helpful.

THE PATIENT HISTORY

The Neurologic History

Obtain the name, age, gender, occupation, and handedness of the patient. Record the chief complaint in the patient's own words and give the duration of the complaint. It is important to record the chief complaint in quotation marks, precisely as the patient provides it.

Give a chronologic sequence of the present illness beginning with the first symptom, and then describe how the symptoms have changed over time. Often patients wish to discuss what other physicians thought about their illness and to mention the many tests that were done. This information is usually not helpful. Make special inquiry about the following complaints:

1. Changes in memory or personality
2. Disturbances of consciousness
3. Convulsions
4. Headaches
5. Loss of vision
6. Diplopia (double vision)
7. Deafness
8. Tinnitus (ringing or roaring in the ears)
9. Vertigo (a sense of movement of the environment or of the patient)
10. Nausea and vomiting
11. Dysphagia (difficulty swallowing)
12. Speech disorders (comprehension, execution, articulation)
13. Weakness, stiffness, or paralysis of the limbs
14. Gait imbalance and falls
15. Pains and paresthesias
16. Disturbances in control of the bowel and bladder

Past History

Obtain a history of previous illnesses, operations, and allergies. List the medications the patient is taking, including the doses. Review the history of symptoms related to the major organs (i.e., heart, lungs, gastrointestinal tract, urinary tract, bones, joints). Inquire about any major trauma to the head or neck. When indicated, obtain a history of birth and developmental milestones. Inquire about the patient's level of education.

Family History

Note the ages of death of the patient's parents, and if indicated, of other family members. Ask whether any family member had a neurologic illness. Include inquiries about paralysis, gait or movement disorders, and convulsions.

Marital and Sexual History

It is important to obtain a history of sexual function in many patients with neurologic problems.

Social History

Inquire about the patient's habits. Include the use of alcohol, caffeine, tobacco, and "recreational" drugs.

Occupational History

Obtain a history of the patient's occupation and how it has changed over time.

THE PHYSICAL EXAMINATION

• • • • • • • • •

Obtain the blood pressure, pulse, and respiratory rate. Examine the heart, lungs, abdomen, and extremities.

THE NEUROLOGIC EXAMINATION

• • • • • • • • •

The neurologic examination usually requires only a few simple materials, including a pen, a blank sheet of paper, a paragraph of material from a newspaper for testing reading, a visual acuity testing card or a Snellen chart, an ophthalmoscope, a pocket flashlight, a reflex hammer, a safety pin, tuning forks of both 128 cycles per second (Hz) and 256 Hz, a tongue depressor, a scent such as mint or cloves, a small wisp of cotton, and a coin.

The neurologic examination is divided into five parts: (1) mental status, (2) cranial nerves, (3) motor system, (4) reflexes, and (5) sensation.

Examination of Mental Status

1. **Orientation.** Ask the patient to state the date, including day, month, and year; where he or she is located (the name of the hospital or clinic); and his or her name.
2. **Attention and state of consciousness.** This assessment is obtained by simple observation. Four levels of disturbances of state of consciousness are described:

   a. Confusional states (shortened attention span, difficulty following commands, minor disorientation, faulty memory)
   b. Delirium (disorientation, fear, irritability, hallucinations)
   c. Stupor (unresponsiveness, arousal only with vigorous and repeated stimuli)
   d. Coma (unarousable unresponsiveness)

3. **Memory.** Test **remote memory** by asking the date of birth, date of marriage, and any other personally important dates. For **intermediate memory**, ask for the events of the prior 5 years. For **recent memory**, ask about the present illness, events since the hospitalization, and events of the last 2 days. Test digit retention by saying seven digits, one per second, and asking the patient to repeat them in sequence, both forward and backward. Most people can remember seven digits forward and five backward. Give the patient a brief sentence and ask him to repeat it. Ask the patient to recall three objects after 5 minutes. Examples include sailboat, basketball, and Webster Avenue (a street name). Tell the patient a brief story and ask the patient to recall the story.
4. **Calculations.** Ask the patient to subtract 7 from 100 in serial fashion. Ask the patient to count from 1 to 20 and then backward to 1. Ask the patient to compute 3×16 or to compute the interest on $200 at 10 percent annual rate for 18 months.
5. **Grasp of general information.** Ask the patient to name the president, vice president, secretary of state, mayor, and governor. Ask for the names of five of the largest cities in the United States. Ask for the dates of Washington's birthday or Christmas. Ask for the dates of the beginning and end of the World Wars.
6. **Interpretation of proverbs and similarities.** Ask the patient to interpret the proverbs "People who live in glass houses shouldn't throw stones," "A rolling stone gathers no moss," "A new broom sweeps clean," or "Every cloud has a silver lining." The patient should provide an abstract interpretation of the proverb. Patients who are demented or mentally retarded often give concrete interpretations. For example, in response to the proverb "people who live in glass houses shouldn't throw stones," a normal individual may say, "Since everyone is vulnerable, people should not be critical of others," whereas demented patients often reply, "You will break the windows."

   Ask for the similarities between an apple and a lemon; a bicycle and an automobile; and a bird and an airplane. The patient should provide abstract interpretations such as "An apple and lemon are both fruit." If the patient gives concrete interpretations such as "An apple and lemon are round," suspect that the patient may have a dementia.
7. **Insight and judgment.** Use the letter test and the fire test. In the letter test, tell the patient that he or she is walking down the street and sees a stamped, addressed, sealed envelope on the ground. What should he or she do with it? The correct answer is to place the letter in a mailbox or give it to a postal employee. In the fire test, tell the patient that he or she is sitting in a theater and sees a fire. Ask what he or she should do. The patient should stand up and walk slowly out.

The patient should not shout "fire!" or run lest he or she start a stampede. Patients with defective insight and judgment may suffer from a dementia.

8. **Affect.** Observe the patient for signs of anxiety, pressured speech, psychomotor retardation, melancholy, or lability of emotional responses. These findings can be particularly important in patients with degenerative disorders such as Alzheimer's disease, demyelinating diseases such as multiple sclerosis, and vascular disease (i.e., stroke). These findings are also important in patients with multiple somatic complaints but few or no abnormal neurologic findings on physical and laboratory examination.

9. **Special tests.** In patients with suspected disorders of higher cerebral function, the following tests should be used.

   a. **Language.** Note the content of the patient's spontaneous speech. When taking the history, determine whether the patient's speech is nonfluent (effortful speech) or fluent (facile, smooth, rapid speech) and assess for dysarthria. A nonfluent aphasia often results from a lesion in the anterior part of the dominant cerebral hemisphere, whereas a fluent aphasia often results from a lesion in the posterior part of the dominant cerebral hemisphere. Dysarthria (difficulty articulating speech) without aphasia often occurs with subcortical, brain stem, or cerebellar lesions.

   b. **Naming.** Ask the patient to name various objects (e.g., pen, thumb, watch, face, belt buckle, colors).

   c. **Repetition.** Ask the patient to repeat a phrase such as "no ifs, ands, or buts" or "the lawyer's closing argument convinced him."

   d. **Comprehension.** Determine the patient's ability to follow commands such as "Close your eyes" or "Pick up the paper, fold it in half, and hand it to me."

   e. **Reading.** Test the patient's ability to read aloud and comprehend a paragraph from a newspaper. A disorder in comprehension of written material in an alert patient often results from disease in the posterior part of the dominant cerebral hemisphere.

   f. **Writing.** Ask the patient to write an original sentence and to copy a sentence. A disturbance of writing in an alert patient usually signifies pathology in the posterior part of the dominant cerebral hemisphere.

   g. **Constructional ability.** Ask the patient to copy a cube or complex figure. Ask the patient to draw a house or a flower. A disturbance of constructional ability in an alert, nonaphasic patient suggests a lesion in the nondominant (usually right) parietal lobe, particularly when the left parts of the drawings are not completed or are ignored.

   h. **Praxis.** Praxis refers to the motor integration used in the execution of complex learned movements. Give the patient commands such as "Show me how to blow out a match," "Show me how to use a toothbrush," "Show me how to wave goodbye." Note the patient's performance. Lesions of the dominant hemisphere often cause apraxias.

Examination of the Cranial Nerves

   I. **Olfactory nerve.** Test the patient's sense of smell with oil of lemon, cloves, or coffee. Do not use alcohol or other noxious vapors; these substances test cranial nerve V, not I. Most clinicians test olfactory sense only when indicated by the history.

II. **Optic nerve.** Test visual acuity with a visual acuity card for bedside use or a Snellen chart. Visual acuity should be tested with and without corrective lenses. Visual acuity is recorded as 20 (the distance to the Snellen chart) over the size of type read (20/20, for example, indicates excellent acuity; 20/200 indicates poor acuity). Test each eye independently. Test the visual fields with bedside confrontation by moving a finger in each of the four quadrants of each field (see Chap. 19 for further details). Test double simultaneous stimulation. If indicated, test the visual fields formally with a perimeter or a tangent screen. Examine the optic fundi with an ophthalmoscope (see Chap. 27).

III, IV, VI. **Extraocular muscle function.** Examine the pupils and note the size, regularity, and equality. Test the reactions to light and accommodation (see Chap. 20). Look for strabismus (lack of parallel alignment of the eyes). Look for spontaneous nystagmus (beating movements of the eyes, either with the eyes looking straight ahead or on lateral or vertical gaze). Look for lid droop or retraction. Test extraocular movements to command and also to pursuit by having the patient follow an object through all four quadrants of movement. Test for ocular convergence. Oculocephalic maneuvers and caloric stimulation of nystagmus are useful in unresponsive patients.

V. **Trigeminal nerve.** Ask the patient to open and close the jaw against resistance. Test the jaw jerk reflex by asking the patient to open the jaw slightly, then tapping lightly over the chin and looking for reflex closure of the jaw. It is often useful to compare the jaw jerk to the spinally mediated muscle stretch reflexes. Test sensation on the face with a light touch of a pin or a cold object such as the tine of a tuning fork. Test the corneal reflexes with a small wisp of cotton (see Chap. 13, Sensory Division of Nerve V).

VII. **Facial nerve.** Examine the face for any asymmetry at rest and examine facial movement with contraction during voluntary effort.

VIII. **Auditory and vestibular nerves.** Whisper a different number in each of the patient's ears and ask the patient to repeat each number. Perform the Rinne and Weber tests as described in Chapter 15. When indicated, use cold water to irrigate the external auditory canal and examine for nystagmus. Before performing this test, be certain that the eardrum is intact (see Chap. 16).

IX and X. **Glossopharyngeal and vagus nerves.** Ask the patient to say "ah" while you look at the palate using a tongue depressor and flashlight. Determine whether the palate elevates symmetrically with phonation to test the motor function of X. Test the gag reflex on each side to test nerve IX (afferent) and X (efferent).

XI. **Spinal accessory nerve.** Test the strength of contraction of the sternomastoid and trapezius muscles. Ask the patient to turn the head to the left and then to the right while you test the strength of muscle contraction by resisting the movement. Turning the head to the left requires contraction of the right sternomastoid, and vice versa. To test the strength of the trapezius muscles, ask the patient to shrug the shoulders.

XII. **Hypoglossal nerve.** Have the patient protrude the tongue and move it rapidly from side to side.

Examination of the Motor System

Inspect the patient's posture at rest, standing, and seated. Look for any asymmetry and for tremor or spasm. Ask the patient to extend the arms with the fingers spread, palms up, and eyes closed and look for drift and pronation of either arm. This occurs with limb weakness and may be a subtle sign of a hemiparesis.

Examine the power of movement and record it on a scale of 0 to 5, as follows: 0 = no contraction; 1 = feeble contraction; 2 = weak contraction insufficient to overcome gravity; 3 = weak contraction able to overcome gravity; 4 = fair but not full strength; 5 = full power of contraction. Note the bulk of the muscles and look for atrophy and fasciculations (twitching movements seen beneath the skin without movement of the limbs). Test coordination in the arms with the finger-nose-finger test as follows. Have the patient touch his or her index finger to his or her nose and then touch your finger, which is held at a full arm's length away from the patient. Test coordination in the legs with the heel-knee-shin test as follows. Have the patient run his or her heel from the opposite knee straight down the shin to the foot, then elevate the leg in the air and repeat the movement. Test rapid alternating movements by having the patient alternately pronate and supinate one hand, touching the palm of the opposite hand. Have the patient perform rhythmical tapping tests as well. Have the patient walk normally and also in tandem, heel to toe. Ask the patient to walk on the heels and then on the toes.

Test the resistance to passive manipulation of the limbs. **Spasticity** consists of the "clasp-knife" phenomenon, in which the examiner feels a free interval, then a catch, and then a release of resistance. **Rigidity** is manifested as increased resistance to passive manipulation of the cogwheel type, commonly seen in Parkinson's disease; the plastic type, with a smooth, even resistance to manipulation; and of the dystonic type, in which there is increasing resistance that mounts as the movement continues. **Hypotonia** consists of decreased resistance to manipulation and is commonly seen in cerebellar disease and in peripheral nerve disease.

Look for involuntary movements, including tremor. A **parkinsonian tremor** usually consists of a 4- to 5-Hz distal tremor with flexion–extension movements of the fingers, wrists, and often, the feet. A **senile (heredofamilial) tremor** often includes a flexion–extension tremor of the head and a fine flexion–extension tremor of the fingers when they are extended. When completely at rest, patients with a heredofamilial tremor have no involuntary movements, whereas parkinsonian patients at rest continue to have tremor. **Cerebellar tremor** consists of a proximal side-to-side tremor found on heel-knee-shin or finger-nose-finger testing. **Athetosis** consists of involuntary, usually slow and writhing movements of the limbs and is commonly seen in cerebral palsy. **Chorea** consists of rapid movements that flow from limb to limb, with sweeping sideward movements of the head, wincing movements of the face, and "piano-playing" movements of the hands. **Hemiballismus** consists of rapid flinging movements of an arm and a leg on one side of the body. **Myoclonus** consists of lightinglike movements of the extremities.

Examination of the Reflexes

Examine the muscle stretch reflexes, including the jaw jerk and the biceps reflex (innervated through the C5-6 reflex arc); triceps reflex (C7); brachioradialis reflex (C5-6); patellar reflex (L3); and ankle reflex (S1). Test the abdominal reflexes, the cremasteric reflexes, and the anal reflex. Examine the plantar response by moving a blunt object such as a key along the lateral border of the sole of the foot. An **extensor plantar response (Babinski's sign)** consists of a dorsal flexion movement of the great toe. A flexor plantar response consists of plantar flexion of the great toe.

Examination of Sensation

Test sensation in areas where the patient has complaints and compare the responses in areas that are symptomatically not affected. Compare left and right sides of the body, and compare distal and proximal parts of the limbs. Compare the face with the body and check sensation from rostral to caudal along the trunk. Test the patient's response to pinprick, using a new pin for each patient. Test light touch with a cotton wisp, and test vibration sense using a 128-Hz tuning fork applied to bony prominences. Test position sense by moving a distal joint up or down and have the patient, with his or her eyes closed, state whether the joint has moved up or down. Test thermal sensation with a tube of cold or warm water. The tine of a nonvibrating tuning fork usually can be used to test for the sense of coldness. When indicated, test discriminatory sensation with two blunt points approximately 1 mm apart on the fingers. Test stereognosis by having the patient, with the eyes closed, determine what size coin has been placed in the palm. Test tactile localization by having the patient, with the eyes closed, point to the part of the limb that the examiner touches. Test for the **Romberg sign** by having the patient stand with the feet together and the eyes open, then ask the patient to close the eyes to determine whether he or she will sway or fall. The Romberg sign is positive when there is a disturbance in dorsal column or peripheral nerve function, resulting in swaying or falling when the eyes are closed.

CHAPTER

29

Neurologic Diagnostic Tests

Many diseases affecting the nervous system can be treated effectively provided a correct diagnosis can be made. The most important methods used by physicians to reach a correct diagnosis are to take a careful history and to perform a complete neurologic and general physical examination. A number of laboratory tests are available to supplement the history and examination.

CEREBROSPINAL FLUID ANALYSIS

Abnormalities of cerebrospinal fluid constituents occur in a number of conditions, including meningitis, encephalitis, syphilis affecting the nervous system, subarachnoid hemorrhage, peripheral neuropathy, brain tumors, stroke, and multiple sclerosis. Samples of cerebrospinal fluid for diagnostic tests are obtained by directing a long needle between the vertebrae at the level of L3–4, L4–5, or L5–S1 and inserting it far enough to reach and pierce the dura mater. There is no chance of striking the spinal cord at this level because the cord terminates rostral to L2, and there is only a slight danger of injuring the nerve roots of the cauda equina that are present at this level. With the patient relaxed and in a recumbent position, the pressure of the spinal fluid should not exceed 200 mm H_2O. Small oscillations of the fluid level in a manometer connected to the needle arise from the transmission of cerebral arterial pulsations. These pulsations indicate that free communication is present. Lumbar puncture is hazardous in the presence of elevated intracranial pressure due to intracranial masses, especially a large mass in one cerebral hemisphere causing midline shift or a mass in the posterior fossa. In this situation, lumbar puncture is dangerous because release of pressure from below may promote herniation of the brain. Herniation of the medial part of the temporal lobe (the uncus) through the tentorium cerebelli can cause coma with decerebrate rigidity from compression of the midbrain, and herniation of the cerebellar tonsils through the foramen magnum can cause death from compression of the medulla and injury to neurons controlling cardiac and respiratory functions. Lumbar puncture is also hazardous with tumors that completely fill the spinal canal because the change in cerebrospinal fluid pressure can cause sudden impairment of spinal cord function.

Spinal fluid also can be obtained by cisternal puncture or lateral cervical puncture. Cisternal puncture is performed by passing a needle at the base of the skull directly through the atlantooccipital membrane into the cisterna magna. No nervous system structures are encountered, but the needle will strike the medulla if it passed too far. Lateral cervical puncture is performed between C1–2 under fluoroscopic guidance. These procedures should be performed only after appropriate training.

After cerebrospinal fluid is removed through the lumbar or cisternal needle, it is analyzed for cellular content, glucose, and total protein. When bacterial meningitis is suspected, a gram stain and bacterial culture are performed. If chronic meningitis is suspected, smears and cultures for tubercle bacilli and fungi are indicated. When multiple sclerosis is suspected, additional helpful information can be obtained from tests for immunoglobulin G, oligoclonal bands, and myelin basic protein.

ELECTROENCEPHALOGRAPHY AND EVOKED-POTENTIAL STUDIES

• • • • • • • • •

Neuronal activity in the brain can be studied indirectly by recording electrical activity from the surface of the scalp **(electroencephalography, EEG)**. This technique is important in evaluating patients with epilepsy, coma, and other disturbances of the state of consciousness. Neuronal activity can also be recorded directly from the exposed cerebral cortical surface (electrocorticography) at the time of a neurosurgical procedure. The electrical responses of large aggregates of neurons can be recorded at sites distant from the origin of the responses because of **volume conduction**, which is the flow of current through extracellular space. Changes in potential within neurons cause current to flow in the extracellular fluid. Although the resistance of this fluid is low, current flow across the resistance is sufficient to cause a potential change. Clinical EEG recordings employ multiple active electrodes located over the surface of the head with an indifferent electrode over one or both ears. The EEG records potential differences between adjacent active electrodes and also differences between each active electrode and an indifferent electrode. Although action potentials are the largest signals generated by neurons, they actually contribute little to EEG potentials because they do not occur simultaneously in large numbers of neurons. Most of the activity recorded in the EEG consists of extracellular current flow associated with summated postsynaptic potentials in synchronously active pyramidal cells of the cerebral cortex.

The frequencies of the potentials recorded from the surface of the scalp vary from 1 to 50 cycles per second (Hz), and the amplitudes range up to 100 µV. The frequency characteristics of EEG potentials are complex, but a few frequencies are observed often. **Alpha rhythm** (8 to 13 Hz) is best recorded from the parietooccipital region and is most prominent during relaxed wakefulness when the eyes are closed. **Beta activity** (14 to 30 Hz) is normally seen over the frontal regions. **Theta** (4 to 7 Hz) and **delta** (0.5 to 4 Hz) activities develop during sleep in the adult.

Evoked potentials result from a change in the ongoing electrical activity of neurons in response to stimulation of a sensory organ or pathway. They are specific for the sensory stimulus that evokes them and are timelocked to the stimulus. Evoked potentials are recorded from the scalp with electrodes and amplifiers similar to those used in EEG recording, but they are too small in amplitude to be discerned in EEG tracings. The averaging of responses from several hundred stimuli is necessary to portray these potentials. Among the evoked potentials used clinically, **visual evoked potentials** are usually elicited by having the patient view a checkerboard pattern that alternates colors, **brain stem auditory evoked potentials** are elicited using clicking sounds, and **somatosensory evoked potentials** are generated with low-amplitude electrical stimuli on the extremities. Each of these provides information concerning the conduction pathway of the modality stimulated. For example, patients with multiple sclerosis tend to develop lesions in the visual system, often involving the optic nerves. At times, lesions that are not detectable on clinical examination will cause an abnormality of the visual evoked potential.

In **polysomnography**, multiple variables, including EEG, eye movements, respirations, cardiac rate and rhythm, and muscle activity, are recorded during sleep. Polysomnography is useful in diagnosing narcolepsy, sleep apnea, and other sleep disorders.

NERVE CONDUCTION STUDIES, ELECTROMYOGRAPHY, AND MUSCLE AND NERVE BIOPSY

• • • • • • • • •

Nerve conduction studies and electromyography are usually performed together as a clinical diagnostic procedure to evaluate the function of peripheral nerves and muscles. **Nerve conduction studies** are performed by applying an electrical stimulus to the skin over a peripheral nerve while recording the electrical activity elsewhere over the nerve or in a muscle supplied by that nerve with an electrode placed on the skin surface. Nerve conduction studies permit assessment of the velocity of conduction through peripheral nerves and the amplitude of the response evoked in muscle. Conduction velocity is usually slower than normal in demyelinating neuropathies (diseases of peripheral nerve that damage the myelin coating, leaving the axons intact) but normal in axonal neuropathies (diseases of peripheral nerve that damage the axons but leave the myelin intact).

In **electromyography**, a needle electrode is inserted into muscle, and the electrical activity is amplified and displayed on an oscilloscope. Muscle activity is evaluated at rest and during active contraction. Normal muscle shows no activity at rest. In denervated muscle, activity appears at rest, including **fibrillations** and **fasciculations**. Fibrillations are action potentials in single muscle fibers, probably occurring spontaneously as a result of denervation hypersensitivity of muscle receptor sites. Fasciculations are thought to represent action potentials involving entire motor units. Fasciculations commonly result from diseases of the anterior horn cells such as **amyotrophic lateral sclerosis**. During increasing muscular contraction, progressively large numbers of motor units are recruited. In muscles suffering from chronic denervation, the responses of motor units are unusually long in duration and large in amplitude, probably because reinnervation causes each nerve fiber to supply an increased number of muscle fibers. In primary diseases of muscle, the responses of motor units are abnormally short in duration and small in amplitude, and the number of motor units is increased in relation to the force exerted.

In patients thought to be afflicted with a muscle disease, muscle tissue can be biopsied. The tissue can be studied with conventional staining materials and with histochemical stains. In some patients with diseases of peripheral nerves, biopsy of the sural nerve can be helpful diagnostically.

ANATOMIC IMAGING STUDIES

• • • • • • • • •

Conventional x-ray studies of the head provide useful images of the skull but furnish little information about its contents. They are performed primarily when clinical findings are suggestive of skull fracture. Spine radiographs are useful for diagnosing a variety of conditions involving the vertebral column, including fractures, dislocations, congenital anomalies, and bone tumors, but they provide little information about the spinal cord.

X-ray computed tomography (CT) provides important diagnostic information about the brain or spinal cord. With CT, x-rays are passed through the head from many different angles, and the attenuation at each point is determined by computer. The results are displayed as cross-sectional layers through the brain, usually at an angle perpendicular to the axis of the body and spaced at 0.5- to 1.0-cm intervals. CT scans are useful for diagnosing a wide variety of conditions, including subarachnoid and intracerebral hemorrhage, stroke, hydrocephalus, and brain atrophy, as well as abnormalities of the skull. Often the scan is performed after intravenous infusion of an iodinated contrast agent. In regions where the blood–brain barrier is disrupted, the contrast agent enters the brain and causes increased x-ray attenuation. Thus, contrast agent infusion increases the sensitivity of CT for detection of tumors and inflammatory conditions.

Magnetic resonance imaging (MRI) employs a strong magnetic field and radiofrequency (RF) waves. The magnetic field orients the spin of protons (hydrogen nuclei) parallel to the magnetic field. A brief RF current disturbs the orientation of the protons, but after the RF current stops, the protons reorient to the magnetic field and emit radio signals that can be detected. The result is an image of the anatomy of the structures under study. MRI portrays greater detail in the brain than CT and is superior for diagnosis of certain conditions, including multiple sclerosis. It has the advantage of being free of exposure to hazardous radiation, but it is more expensive and less readily available than CT.

Imaging of the cerebral vessels can be performed with **Doppler ultrasound, MR angiography**, and **cerebral arteriography**. Doppler ultrasound studies of the neck are useful for imaging the extracranial carotid arteries to detect surgically correctable stenosis (narrowing) caused by atherosclerosis, which occurs most commonly near the bifurcation of the common carotid into the internal and external carotid arteries. Transcranial Doppler ultrasound studies permit visualization of the intracranial vessels as well. Magnetic resonance angiography, in which vessels are imaged by detection of the motion of hydrogen nuclei between RF stimulus and the RF response, is useful for studying both the extracranial and intracranial vessels. Cerebral arteriography is usually performed by injecting iodinated dye through a catheter passed from the femoral artery to the carotid and vertebral arteries while x-ray images are taken in rapid sequence. Cerebral arteriography has better resolution and reliability than Doppler ultrasound and MR angiography, but it is an invasive procedure and entails a small risk of stroke. Cerebral arteriography is performed to confirm abnormalities of the extracranial vessels suggested by other techniques and to detect disorders of the intracranial vessels such as stenosis, aneurysms, and vasculitis.

Imaging the spine and spinal cord can be carried out with MRI, CT scanning, and myelography. Currently the preferred method of imaging the vertebral column and spinal cord is with MRI when clinical evidence suggests disorders of these structures. CT scanning also provides reliable information when MRI is contraindicated or unavailable. CT scanning coupled with myelography is often used to obtain precise delineation of areas in the spinal cord involved by tumors, abscesses, and other mass lesions. Myelography is performed by injection of a small amount of an iodinated dye into the subarachnoid space by lumbar puncture or lateral cervical puncture. The patient lies on a table that can be tilted to cause the dye to move up and down the spinal canal. The dye is visualized fluoroscopically and permanent images are made with conventional radiographs or CT images. Myelography is performed when additional information is needed to supplement that obtained by MRI or when MRI is contraindicated or unavailable.

PHYSIOLOGIC IMAGING STUDIES

● ● ● ● ● ● ● ● ●

CT and MRI provide excellent information about brain structure, but **positron emission tomography (PET), single photon emission computed tomography (SPECT)** and **fast MRI** can provide quantitative information about brain function.

For **PET**, a positron- (a positively charged electron) emitting nuclide of fluorine, carbon, nitrogen, or oxygen is produced in a cyclotron. This nuclide can be incorporated into metabolic substrates and pharmaceuticals. The resulting radiopharmaceuticals are injected intravenously. Decay of the radionuclides releases positrons, which react with electrons present in tissue (a matter-antimatter reaction) to produce two gamma rays. The gamma rays are detected with a scanner that portrays the distribution of the radionuclide through the brain. PET is most commonly used to display images of local metabolic rate for glucose throughout the brain, but it can also be used to evaluate cerebral blood flow, oxygen metabolism, and neurotransmitter receptor density. It may prove most useful for detection of epileptic foci in the brain and for the diagnosis of degenerative conditions such as Alzheimer's disease.

Activation scans permit the mapping of brain regions with enhanced activity due to cognitive tasks, motor tasks, or sensory stimulation. In PET activation scans, a blood-flow tracer is injected during the activation, and the resulting scan is compared to a scan performed without activation. Brain regions participating in the neural processing are demonstrated as areas of increased blood flow.

SPECT is similar to PET in many ways, but it provides slightly less detail, and the available nuclides, including technetium and iodine, are of less biological interest. However, SPECT is less expensive and more widely available than PET. SPECT is most promising for evaluation of cerebral blood flow.

Fast MRI is a newly introduced technique that permits visualization of changes in local cerebral blood flow without injection of radioactive substances. Fast MRI can be used to study brain activation.

SUGGESTED READING

Adams, JH and Duchen, LW: Greenfield's Neuropathology, ed 5. Oxford, New York, 1992.

Adams, RD and Victor, M: Principles of Neurology, ed 5. McGraw-Hill, New York, 1993.

Asbury, AK, McKhann, GM, and McDonald, WI (eds): Diseases of the Nervous System, ed 2. WB Saunders, Philadelphia, 1992.

Baloh, RS and Honrubia, V: Clinical Neurophysiology of the Vestibular System, ed 2. FA Davis, Philadelphia, 1990.

Bradley, W, Daroff, R, Fenichel, G, and Marsden, CD: Neurology in Clinical Practice. Butterworth-Heinemann, Boston, 1991.

Byrne, TN and Waxman, SG: Spinal Cord Compression. FA Davis, Philadelphia, 1990.

Cooper, JR, Bloom, JE, and Roth, RH: The Biochemical Basis of Neuropharmacology, ed 6. Oxford University Press, New York, 1991.

Cumings, JL: Clinical Neuropsychiatry. Grune & Stratton, Orlando, FL, 1985.

Cumings, JL and Benson, DF: Dementia: A Clinical Approach, ed 2. Butterworth-Heinemann, Boston, 1992.

Dyck, PJ, Thomas, PK, Griffin, JW, Low, PA, Poduslo, JF (eds): Peripheral Neuropathy, ed 3. WB Saunders, Philadelphia, 1993.

Engel, AG and Franzini-Armstrong, C: Myology, ed 2. McGraw-Hill, New York, 1994.

Fishman, R: Cerebrospinal Fluid in Diseases of the Nervous System. WB Saunders, Philadelphia, 1984.

Fuster, JM: The Prefrontal Cortex, ed 2. Raven Press, New York, 1989.

Gilman, AG, Goodman, LS, Rall, TW, and Murad, F (eds): Goodman and Gilman's The Pharmacological Basis of Therapeutics, ed 8. Macmillan, New York, 1990.

Gilman, S, Bloedel, JR, and Lechtenberg, R: Disorders of the Cerebellum. FA Davis, Philadelphia, 1981.

Haerer, AF: DeJong's The Neurologic Examination. JB Lippincott, Philadelphia, 1992.

Hille, B: Ionic Channels of Excitable Membranes, ed 2. Sinauer Associates, Sunderland, MA, 1992.

Ito, M: The Cerebellum and Neural Control. Raven Press, New York, 1984.

Iyengar, R and Birnbaumer, L: G Proteins. Academic Press, New York, 1990.

Kandel, ER, Schwartz, JH, and Jessell, TM (eds): Principles of Neural Science, ed 3. Elsevier, New York, 1991.

Leigh, RJ and Zee, DS: The Neurology of Eye Movements, ed 2. FA Davis, Philadelphia, 1991.

Martin, JB and Reichlin, S: Clinical Neuroendocrinology, ed. 2. FA Davis, Philadelphia, 1987.

Mazziotta, JC and Gilman, S (eds): Clinical Brain Imaging. FA Davis, Philadelphia, 1992.

Mendelsohn, FAO and Paxinos, G (eds): Receptors in the Human Nervous System. Academic Press, San Diego, 1991.

Mesulam M-M: Principles of Behavioral Neurology. FA Davis, Philadelphia, 1985.

Nieuwenhuys, R: Chemoarchitecture of the Brain. Springer-Verlag, Berlin, 1985.

Nieuwenhuys, R, Voogd, J, and van Huijzen, Chr: The Human Central Nervous System, ed 3. Springer-Verlag, Berlin, 1988.

Parent, A: Carpenter's Human Neuroanatomy, ed 9. Williams & Wilkins, Media, PA, 1996.

Paxinos, G (ed): The Human Nervous System. Academic Press, San Diego, 1990.

Rowland, LP (ed): Merritt's Textbook of Neurology, ed 9. Williams & Wilkins, Baltimore, 1995.

Shepherd, GM (ed): The Synaptic Organization of the Brain, ed 3. Oxford University Press, New York, 1990.

Shepherd, GM: Neurobiology, ed 3. Oxford University Press, New York, 1994.

Siegel, GJ, Agranoff, BW, Albers, RW, and Molinoff, P (eds): Basic Neurochemistry, ed 5. Raven Press, New York, 1994.

Squire, LR: Memory and Brain. Oxford University Press, New York, 1987.

Steward, O: Principles of Cellular, Molecular, and Developmental Neuroscience. Springer-Verlag, New York, 1989.

Stuss, DT and Benson, DF: The Frontal Lobes. Raven Press, New York, 1985.

Westmoreland, BF, Benarroch, EE, Daube, JR, Reagan, TJ, Sandok, B: Medical Neurosciences, ed 3. Little, Brown, Boston, 1994.

Whitehouse, PJ (ed): Dementia. FA Davis, Philadelphia, 1993.

INDEX

An "f" following a page number indicates a figure; a "t" following a page number indicates a table.